BRAIN
MENTAL HEALTH

*7 Books in 1:
Vagus Nerve, Cognitive Behavioral Theraphy for Anxiety, Overthinking, Strategies to Overcome Stress, Meal Prep Cookbook, Emotional Eating, Autophagy.*

By

Albert Dales
&
Alan Dieter

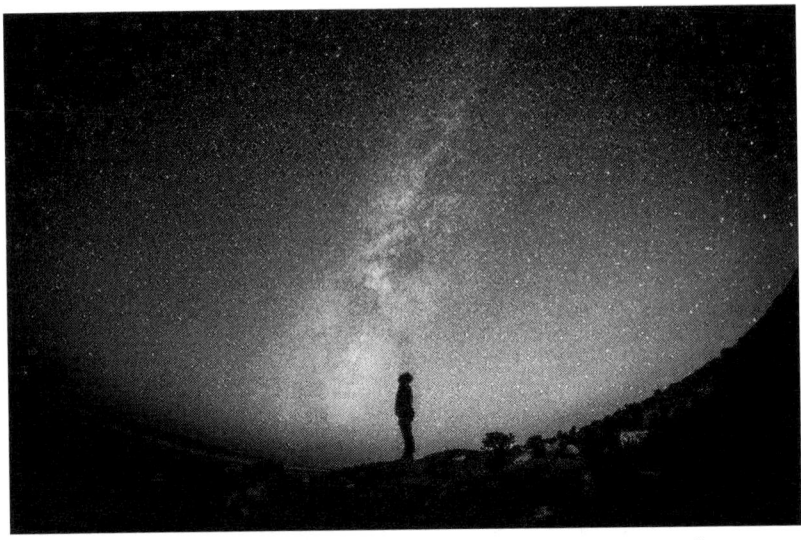

© **Copyright 2020 by Albert Dales - All rights reserved.**

The content contained within this book may not be reproduced, duplicated or transmitted without direct written permission from the author or the publisher.

Under no circumstances will any blame or legal responsibility be held against the publisher, or author, for any damages, reparation, or monetary loss due to the information contained within this book. Either directly or indirectly.

Legal Notice:

This book is copyright protected. This book is only for personal use. You cannot amend, distribute, sell, use, quote or paraphrase any part, or the content within this book, without the consent of the author or publisher.

Disclaimer Notice:

Please note the information contained within this document is for educational and entertainment purposes only. All effort has been executed to present accurate, up to date, and reliable, complete information. No warranties of any kind are declared or implied. Readers acknowledge that the author is not engaging in the rendering of legal, financial, medical or professional advice. The content within this book has been derived from various sources. Please consult a licensed professional before attempting any techniques outlined in this book.

By reading this document, the reader agrees that under no circumstances is the author responsible for any losses, direct or indirect, which are incurred as a result of the use of the information contained within this document, including, but not limited to, — errors, omissions, or inaccuracies.

Vagus Nerve

Self-healing Techniques for Stress, Anxiety, Depression, Panic Attacks. ADHD, Chronic Illness and Inflammation. Relax Your Nervous System and Heal Your Body Through Mind-Gut Connection

By Albert Dales

Table of Contents

Introduction 6
PART I: THE NERVOUS SYSTEM **8**
Chapter 1: The Central Nervous System 8
    Parts of the CNS   8
Chapter 2: The role of nerves in the CNS 11
Chapter 3: The Peripheral Nervous System 14
    The Somatic Nervous System   14
    The Autonomic Nervous System   15
    The Sympathetic Nervous System   15
    The Parasympathetic Nervous System   16
Chapter 4: Stress and the Nervous System 17
    Stress hormones   18
    Burnout   18
    Recovering from stress   19
PART II: THE VAGUS NERVE **20**
Chapter 5: The Vagus Nerve 20
    The Pneumogastric Nerve   20
    The Ventral Branch of the Vagus Nerve   22
Chapter 6: Functions of the Vagus Nerve 25
    Main functions of the vagus nerve   25
    The Visceral Somatic Function   26
    The Physical Motor Function   27
    Essential biological functions   28
Chapter 7: Dysfunctions of the Vagus Nerve 29
    Anxiety   29
    Depression   30
    Panic attacks   31
    Inflammation and Autoimmune diseases   32
    Chronic conditions – Fibromyalgia   33
    Headaches and migraines   34
    Breathing conditions   35
    Digestive System Dysfunction   36
    Dysfunction of the Microbiome   37
    Cardiac dysfunction   38
    Hepatic Dysfunction   39
    Chronic Stress   39
    ADHD and Hyperactivity   39
    Chronic Fatigue Syndrome   40
    Sleep Issues and Circadian Rhythm Disruption   41
    Antisocial Behavior and Lack of Social Interaction   42
PART III: THE MIND BODY CONNECTION **44**
Chapter 7: The Physical and Emotional Connection Between the Mind and the Body 44
Chapter 8: How the Mind Talks to the Gut 47
Chapter 9: About Gut Feelings 49
Chapter 10: How the Gut Talks to the Brain 51
    Diet   51
    Fiber   52
    The Mouse Model   52
    Meat   53
    How Communication Takes Places   54
Chapter 11: How to Improve Brain-Gut Health 55
    Investigate What Your Digestive Symptoms Can Teach You   55
    Keep away from Negativity to Heal Your Gut   55
PART IV: STIMULATING THE VAGUS NERVE **57**
Chapter 12: The Benefits of Vagus Nerve Stimulation 57

A Natural Way to Stimulate the Vagus Nerve — 57
Chapter 13: Vagus Nerve Stimulation Techniques and Exercises 60
Self-healing through Yoga — 60
Chapter 14: The Polyvagal Theory 63
Chapter 15: The Healing Power of Polyvagal Theory 64
Conclusion 66

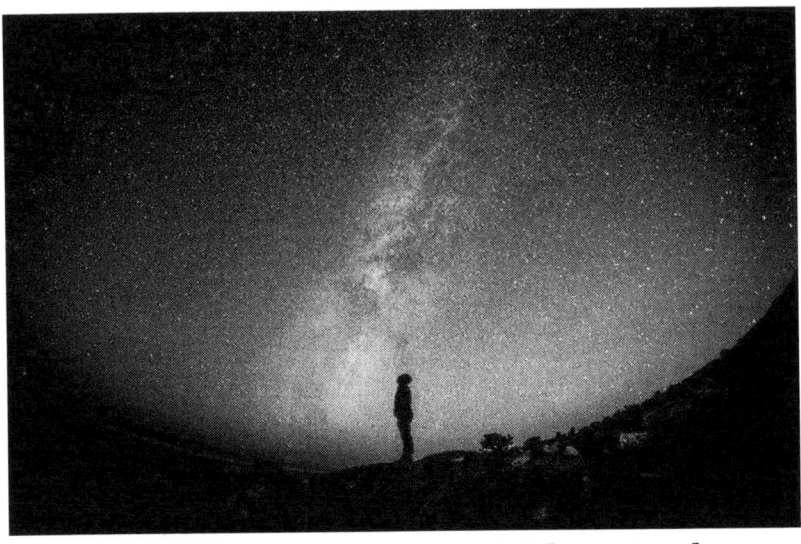

© **Copyright 2019 by Albert Dales - All rights reserved.**

The content contained within this book may not be reproduced, duplicated or transmitted without direct written permission from the author or the publisher.

Under no circumstances will any blame or legal responsibility be held against the publisher, or author, for any damages, reparation, or monetary loss due to the information contained within this book. Either directly or indirectly.

Legal Notice:

This book is copyright protected. This book is only for personal use. You cannot amend, distribute, sell, use, quote or paraphrase any part, or the content within this book, without the consent of the author or publisher.

Disclaimer Notice:

Please note the information contained within this document is for educational and entertainment purposes only. All effort has been executed to present accurate, up to date, and reliable, complete information. No warranties of any kind are declared or implied. Readers acknowledge that the author is not engaging in the rendering of legal, financial, medical or professional advice. The content within this book has been derived from various sources. Please consult a licensed professional before attempting any techniques outlined in this book.

By reading this document, the reader agrees that under no circumstances is the author responsible for any losses, direct or indirect, which are incurred as a result of the use of the information contained within this document, including, but not limited to, — errors, omissions, or inaccuracies.

Introduction

Congratulations on purchasing Vagus Nerve: Self-healing Techniques for Stress, Anxiety, Depression, Panic Attacks. ADHD, Chronic Illness and Inflammation. Relax Your Nervous System and Heal Your Body Through Mind-Gut Connection and thank you for doing so.

If you are reading this book it is because you are keen on learning more about how you can improve your overall health and wellbeing by improving your understanding of how the body works. In particular, your understanding of the nervous system will enable you to gain a deeper insight into the way your body is able to process many of the situations that it encounters on a daily basis.

The vagus nerve is one, if not, the most important neural network in the human body. It controls a number of systems which are vital to the overall functioning of the body's essential biological functions. That means that if the vagus nerve does not perform up to its optimal capabilities, the effects on the overall functioning of the body can be significant. Hence, there is a great need for everyone to understand how it works, what it does and what can be done to ensure that it functions up to its full potential.

Moreover, the vagus nerve is not fully understood. Its incredible power hasn't been fully understood until recently. Modern research has revealed the importance of this nerve and the need for its care. This has given way to a score of approaches with the aim to keep the vagus nerve in peak performance. In this book, we will discuss these approaches as a means of ensuring that we are able to maintain optimal health and wellbeing, both of the vagus nerve itself, and by extension, the body systems that it controls.

This book has been written with the intent to inform the general public on this topic. So, even a novice in the topic of the nervous system will be able to make the most of this important issue. After all, we are not here to provide complex information; rather, our intent is to provide you with information you won't easily find anywhere else.

As such, this book has been written with the aim of allowing anyone who is interested in learning about the topic the opportunity to do so in plain language. This book isn't an attempt at trying to sound smart; it is an exercise in helping the average individual learn as much as they can in a clear and concise manner. That means that we are going to be getting down to the meat and potatoes of this topic straight from the get-go.

This is an important consideration especially since the vagus nerve is indeed the body's main control module. Also, given the fact that we tend to know very little about it, we end up ignoring its relevance in our overall health and wellbeing. When we understand what this nerve does in our body, we are able to make a conscious choice to ensure its health. In doing so, we can keep a good level of physical wellbeing.

It should also be noted that our emotions also play a key role in maintaining the health of the vagus nerve. So, we need to be keen on understanding how we can address our emotional life in benefit of our overall body's performance. With this book, you will be able to get a working knowledge of how this can be achieved. It really is possible however unlikely it may seem.

Best of all, the information provided herein is intended to help you get off the ground and into a great physical condition. So, let's jump right on in and discuss how you can use the information we will discuss throughout to improve your overall quality of life. You will surely find that improving your physical health and emotional wellbeing isn't nearly as complicated as you might have thought. Indeed, you will have the power and the knowledge you need to improve your quality of life by the end of this book.

So, thank you once again for taking the time to read this book. We are certain that you will find the information contained herein to be both useful and informative. And don't worry if you haven't heard much about the topic. The fact is that the research discussed throughout this book is quite new. Thus, it hasn't quite made its way into the mainstream media. Over the next few years, you can expect more and more information to trickle its way into the mainstream. In the meantime, you have a primer at hand. In a manner of speaking, you are getting a look at the full movie well before it premieres at the cinema. So, sit back and enjoy the topic at hand. We do hope it will help you achieve a healthier version of yourself and your loved ones.

Let's get started!

PART I: THE NERVOUS SYSTEM

Chapter 1: The Central Nervous System

The starting point in this book is a discussion on the Central Nervous System (CNS). The CNS is perhaps the single most important component of the entire human body. It is the control center of the entire body's functioning. It essentially controls everything that happens throughout the body. As such, there is no function that is not controlled, one way or another, by the nervous system.

Generally speaking, the CNS is comprised of the brain and the main control unit and the spinal cord. The spinal cord then branches out into the millions of individual nerves that control the information sent from the brain and into each body component.

It is safe to say that without the CNS and its neural network, none of what we do would be possible. Think about a person who has been in an accident. If the suffer significant trauma to the brain, or perhaps the spinal cord, they may lose control over certain body parts. For instance, a severed spinal cord at the base of the neck will essentially mean that a person can be completely paralyzed from the neck down.

However, despite the loss of body movement, it is still possible for the Autonomic Nervous System (ANS) to function thereby maintaining essential body functions such as breathing, digestion, and blood flow. While we will discuss the ANS later on, it is worth mentioning that significant trauma to the brain and spinal cord does not necessarily mean a death sentence for the sufferer. In fact, modern science has made great advancements in the regeneration of the nervous system to the point where once paralyzed individuals are now able to regain much of their body's original functions.

Parts of the CNS

The CNS mainly consists of two parts, the brain, and the spinal cord. So, let's take a look at what each one of these parts does and how they are comprised.

The brain

The main processing unit of the entire CNS is the brain. The brain houses cells called neurons. Neurons are the cells which are responsible for relaying information back and forth. As such, the brain serves as one immense messaging center. Millions of messages are relayed at any given moment. These messages control everything from voluntary movements, such as reaching out for a cup of coffee, to all of the involuntary movements such as breathing. These involuntary functions are vital. After all, if you stop breathing, you would die.

The brain is also believed to control thoughts and emotions. While mythological and cultural beliefs contend that emotions are housed in specific organs (for example love is believed to reside in the heart) the fact of the matter is that emotions are a psychological response to the stimuli around us.

The brain mainly consists of four parts:

- The frontal lobe
- The temporal lobe
- The parietal lobe
- The occipital lobe

The sum of these four lobes is known as the cerebrum. In addition, the brain is divided into two hemispheres.

While there is much research still ongoing, much of the brain's overall functioning remains a mystery. Of course, science has decoded the brain's main workings, but it is the finer points of the brain which we still struggle to comprehend. For instance, the nature of thought, which is believed to be housed in the brain, largely remains unclear.

That being said, the various parts of the brain are in charge of various functions. So, it is certainly worth digging deeper into them.

The frontal lobe is responsible for the majority of human cognitive skills such as emotional expression, memory, linguistic skills, problem-solving abilities, and even sexual behavior. It is indeed one of the most important parts of the brain for modern homo sapiens.

The temporal lobe is in charge of managing key features such as language, speech and comprehension skills. A significant lesion to the temporal lobe may leave the sufferer unable to communicate appropriately. As such, blows to the head may result in impaired cognitive abilities.

The parietal lobe can be found behind the frontal lobe. Its main function is the processing of sensory input, that is, information that enters from the five senses. This information is decoded by the parietal lobe and transformed into usable knowledge that the individual can then use as a part of daily life.

The occipital lobe is found at the back of the head. Its main purpose is to process visual information. As such, this information is taken from visual input (the eyes) and then transformed into working data which is perceived by the mind as a visual representation of stimuli. A good example of this is how light is decoded by the brain to reveal the color.

The spinal cord

The spine is one of the distinguishing characteristics of homo sapiens. Firstly, humans are able to walk upright. While this trait is not exclusive to humans, it is very uncommon in nature. Only a handful of mammals are capable of walking upright. As a result, the spine enables the human body to maintain its upright structure.

Furthermore, the spine is also the hub for the entire neural network that runs throughout the body. This is why lesions to the spine may lead to severe disruption of bodily functions. In addition, the spine is also divided into parts that govern the functioning and movement of the body.

The bones which make up the spine are called vertebrae. Each vertebra has a form of a disc. Each disc is insulated with a gelatin-like substance. This substance can wear down over time. When this happens, individual nerves may get caught in between two vertebrae. This may cause excruciating pain, issues with mobility or even paralysis. In general, such situations may be remedied by surgery though the outcome isn't always assured.

The junction at which the brain is joined to the spinal cord is known as the brain stem. This is the most sensitive part of the CNS as the entire neural network passes through this section. As such, a serious injury to the neck could prove catastrophic to an individual.

The layers which cover the brain and the spinal cord are known as meninges. These layers serve as insulation so that the brain and spinal cord are isolated from bacteria and infection. Also, deep inside the spine is the spinal fluid. This fluid is responsible for nourishing the spine and the brain.

Lastly, it should be mentioned that proper blood flow throughout the CNS is vital in order to ensure proper functioning. If insufficient amounts of oxygen circulate in the blood, potential damage can be sustained. If the supply of oxygen is cut off completely, irreversible damage may be caused to the CNS leading the sufferer to experience anything from cognitive dysfunction to physical limitations.

Chapter 2: The role of nerves in the CNS

The CNS communicates with the entire body through an intricate network of nerves. As such, nerves as thread-like membranes that run through every part of the body. This is the means of communication that the body maintains with individual body parts.

Here is a good example of how this communication takes place.

One of the most important responses that the CNS produces is pain. Pain is the body's natural way of signaling that there is a potentially destructive situation underway. For instance, a person has stubbed their toe on their coffee table. The blow is recorded by the nerve receptors in the toe. The sensation is relayed through the nerves and up to the brain. The brain then decodes the information and sends back a signal indicating that this is pain. The toe then receives the information and decides that this is not good. As a result, the individual feels tremendous pain which is meant to be taken as a signal of damage to that part of the body.

A further nervous response could be swelling in the toe. This inflammation is the body's natural way of isolating an injured body part. In a way, it is like sending the police to close off the area and ensure that help gets to where it needs to.

This entire process seems like a long one; and in reality, it is. However, it takes place in a matter of nanoseconds. The body's processing capabilities far exceed any capability that computers are currently able to display.

That being said, the CNS is made up of four main types of nerves. This is important to note as nerves are a one-size-fits-all proposition. Nerves are highly specialized so that they are able to relay the right messages as accurately as possible.

The reason for dedicated neural networks can be attributed to evolution. The evolution of the human brain required the development of specialized types of nerves, cells, and receptors. Give the fact that humans are highly complex machines, certainly much more complex when compared to other mammals, the need for specialized and dedicated neural networks becomes evident.

Cranial nerves

Cranial nerves are located within the cranium, that is, the head. These nerves are essentially dedicated to the processes that occur within the head and are associated to the eyes, mouth, ears, nose and any other process that occurs directly within the cranium. They are highly important as they control four of the five senses. In addition, the facial muscles are the most complex muscle system in the body. Facial muscles are comprised of minuscule groups that enable humans to use their faces to express feelings and communicate non-verbally.

Furthermore, the cranial nerves process sight, sound, taste, and smell. Indeed, they are constantly working in overdrive thereby enabling a person to perceive the environment around them in the most efficient manner possible.

Central nerves

The central nerves run from the brain and down the spine. In a manner of speaking, they are the main highway from which individual side roads branch off to specific destinations. This implies that central nerves need to be the most robust nerves in the body as they must tend to thousand and thousands of messages per second. Their capability enables the body to make any number of movements simultaneously. If central nerves happen to become damaged, for example as a result of infection, then a person's motor development may become impaired.

Peripheral nerves

The periphery of the CNS is associated to the nerves which control messaging in the limbs. This is what enables, arms, legs, feet, toes, hands, and fingers to move with ease. It should be said that this neural network develops as we progress from childhood to maturity. Therefore, it is of the utmost importance for children to engage is as much physical activity as possible. A lack of physical activity during childhood may lead to decreased motor skill development.

Autonomic nerves

This neural network is the unsung hero of the human body. These nerves control the involuntary movements that keep the body alive. These nerves ensure the functioning of the heart, lungs, brain, digestive system, among other essential biological functions. Moreover, these nerves are so specialized, that they cannot be easily repaired by the body. That is why any neural damage to this particular network, such as the result of an illness like diabetes, may lead to irreversible consequences. That is why renal failure is common among diabetics much the same way that prolonged hypertension damages blood vessels, the heart muscle, and autonomic nerves.

Neurons

The last component of the CNS is known are the neuron. Neurons are cells that resemble worker bees; they do the yeoman's work of the entire nervous system in such a way that they enable to transmission of information from one part of the body to another. It is safe to say that if neurons should fail for whatever reason, the body may encounter grave complications.

In essence, neurons work on electrochemical impulses that transmit information by means of relays. So, while the nerves themselves act as a highway, the neurons in the brain work on a relay system. What this enables the brain to do is process a multitude of operations in a matter of nanoseconds. Each neuron is composed of the cell body, dendrites, and axon. The dendrites are tiny branches that receive sensory information. Then, the axon takes that sensory information and passes it on to another cell. This is a thread-like branch that enables communication among cells.

There are three main types of neurons.

- Multipolar neurons contain one axon and a number of dendrites. They are commonly found in the spinal cord and the brain. They serve to relay all sorts of information to the nerves where they need to go.
- Bipolar neurons contain a single axon and a single dendrite. These can be seen in the retina of the eye, in the nose (olfactory cells) and in the inner ear. These are highly specialized neurons.
- Unipolar neurons focus on one type of process throughout the body. This single process has part of the cell functioning as an axon and another as a dendrite. They are commonly located within the spinal cord.

It should be noted that there are millions of neurons allotted to the brain. In the past, it was believed that we were all born with a fixed lot of neurons. As we age, these neurons would deplete thereby leading to cognitive decline over time. However, modern research has shown that neuron does regenerate. Yet, what leads to cognitive decline over time, is "gunk" that builds up in the brain. This gunk is the byproduct of the electrochemical processes that happen in the brain and is cleaned up every night when we go to sleep. Therefore, it is vital to get enough sleep. That way, the brain can go about its maintenance process thereby preserving optimal performance.

Chapter 3: The Peripheral Nervous System

At the outset of this book, we focused on the CNS. The CNS is the essential unit that controls the functioning of the entire nervous system. As we have also established, the CNS plays a pivotal role in ensuring that the body is able to sustain life, repair itself and go about daily chores and activities.

At this point, we are going dive into the Peripheral Nervous System (PNS). The PNS is responsible for a myriad of functions and activities. Hence, it is just as important as the CNS, though with a more specialized task.

The PNS is made up of two main components: the somatic nervous system (SNS) and the autonomic nervous system (ANS). Each one of these individual nervous systems provides specific functions to the CNS. As such, they are significant insofar as providing the brain with the information it requires on the movements of the body and essential biological functions.

The Somatic Nervous System

The SNS has a very specific task, that is, to relay information from the limbs to the CNS. The SNS is made up of a network of nervous fibers that allow the brain to control the movement of the limbs. This is what enables walking, sitting, typing, eating, playing sports and so on. Without this network, the brain would be unable to control voluntary movement. Therefore, a person would not be able to move voluntary. Since this is not the case, we can only speculate as to how the body would be controlled.

The SNS controls muscles and their movements through a series of voluntary responses, either stemming from an individual's desire to carry out a specific activity, or as a result of the response which emanates from an external stimulus.

Consider this example:

First, an individual wants to grab an apple. This is a voluntary movement that requires the brain to signal the limbs (arms and hands) to reach out and grab the apple.

Next, the brain receives input from a visual stimulus. The brain has perceived there is a fire. As such, the brain sends a signal to the legs to get moving and hightail away from the fire. In this case, this is a matter of responding to the external stimulus.

Now, it should be noted that the reaction to the fire is part of the ANS, it is worth mentioning that without the SNS, the legs would be unable to make any kind of movement whatsoever. So, the SNS plays a crucial role in survival.

The Autonomic Nervous System

The ANS is incredibly important in the body's sustainment of life. Without it, the essential biological functions, the involuntary kind, would be impossible to carry out. After all, imagine how hard life would be if you have to remember to keep breathing or make a conscious decision to digest food.

As such, the ANS is commonly associated with biological functions that are broken up into two main categories: the sympathetic nervous system and the parasympathetic nervous system.

The Sympathetic Nervous System

The Sympathetic Nervous System is associated with the fight-or-flight response that virtually all living beings have. In humans, this is a response to an external stimulus. In the example of the fire, the reaction to the perceived threat is generated by the Sympathetic Nervous System. This system sends a signal to the CNS which then sends an order to the SNS to get moving.

Also, the Sympathetic Nervous System is considered to be on stand-by and comes into action generally when levels of stress increase. The hormone known as cortisol plays a key role in this situation. When the body detects higher levels of cortisol, the Sympathetic Nervous System kicks into gear.

Here are the main attributes of the sympathetic nervous system:

1. The bronchioles in the lungs are expanded to permit more air into the lungs, which build the oxygenation of the blood and stay aware of the increased blood flow through the lungs as a result of the expanded heart rate.
2. Bladder and sphincter control. This part of the nervous system is associated with bladder and sphincter control at a conscious level. In fact, loss of control of these two functions can be traced back to some kind of damage in this biological function. As a result, care needs to be taken to avoid any potential issues with these functions.
3. The pupils of the eyes become dilated. Since the sympathetic nervous system is regularly enacted when individuals are under stimulation, the dilation of eye pupils is a clear sign of some type of increase in the nervous system's response to the stimulus in question.
4. Increased heart rate. When the heart increases, whether as a result of physical exertion or a stress response, the flow of blood increases thereby leading to greater amounts of oxygen flowing through the body.
5. The digestive system is slowed as a result of the increased response to stress, among other biological functions which are slowed down. This slowdown is the result of the body's need to prioritize resources with regard to the physiological response that is in course.
6. The adrenal organs epinephrine and norepinephrine. The adrenals are a couple of hormone-creating glands situated over the kidneys that react to stress. Together, the epinephrine and norepinephrine discharged by the adrenal glands have an essential impact on the sympathetic nervous system by increasing heart rate, expanding the bronchioles, and increasing glucose discharge from the liver. Moreover, norepinephrine is likewise known to increase alertness. It might appear to be repetitive that these hormones have indistinguishable activities from the sympathetic neurons, however, hormones have longer enduring impacts than nerve driving forces, so while the underlying battle or flight

reaction is interceded by neurons, these hormones serve to fortify and support the reaction.
7. The liver discharges glucose into the circulatory system giving the body an increased caloric supply that will be prepared to control the muscles in the event that it is required.

The Parasympathetic Nervous System

The Parasympathetic Nervous System plays an active role insofar as keeping essential bodily functions moving. As such, the parasympathetic nervous system is commonly called the "feed and breed" system since it controls common procedures that are indispensable for the sustainability of ordinary life. The elements of this system include lowering pulse and heart rate after a spike of the fight-or-flight reaction, regulation of stress hormones such as cortisol and the blood pressure control in addition to biological functions such as breathing, circulation, digestion and sensory management.

Parasympathetic nerves begin in the spine, emerging from the spinal nerves of the central nervous system. The axons of this system are generally very long and stretch out into ganglia throughout the remainder of the body. These ganglia are commonly situated in, or close to, organs, enabling the parasympathetic nervous system to quickly send and receive messages from all over the body. Since the parasympathetic nervous system starts in the spine, it does not ordinarily require conscious thought to activate its functions.

The parasympathetic nervous system begins from average medullary locales (core vague, core tractus solitarius, and dorsal motor core) and is regulated by the nerve center. Vagal efferents reach out from the medulla to postganglionic nerves that innervate the atria by means of ganglia situated in cardiovascular fat cushions with neurotransmission that is adjusted through nicotinic receptors. Postganglionic parasympathetic and sympathetic cholinergic nerves at that point influence heart muscarinic receptors.

Parasympathetic enactment can influence atrioventricular nodal conduction intervened prevalently through the left vagus nerve. Besides, muscarinic receptors on vein dividers can cause vasorelaxation through nitric oxide (NO), regulated pathway however can likewise cause vasoconstriction by legitimately enacting smooth muscle. Subsequently, in spite of the fact that the sympathetic nervous system affects cardiovascular physiology in an all-or-none kind of reaction, the parasympathetic nervous system can have a specific balance at different levels.

Vagus nerve afferent actuation, beginning incidentally, can adjust efferent sympathetic and parasympathetic capacity centrally and at the degree of the baroreceptor.

Efferent vagal nerve actuation can have tonic and basal impacts that hinder the sympathetic initiation and arrival of norepinephrine at the presynaptic level. Acetylcholine discharge from parasympathetic nerve terminals will initiate ganglionic nicotinic receptors that thusly enact muscarinic receptors at the cell level. Cardiovascular impacts incorporate pulse decrease by the hindrance of the sympathetic nervous system and by direct hyperpolarization of sinus nodal cells.

Chapter 4: Stress and the Nervous System

Stress is undoubtedly one of the most widely discussed topics in modern society. The hustle and bustle of everyday life make it hard for us to get a grip on our feelings and the environment around us.

The fact of the matter is that no matter how many coping strategies we may have, stress will eventually catch up to us. Furthermore, tolerance to stress varies greatly from person to person. For some folks, stress is a part of daily life. As such, they are more accustomed to dealing with prolonged periods of stress. In contrast, others may feel more overwhelmed especially when stress moments spike at any given point.

For all of the negative press that stress receives, the truth is that stress is a very useful response as it is an evolutionary trait that humans developed over time. The reason why stress exists is to help ensure survival. Plain and simple.

If we go back to the early days of humanity, early humans had to contend with the elements, large predatory animals and an endless shortage of food and water. That is why stress emerged as a response to external stimuli. The human body needed some type of signal to alert the individual that something wasn't right, and action needed to be taken.

For instance, is a human encountered a bear, such an encounter would hardly be pleasant. In fact, the bear might feel threatened and its fight or flight mechanism would spur it to attack. Such an encounter could lead to loss of life on the human's part, or in the best of cases, a very good run while attempting to get away from the bear.

This example underscores the function of stress as part of the human condition. As humans began improving agricultural techniques and the domestication of animals, hunter-gatherer civilizations gave way to agricultural-based ones. Then, as civilization flourished in various parts of the world, the need to engage other large predators diminished. Fast forward to our time, and the need to engage the fight or flight mechanism is limited to instances of potential harm such as a robbery, physical violence and so on.

So, human civilization has moved away from those elements which induced the evolution of stress, yet the stress remains hardwired in the human body. Perhaps we might go through another evolution in which the stress response becomes more attuned to a less stressful environment. In the meantime, we have the nervous system that we inherited from our ancestors.

Stress hormones

Stress hormones are unleashed when a perceived threat is processed by the brain. The brain then signals the body to begin production of several hormones. One of the most common hormones is adrenaline.

Adrenaline is a hormone which kicks the body into high gear. It stimulates the response from the immune system, locks down the digestive tract and improves blood circulation and airflow to the brain. This is the rush that most people get when they practice extreme sports and other types of dangerous activities. It is also the same rush that a person gets when they feel their life might be in danger.

Another hormone that plays a key role in stress is called cortisol. This hormone isn't normally produced by the body unless there is a stress response to some kind of stimulus. Cortisol signals the body to hoard energy and enter "survival mode". In fact, when a person engages in a crash diet in which they drastically reduce the caloric intake in a short period of time, the body may begin to emit cortisol as a stress signal, an SOS if you will, and thereby force the metabolism to go on lockdown. This means that the individual plateaus in their diet and no matter how long they stay on it, they lose weight.

Burnout

When a person is exposed to prolonged periods of stress, such as months or even years, a condition known as "burnout" may take place. Burnout is a condition in which the nervous system becomes so overloaded by stress that it simply begins to shutdown as a means of protecting the body.

In this condition, the individual may begin to feel chronic fatigue, pain, and constant illness. The nervous system may become permanently damaged leading to irregular sleep, digestive and metabolic disorders in addition hypersensitivity to stress. One associated condition to prolonged stress is insulin resistance which is a common marker for diabetes.

Burnout may also result from a single event in which the nervous system becomes completely overwhelmed. Think of a traffic accident, a violent incident or perhaps the loss of a loved one. In this circumstance, Post-Traumatic Stress Disorder (PTSD) may ensue thus leaving the individual with "frayed nerves".

In olden times, frayed nerves were equated to a "nervous breakdown". A nervous breakdown in an incident in which a person has been exposed to stress, usually intense stress over a short period of time, thereby leaving the individual exhausted and in need of recovery. Think of an individual working long hours, over a period of several weeks in order to get a project done. This intense regimen will leave the person in need of recovery from such an event, but without the long-term effects that may emerge as a result of months or even years of prolonged stress.

Recovering from stress

Recovering from stress may be a combination of nutrition and medication. For folks who are under intense periods of stress, such as suffering from PTSD, antidepressants may be prescribed. In other cases, some type of psychotherapy may be recommended.

The fact of the matter is that recovery from stress may necessitate complete isolation from the source of stress. Furthermore, the individual may need extended periods of rest, sleep and recreation in order to level out hormone production. Ultimately, the individual can make a full recovery from the effect of stress, but it may require a complete lifestyle overhaul especially when the individual has been immersed in a violent and/or abusive environment.

If you, or a loved one, are going through a prolonged period of stress, it is best to consult your physician about the treatment options available to you. It is best to address this issue sooner rather than later. That way, you can avoid the development of potentially serious long-term effects.

PART II: THE VAGUS NERVE

Chapter 5: The Vagus Nerve

After discussing the nervous system and its components, we will now focus on one of the most interesting elements that comprise the nervous system: the vagus nerve.

If you haven't heard about this nerve before, don't worry. While its existence has been known for some time, doctors and researchers didn't really understand it until recently. Modern research conducted on this nerve has led to many interesting discoveries.

So, what is the vagus nerve?

The name "vagus" is Latin for "wanderer". This means that the vagus nerve wanders and meanders throughout the body. It is a cranial nerve that runs throughout the entire body. It is associated to the parasympathetic nervous system (PNS). As such, it is the main highway by which the Central Nervous System (CNS) communicates with the PNS. As such, it is tremendously important in regulating all of the essential bodily functions that the PNS regulates.

Given the fact that it is so important, it is surprising just how overlooked this nerve actually is. That is why this section is dedicated to understanding what it is and what it does. In addition, we will be discussing how your understanding of this nerve can help you increase your overall health and wellness. So, sit tight because we are going to be discussing quite a bit of information here. You will surely find this to be insightful as well as fascinating.

We will begin by looking deep into two crucial components of the vagus nerve, the Pneumogastric Nerve and the Ventral Branch of the vagus nerve.

The Pneumogastric Nerve

Before modern research on the vagus nerve was conducted, the name it commonly received was the "pneumogastric nerve". It had earned this designation since the vagus nerve is responsible for the regulation of the heart, lungs and digestive tract.

As the pneumogastric nerve is responsible for ensuring the proper functioning of these systems through the PNS. The PNS relies on the pneumogastric nerve to relay the right information to and from the CNS and the brain. Yet, the fact that the pneumogastric nerve starts in the brain and works its way down into the lungs, heart and digestive tract, it essentially becomes one of the most important neural networks in the body. Needless to say, that if something goes haywire in the pneumogastric nerve, it can lead to serious consequences in the rest of the body.

The pneumogastric nerve begins in the brain and leaves through the medulla oblongata. Then, it basically runs straight through the middle of the body down the neck, chest and into the abdomen. The pneumogastric nerve has ramifications, or branches, that touch upon the main organ systems described earlier.

First, the pneumogastric nerve connects into the laryngeal nerve and then curves around the subclavian artery so that it emerges between the trachea and the esophagus. This is where it is able to regulate the functioning of the lungs. As such, this nerve enables the PNS to regulate breathing.

Next, the nerve runs down from the subclavian artery into the superior vena cava. From there, it moves on onto the bronchus before settling into the vagal trunk that passes through the diaphragm. It also connects into the carotid artery in which then allows it to link with the cardiac tissue. This is the point at which the pneumogastric nerve enables the PNS to hook up with the heart.

As the pneumogastric nerve makes its way down the esophagus and through the diaphragm, it is now able to link up with the digestive tract. This is what permits the PNS to regulate digestion.

As you can see, the pneumogastric nerve is truly an intricate piece of hardware which enables the PNS to regulate some of the most complex bodily functions. Needless to say, the body would not be able to function adequately without the pneumogastric nerve.

The pneumogastric nerve has the following branches which serve as means of communication among the entire routing of this nerve:

- Anterior vagal trunk
- Branches to the esophageal plexus
- Branches to the pulmonary plexus
- Hering-Breuer reflex in alveoli
- Inferior cervical cardiac branch
- Pharyngeal nerve
- Posterior vagal trunk
- Recurrent laryngeal nerve
- Superior cervical cardiac branches of vagus nerve
- Superior laryngeal nerve
- Thoracic cardiac branches

These branches are what enables the pneumogastric job to do its job effectively. When the system is firing on all cylinders, the communication flows effortlessly and regulation happens without a hitch. However, when there is a disruption in communication, or if the pneumogastric nerve becomes altered in any fashion, disruptions may occur leading to any number of potential medical conditions. Later on, we will dig deeper into these conditions.

The Ventral Branch of the Vagus Nerve

The emergence of Polyvagal Theory has allowed for a deeper understanding of the nervous system and its effects on the overall wellbeing of the body. Generally speaking, the vagus nerve is considered as one mega-unit which regulates a number of vital biological systems. We have covered this in-depth throughout the book.

At this point, we can dive straight into the discussion of Porges' Polyvagal approach explains the effect of the vagus nerve on the body. Since the vagus nerve is at the forefront of the PNS, it has a calming effect on the SNS.

Let's elaborate on that point further.

For instance, a person has been involved in a minor car accident, a fender-bender if you will. The incident itself is rather stressful though it does not bear any major consequences. As such, the individual is just shaken up and in need of some rest in order to get over what has occurred. In this example, the SNS kicked into high gear at the occurrence of the accident since the brain perceived a potential threat, that being the car accident. After closer inspection, there were no injuries, and everything proved to be rather innocuous.

If the PNS did not exist, there would be no way for the SNS to essentially shut off; the individual would remain at a constant state of stress and anxiety. Needless to say, they would not be able to sleep or eat due to the stress on them. This harkens back to the point we made earlier about prolonged stress and the effect it has on the overall nervous system.

After the brain has perceived that the threat is over, the PNS takes over and begins to bring back bodily functions down to normal parameters. This means that pulse and heart rate return to normal, blood pressure decreases, and the metabolism resumes normal operations. In the theory, all is well, and the individual makes a full recovery after a good night's sleep.

As a corollary, it is important to highlight the fact that sleep is a great equalizer. This is why you tend to feel sleepy after a significant spike in stress. Sleep allows the PNS to regulate body functions and bring the entire system back to normal. If you are unable to sleep, then the lasting effects will take much longer to become subdued thereby leading you to feel as if you had been hit by a train.

Based on the previous example, the ANS was seen as a mix of both active and passive roles. Of course, the active part only springs into action when there is the need for it, while the passive role hums along in the background.

That being said, the Polyvagal theory suggests that there is a third component of the system. A component which Porges called the "social engagement" system. In a way, this is a smart system that requires the removal of any perceived threat. What this implies is that we need to be able to discern when there is a threat and when there is not. When this discrimination occurs, it is not the "passive" side that takes over, but rather, it is the social engagement side of the equation.

So, how do these three systems work in tandem?

The SNS kicks into gear when there is a threat. Everything goes into high gear. The threat subsides and the brain determines the threat is over. Then, the social engagement system kicks in and alerts the SNS giving it the "all clear" signal. As such, the only thing that the SNS does is regulate the parameters of bodily functions; the SNS and the social engagement system work in an on/off basis. It should be noted that the default setting for the body is the activation of the social engagement system. The SNS is meant to be used only in case of emergency.

The ventral branch comes into play when the social engagement system is in control. The ventral branch essentially regulates everything that happens above the diaphragm in such a manner that the body is able to continuously regulate its responses.

In other words, the brain perceives a potential threat but then quickly discards it. The social engagement system clicks off and clicks back on almost instantly.

How does such a thing work?

For example, you are walking down the street at night and a person approaches. You are concerned that this may be a stranger who means harm. As you get closer, you realize it is a friendly neighbor. The warning issued by the brain did not last long enough for the social engagement system to be shut off and the SNS activated. However, the brain did issue a warning with alerted the social engagement system to be on standby. If the warning was real, then the SNS would kick in and the appropriate response would ensue.

According to this example based on the Polyvagal theory, the social engagement system is the default system for the human body. Consequently, this brings to light the fact that the SNS is only meant to be active for very brief periods of time. As a result, we can infer that prolonged periods of SNS activation can lead to a serious drain on the body's overall energy and wellbeing. Hence, it is vitally important to help the body calm down.

As we will discuss later on, this calming, or soothing effect can be achieved through the right stimulation of the vagal nerve. Moreover, it is helpful to look at this stimulation at a broader level insofar as the calming and soothing of the entire nervous system thereby leading the body to achieve proper balance among all of its functions.

One other important consideration to take into account is that prolonged stress on the nervous system can lead to some of the disorders which we will discuss in an upcoming chapter. That is why we would like to point out the importance of calming the nervous system throughout this book. That way you can begin to see immediate results. In fact, just by being able to take some time away from the main sources of stress in your life, you will be able to see a quick turnaround in the way you feel and the way your body reacts to the various stimuli around you. Of course, we will delve deep into this topic in due time.

In the meantime, it is highly recommended that you make an assessment of the various aspects that may be causing you to feel stressed out. Sure, there may be a stressor which you have little control over. For example, you may have very little control over your job. Still, you have control over the ways in which you can dissipate that negative energy that may be overloading your nervous system, in particular, the SNS thereby leading you to walk around with an overloaded PNS.

Chapter 6: Functions of the Vagus Nerve

In earlier chapters, we have mentioned the main function of the vagus nerve. As such, we have pointed out the importance of the vagus nerve and its pivotal role in keeping the entire body's biological system humming along.

In this chapter, we are going to focus on the specific functions of the vagus nerve and highlight the points in which the vagus nerve may be vulnerable. Thus, we would like to further underscore the importance of taking proper care of the nervous system thereby ensuring proper functioning of the vagus nerve and associated biological systems.

Main functions of the vagus nerve

The vagus nerve is one large highway that conducts the flow of information from the biological systems that it controls up to the CNS. This is the main raison d'etre of the vagus nerve. In a manner of speaking, the vagus nerve is like a central command post in which the information comes and goes. Consequently, the vagus nerve provides the CNS with all of the data it needs to keep the body alive.

Let's assume that the vagus nerve simply stops working for whatever reason. In such a situation, the person would simply die. How so? If the vagus nerve stops sending information to the CNS, the CNS may conclude that the heart and lungs have stopped functioning. Therefore, the brain may have no choice but to begin shutting down other organ systems as well. This type of response may lead doctors to place a patient on life support.

This example highlights the importance that the vagus nerve has on the body's overall ability to sustain life. Now, let's assume that the vagus nerve is functioning properly, but there is some kind of damage to one of the organ systems. In that case, the vagus nerve relays the data on the damage to the organ system back up to the CNS. The brain then sends back the information through the vagus nerve and adjusts accordingly. For instance, if one lung is severely damaged, the brain may choose to shut down that lung and shift all of the breathing functions to the other healthy lung. This is enough to keep the body alive though not necessarily at peak performance.

In addition, the vagus nerve is the main command post for the digestive system. This is a crucial function to consider since the digestive system provides the body with the nutrition it needs to repair itself, fuel movement and keep cells running along. Hence, the digestive system needs close attention. This causal link between the digestive system and the CNS explains why folks who have undergone a traumatic experience often experience digestive distress. When the nervous system suffers a significant jolt, it is not uncommon to see that it has serious repercussions on the entire network controlled by the vagus nerve.

So, let's move on and take a deeper look at the specific functions that are associated with the vagus nerve.

The Visceral Somatic Function

Given the fact that the vagus nerve is part of the Autonomic Nervous System (ANS), it is inextricably linked to the entire body. Think of it as a main highway that receives traffic from all over the region even if the majority of motorists don't actually plan to stay in that particular area. In a way, the main traffic is just passing through.

Based on that premise, any disruption in the flow of traffic in that area may lead to disruption in the flow of traffic in other seemingly unrelated areas. The same goes for the nervous system and biological functions.

When we refer to a somatic function, we are talking about the reaction that comes as a result of the stimuli in the environment surrounding an organism. In this case, the human body is the organism immersed in a given environment. We have also discussed ad nauseum how the body reacts to stimuli by enacting the SNS at the sight of a perceived threat.

As such, the somatic function that the vagus nerve plays is one of constant monitoring and regulation. Think of it as one large pressure valve that looks to regulate the build-up within a large engine. If too much pressure builds up, then the engine may explode. The same goes for the nervous system.

With that in mind, there is one interesting bit of good news... if we could call it that. The body is adept at adjusting to its environment. So, if the individual finds themselves consistently inundated by stressful situations, there is the possibility that the body will become adjusted to such levels of stress. In a way, it creates a "new normal".

An example of this attitude can be seen in the so-called "adrenaline junkies". These people become addicted to extreme sports due to the exhilaration that they get from engaging in a dangerous activity. However, they consistently need to up the ante since their nervous system constantly adjusts to the level of danger in each activity. So, in order to get the same rush, they need to overload their nervous system more and more. Otherwise, they may not find the same amount of enjoyment in the same activities.

As far as the visceral function is concerned, the vagus nerve is constantly tracking the performance of the body's internal organ systems. As a matter of fact, it is designed with a number of automatic switches that are intended to protect the body from grievous damage. Think of these switches like circuit breakers in an electrical system. When the system is overloaded by the electrical current, the circuit breaker is tripped thereby protecting the entire system. If no such breaker existed, the wiring would overheat potentially causing a fire.

The vagus nerve has built-in parameters that prevent the body from overexerting itself to the point where permanent damage is done to organs. Consider this situation:

A person who has been working non-stop for a week may find that after going on little to no sleep, they simply crash and sleep for an extended period of time. This reaction is triggered in the nervous system in order to prevent the heart from literally burning out. This is why drug consumption, the kind that disrupts the nervous system, making it prone for individuals to suffer from cardiac arrest. Since the substance wreaks havoc with the PNS natural regulation mechanisms, the body keeps going until it eventually shuts down.

A good example of this can be seen in modern cars. The car's computer shuts the engine down when it diagnoses a potentially serious problem in the engine. The car's control computer module shuts off the flow of gas, for example, in order to keep the engine from completely failing. The car will restart once the issue has been corrected.

So, just like a car's control module, the vagus nerve serves as the body's main regulation unit. This protects the body's vital organs from failing altogether at which point death would ensue. This is why optimal performance from the vagus nerve is essential to ensuring the body's overall optimal performance.

The Physical Motor Function

Since the vagus nerve is part of the overall ANS, it is also connected to the body's peripheral nervous system which controls the movement of limbs. As such, the vagus nerve is involved in the motor functions of the body.

Now, the vagus nerve itself does not regulate movement, but it does regulate the biological functions that aid movement. The following example will illustrate this point.

When a person engages in physical activity, the CNS broadcasts the necessary signals to the limbs for movement, be it running, swimming, and so on. However, the heart is also responsible for supply blood to the muscles while the lungs need to provide oxygen. Furthermore, there is an increased metabolic response as the body needs to create the energy it requires to sustain the level of physical activity. If the activity exceeds the heart's capacity to pump blood and the lungs' ability to provide oxygen, then the individual may simply get tired and stop moving.

This example highlights how important the vagus nerve is when taking movement into account. High-performance athletes have trained not only for their sport, but also develop stamina. Now, you may have heard of this term, yet it is generally associated to endurance, that is, sustaining physical activity over longer periods of time. But the fact of the matter is that stamina is the body's ability to provide the elements the body needs to sustain prolonged periods of physical activity.

Consequently, the vagus nerve is able to recognize these increased levels of physical activity and make the necessary adjustments so that muscles get the elements they need in order to keep going. It should be noted that the vagus nerve will also recognize when an athlete is becoming overexerted. At which point, the athlete may feel like they can't go on anymore. This is the body's protective measures that keep it from causing serious damage.

This last point illustrates the importance of keeping a balanced nervous system so that the vagus nerve can perform its functions appropriately thereby allowing the body's organ systems to provide the elements that the body requires.

Essential biological functions

At this point, we have widely discussed the essential biological functions that the vagus nerve regulates. These functions are what basically keeps the body alive. After all, if your heart stops breathing, then chances are you are not going to make it.

With that in mind, it is important to note that when the vagus nerve is not functioning at 100%, that is, when there is some kind of disruption, the essential biological systems may begin to go haywire. In some cases, it might be a slow and progressive disruption while in other cases it may be a sudden and shocking disruption.

Let's consider two possible scenarios:

An individual who has been working a stressful job begins to feel the effects of chronic stress over months or even years of accumulated stress. Suddenly, they may develop cardiac conditions, anxiety or even chronic digestive disorders. Yet, the progression of these conditions was so subtle that the person didn't really feel much of a difference.

On the flip side, there is a person who underwent a major traumatic incident, for instance, the loss of a loved one. The stress caused by the sudden loss of a dear person may cause a sudden overload to the nervous system. This sudden overload may lead to the onset of any of the aforementioned conditions. This may prompt swift intervention by medical professionals in order to address the onset of the symptoms the person is experiencing.

In either case, the vagus nerve can come under attack. At this point, there is s serious need for treatment which can correct the imbalances in the nervous system thus promoting recovery from the overwhelming effects on the nervous system. Given these considerations, the following chapter will go into great detail about the conditions that are beset by disruptions in the vagus nerve's proper functioning. In fact, you may be surprised that some of the most common conditions that you may be familiar with can be addressed by balancing out the vagus nerve's functions.

Chapter 7: Dysfunctions of the Vagus Nerve

Thus far, we have focused heavily on the functions of the vagus nerve and what it is intended to do. However, we have only briefly touched upon the various consequences of a dysfunctional vagus nerve.

The vagus nerve, on its own, does not break down or show signs of dysfunction on its own. Barring some sort of physiological issue in which a person is born with a dysfunctional vagus nerve, the dysfunctions that may occur to it are generally the result of the strain the nervous system is put under. This is important to note as the nervous system is designed to take its share of wear and tear. Nevertheless, even something as strong and robust as the nervous system can, and will, eventually begin to break down.

Unless the individual is faced with a sudden shock, say an accident, in which the vagus nerve is severely damaged, the dysfunctions of the vagus nerve occur after a prolonged period of strain. Therefore, the wear and tear that the vagus nerve suffers is a progressive condition. In fact, it can be so subtle, that a person may not know that something is wrong until it is too late. For example, a person may not be fully aware of the stress he has in his body, until he has a heart attack. At this point, doctors may discover that there is something wrong with the person's nervous system. By that point, the results may be irreversible.

This is why we can infer that, barring physiological causes, the vagus nerve becomes damaged as a result of prolonged periods of stress and overwhelming strain on the nervous system. As such, it is important to address nervous system health at once. In a later chapter, we will focus on specific means of stimulating the vagus nerve. Nevertheless, it is worth mentioning that adequate rest, sleep and proper nutrition are the core tenets of building a healthy nervous system. In doing so, you will get a leg up on recovery from any of the conditions that we will mention in this chapter.

So, let's take a closer look at the various conditions that may be onset by dysfunctions of the vagus nerve.

Anxiety

Anxiety is a condition that affects people from all walks of life. It affects men and women alike, while it affects children, teens, and adults just the same. The root cause of anxiety is stress. As such, it is important to determine the sources of that stress.

Stressors abound in the world around us. These can range from purely emotional causes to physiological causes. That is why we are going to explore both angles. That way, we can gain a broader perspective on anxiety and its relation to the vagus nerve.

As we have mentioned throughout this book, the vagus nerve is part of the PNS. The PNS is charged with the task of bringing the body's bodily functions back to within acceptable parameters. When the nervous system is maxed out, the PNS may have trouble regulating the body back to normal parameters.

Consider this situation:

A person who is consistently under stress due to a violent environment in which he lives. This could be a country at war, a rough neighborhood, or a break down in the law and order of a place. The person is constantly fearing for his safety and that of his loved ones. Such people are constantly worried about attacks, gunfire or any other type of violent attack. Since the fight or flight response is active all the time, there will come a time with the PNS will be unable to regulate the nervous system. Eventually, the vagus nerve begins to suffer the effect of this overload. So, once the person is finally removed from this violent environment, he may be unable to return to normal. He may suffer from chronic anxiety and require medication in order to help him get back to normal.

There is an individual who recently lost his job. While he had a comfortable financial position, now he feels at a loss. He feels like his skills and talents have not been appreciated. This state of loss leads to overloading the nervous system. Since the person is unable to get over the loss of his job, he can't seem to get any peace. In the end, the vagus nerve begins to pay the price since the individual cannot get back on track. In the end, a condition of chronic anxiety may ensure especially since it doesn't seem to be any respite from the feelings produced by this event.

Both of these events, although somewhat extreme, serve to show how the PNS eventually becomes overwhelmed and unable to regulate the body back to its normal parameters. As such, the anxious state becomes the "new normal" for the body. At this point, the individual may have no choice but to go on medication. Nevertheless, addressing the damage done to the vagus nerve may very well be enough to sort out the issue and help the individual get back on track.

Depression

Depression is usually associated to anxiety though depression is not necessarily the consequence of anxiety. In fact, a person may suffer from both depression and anxiety given the circumstances they are forced to endure. Under this consideration, depression can be differentiated from anxiety insofar as depression is a constant state of sadness and gloom. The individual suffering from depression may feel there is nothing to live for. If unattended, depression can lead to thoughts of harming oneself. In the worst of cases, depression may lead to suicide.

Just like anxiety, the causes for depression may vary from a purely physiological one, such as irregular brain chemistry, to purely psychological ones such as feelings of profound sadness as a result of the loss of loved one, significant life changes and even untreated anxiety.

In such cases, depression may reach a point in which psychotherapy and medication may be insufficient to help an individual return to normalcy. In fact, some folks may require hospitalization in a proper mental care facility especially when they have shown signs of harming themselves.

The onset of depression generally has its origins in an overloaded nervous system. When the individual is not removed from the environment which is causing them significant stress, they may end up suffering from physical effects such as chronic fatigue, low immune response, or even impaired cognitive ability. All of these physical conditions can be traced back to poor regulation from the vagus nerve.

Hence, the need for proper regulation from the vagus nerve will ensure that the nervous system has the opportunity to recover from the stressful events that caused it to become overloaded in the first place. However, this is a personal decision that every individual needs to make. It might seem like a no-brainer, that is to extricate oneself from a stressful environment, but the fact of the matter is that it may not always be possible to do so.

Depression is generally treated with a combination of medication and psychotherapy. But the fact is that medication only helps to manage the symptoms but does very little to address the root cause of the depression itself. This is what psychotherapy is for. Yet, the process of therapy may be even more stressful as the patient is asked to confront the stressful events causing depression. For instance, if the depression can be traced back to a traumatic event in childhood, the patient may have a major episode when asked to relive this event.

While both medication and therapy are viable means of dealing with depression, doctors often look at the importance of treating the vagus nerve. When this vagus nerve is addressed, many of the symptoms of depression begin to subside. For example, mindfulness and meditation have been known to help depression sufferers. Now, meditation in itself is not the solution. The apparent solution lies in the fact that meditation has a soothing effect on the nervous system. Thus, it is this soothing effect that helps the vagus nerve return to normal operations.

Panic attacks

Another condition associated with vagus nerve dysfunction is known as panic attacks. Panic attacks allude to repetitive, sudden episodes that include unpleasant physical, intellectual manifestations, and social signs. These episodes involve anxiety rising to the level in which the individual is unable to cope with the overwhelming emotions that overcome them. As a result, they may feel completely inundated with worry and stress that goes beyond any coping mechanism they may employ.

The following signs are indicative of a panic attack:

- Significant conduct changes identified with the attacks (for instance, evading activity or spots due to being paranoid about having a panic attack).
- Consistent worry about having another panic assault or the outcomes of a panic assault (for example, having a heart attack).

- A panic attack is an unexpected inclination of serious dread or distress that spikes in a matter of minutes. It incorporates distressing physical and psychological manifestations just like behavioral signs.
- Panic disorder alludes to repetitive, unforeseen panic attacks (e.g., heart palpitations, perspiring, trembling) trailed by in any event one month.

Specific physical symptoms may include:

- Feelings of warmth or cold
- Chest torment or uneasiness
- Dizziness and lightheadedness
- Gag reflex
- Increased heart rate
- Perspiration
- Feelings of loneliness and isolation
- Shortness of breath
- Trembling or shaking

These symptoms fuel a negative feedback loop in which the individual feels terrible to be with, and the addition of these symptoms only makes the individual feel worse thereby fueling the attack to even greater depths. As a result, the onset of a panic attack is enough to keep the sufferer in a constant state of anxiety.

Much like depression and anxiety, panic attacks can be treated with a combination of medication and therapy. Generally speaking, this course of treatment is effective although it should be noted that treatment alleviates the symptoms that lead to the onset of a panic attack but not the root cause itself. Medication is quite adept at helping regulate brain chemistry but does little to aid the nervous system in regulating essential functions such as those related to the PNS. As a result, feelings and symptoms subside but little is actually done to promote the health of the individual sufferer in the long run.

Furthermore, conventional treatments don't do very much in terms of helping the vagus nerve recover to its full capacity. So, even if the individual strives to make a full recovery, the fact that the vagus nerve tends to be overlooked makes a full recovery rather complicated. As such, it is important that treatment also is centered on helping the vagus nerve bounce back to its normal state.

Inflammation and Autoimmune diseases

Inflammation is a condition in which tissue swells up in an attempt to isolate an area that is affected by some sort of aggressor. One of the most common areas of inflammation is the digestive system. Inflammation of the digestive system is common as a result of food allergies or overconsumption of certain types of foods.

Nevertheless, inflammation can happen in any part of the body. This also affects the nervous system as it is quite possible for the CNS to experience inflammation as a result of excessive periods of stress. Swelling in the brain may occur, not just as a consequence of a severe blow to the head, but also of prolonged periods of sleep deprivation, substance abuse (drugs, alcohol, caffeine, painkillers, and so on) and high levels of stress.

When the nervous system becomes overwhelmed, the brain sends a distress signal to the immune system to begin a lockdown on the afflicted parts of the body. However, inflammation in the nervous system is nothing compared to inflammation in a local part of the body. For instance, if you fall and sprain your ankle, the body uses inflammation to protect the sprained ankle.

In the case of the nervous system, we are talking about a significant amount of the body that is affected. Furthermore, the nervous system runs the entire body. Consequently, inflammation of the nervous system means inflammation throughout the entire body. Needless to say, this can lead to all sorts of conditions ranging from mild pain and discomfort to serious conditions which may end up becoming chronic.

When the nervous system is out of whack, the immune system, the body's line of defense against illness, also goes out of whack. When the immune system is not fully online, a recurring illness may set in. But beyond getting constantly sick, the immune system may trigger what is known as an "autoimmune disease".

Autoimmune diseases, by definition, are when the immune system believes that a healthy part of the body is somehow causing the body harm. So, it attacks the body causing damage to an area that it's supposed to protect. If that sounds contradictory, it really is.

The nature of autoimmune diseases is not quite understood by modern medical science. There is any number of causes for such ailments. But almost all of them can be traced back to some sort of issue within the nervous system. Again, unless there is some underlying physiological or genetic factor causing the illness, autoimmune afflictions are almost always caused by dysfunctions in the nervous system.

Examples of such illnesses include Lupus, Psoriasis, Sjogren's Syndrome, Rheumatoid Arthritis and Irritable Bowel Syndrome, among others. Autoimmune diseases lead to degenerative conditions that are almost always irreversible. One such example is the kidney damage that Lupus causes its sufferers. Lupus attacks healthy tissue in the kidneys to the extent of rendering them useless. The ultimate consequence is chronic renal failure. Transplant in Lupus patients is highly risky as the immune system not only tends to reject the new organ but may also require the patient to be on lifelong immunosuppressor treatment. Thus, autoimmune diseases are certainly to be taken seriously.

Chronic conditions – Fibromyalgia

One of the points we have made about dysfunctions of the vagus nerve is the emergence of chronic conditions. By chronic, we understand that these are conditions that are not going away any time soon. In fact, chronic conditions are generally ailments which the person must live with for the rest of their lives. Needless to say, this is not a fun situation to be in.

One of the most common chronic conditions that develop as a result of dysfunctions in the vagus nerve is Fibromyalgia. Fibromyalgia is a disorder described as widespread musculoskeletal torment highlighted by weakness, pain, memory issues, and psychological distress. Specialists accept that Fibromyalgia amplifies difficult sensations by influencing the manner in which the brain processes pain.

Side effects now and again start after a physical injury, medical procedure, contamination or significant mental pressure. In different cases, side effects progressively build up after some time with no single trigger activating an onset of the condition.

While there is no remedy for fibromyalgia, an assortment of prescriptions can help control manifestations. Exercise, unwinding and stress-decrease measures likewise may help. This underscores the need that the vagus nerve requires.

Indications of Fibromyalgia include:

- **Exhaustion**. Individuals with Fibromyalgia regularly feel drained, despite the fact that they report getting regular sleep. Rest is regularly disturbed by agony, and numerous patients with fibromyalgia have other disruptions, for example, fretful legs or even sleep apnea.

- **Far-reaching discomfort**. The unpleasantness related to Fibromyalgia frequently is depicted as a consistent dull pain that has gone on for three months or more. To be viewed as far-reaching, the discomfort must happen on both sides of the body and specifically underneath in the lower body such as the legs.

- **Mental distress**. A side effect generally alluded to as "fibro-mist" which weakens the capacity to concentrate, focus and conduct mental tasks.

Fibromyalgia frequently exists together with other uncomfortable conditions, such as:

- Interstitial cystitis or unpleasant bladder discomfort
- Temporomandibular joint disorders
- Headache leading to possible migraines

As per the definition of chronic conditions, chronic pain doesn't go away on its own. In fact, the individual may experience such conditions for months or even years. Painkillers only mask the symptoms while hardly addressing the actual root cause of the ailment. This is why a closer look at the nervous system may reveal the potential root cause and pathway to relief.

Additionally, vagus nerve dysfunctions manifest themselves throughout the body. So, if a person is suffering from Fibromyalgia, they may not just experience pain the lower extremities but may experience this situation in their hands and arms. For instance, sufferers of this condition often complain of numbness in their hands. This is especially disconcerting when the individual is unable to complete tasks they usually would. As a result, the ailment only fuels the negative feedback loop that is created by the chronic condition itself.

Headaches and migraines

When most individuals hear the term "headache" they regularly think about an extreme headache. What they cannot deny is that headache is a neurological sickness and that there are various different subtypes of headache. Get some answers concerning the different sorts of headache underneath.

Given the fact that it is neurological in nature, it is related to the nervous system in one way or another. Headaches that are not related to stress, such as after a long day at work or school, can be traced back to some sort of nervous system dysfunction. Now, it is entirely possible that headaches can be caused by physical injury such as a concussion sustained in an accident. But beyond clearly identifiable physiological causes, there is little room to doubt that headaches have an origin in neurological causes.

Generally speaking, headaches are discomfort and pain located in the cranial region. In other cases, headaches may extend to the neck and even shoulders. In other cases, a headache may be located in one specific part of the head while in other cases it may simply be a blanket pain that covers the entire head. Regardless of the nature and location of the pain, the main thing to keep in mind is that it is there to being with.

Migraines are generally distinguishable from regular headaches in that they have specific triggers. These triggers may vary from being in crowded places to hearing certain types of sounds. Others may experience migraines when they find themselves inside a movie theater in the midst of a loud action sequence.

Migraines are generally described as stronger than usual headaches that may be accompanied by blurry vision, sensitivity to light and/or sound, nausea, and even digestive distress. For some folks, migraines can be so debilitating that they cannot think properly and are unable to visually focus on any object. This makes tasks such as driving virtually impossible.

Prolonged exposure to stress is also another common source of headaches and migraines. When a person is subject to long hours, little rest and sleep deprivation, headaches may become chronic. It should be noted that the headache itself is not caused by the stress that is being experienced; it is caused by the overload the nervous system is underway. In that case, the vagus nerve's inability to properly regulate the PNS may lead to the sufferer being unable to control the triggers that set off headaches. As such, a chronic condition may be diagnosed if the individual finds themselves suffering from headaches at least 3 days a week, or 14 days out of a month. In the worst of cases, a sufferer may find themselves going consecutive days with headaches. In such situations, medication is almost always the only course of treatment.

Alternative forms of treatment for headaches include meditation and relaxation. This treatment is considered successful since it is aimed at helping the nervous system calm down and help the PNS regulate bodily functions back to normal.

Breathing conditions

Considering that the vagus nerve controls the lungs and heart, it is safe to assume that any dysfunctions in the vagus nerve may lead to breathing issues. In short, breathing issues as a result of the vagus nerve being out of whack can be seen in improper breathing. What this implies is that the body cannot produce enough oxygen for the entire body's functions. When this occurs, the blood cannot carry enough oxygen to the brain and other parts of the body.

The end result may be poor cognitive skills and inadequate cell regeneration. If this should be the case, then the suffering may not be able to recuperate well illness and have difficulty sleeping.

Symptoms of poor breathing include:

- Shallow breathing
- Shortness of breath
- Constant labored breathing
- Poor stamina when engaging in physical activity
- Improper circulation
- Lightheadedness and dizziness

While this list is not exhaustive, it serves to prove that poor breathing can be truly disruptive in a person's day to day routine. Moreover, inadequate breathing can lead to long-term cognitive impairment as the brain cannot function properly on low levels of oxygen. Consequently, it is necessary for the brain to be fully oxygenated.

The vagûs nerve must then be repaired in order to ensure that proper oxygen absorption takes place. In addition, when the vagus nerve is out of balance, it can lead to cardiac issues solely based on the lack of oxygen in the blood. As such, it is important to pay close attention to breathing.

Long-term pulmonary damage may also ensue as a result of improper breathing. The lungs may be forced to work overtime in order to extract as much oxygen as possible from the air that it receives. Consequently, this may place undue stress on the lungs. If the person happens to live in a place with poor air quality, this may also lead to other degenerative conditions. So, exposure to fresh air is a must especially for those living in large areas.

Breathing techniques are almost always the best way to improve the quality of breathing. Meditation and yoga are great ways of helping in this case. However, the broader issues affecting the nervous system need to be addressed in order to fully guarantee that the person can find the right way to improve their breathing and oxygen absorption.

One other important condition to consider when dealing with vagus nerve-related breathing issues is asthma. While asthma has a clear physiological link to it, the vagus nerve is almost always associated to its worsening or improvement. Hence, is it certainly worth digging deeper into the status of the vagus nerve and addressing any potential issues with it? Experience has shown that improving vagus nerve function has a significant effect in alleviating some of the most debilitating symptoms associated with asthma.

Digestive System Dysfunction

Just like breathing issues, digestive dysfunction is almost a given when the vagus nerve is not functioning to its optimal levels. Since the vagus nerve regulates the digestive system, it is only logical to assume that the vagus nerve needs to be properly tended to in order to ensure that nothing is out of sorts.

Granted, digestive disorders are not exclusively the result of issues with the vagus nerve. There might be a number of reasons why a person would suffer from digestive issues. For instance, digestive issues may be related to physiological causes such as food allergies. It is quite common for people to go for years suffering from poor digestion until they realize that they are allergic to gluten, or some other type of foodstuff.

In other cases, there might be genetic conditions at play such as Crohn's disease. In these cases, dysfunctions of the vagus nerve may serve to aggravate the condition but not actually cause it. Furthermore, treating the vagus nerve would improve the treatment of the condition but not necessarily cure it.

One particular condition that is related to the vagus nerve is gastroparesis. With gastroparesis, it is also common to see Vasovagal Syncope in tandem with this condition.

Gastroparesis is where the stomach cannot void nourishment typically. Actually, it can be defined as a "loss stomach of motion." It can cause acid reflux, queasiness, vomiting, and might be treated with meds or medical procedures. Gastroparesis is a typical condition among individuals who have had diabetes for quite a while however can likewise happen in individuals without diabetes.

It is possible to actually have gastroparesis and not experience any direct symptoms. However, when symptoms do become manifest, the condition may have advanced far enough to where medication is only able to quell them. Here are some of the most common symptoms:

- Stomach distress or swelling (bloating)
- Queasiness
- Alteration of glucose levels
- Feeling full immediately when eating
- Indigestion/Acid Reflux/Gastrointestinal Reflux (GERD)
- Loss of appetite / weight loss / Malnutrition
- Vomiting

Some of these conditions may be indicative of other potential ailments and may not necessarily be traced back to the vagus nerve. But just like in the case of asthma, the vagus nerve can play a significant role in improving the symptoms of the illness as opposed to actually curing them. In that case, it is conceivable that conventional treatments would be enhanced by improving the overall functioning of the vagus nerve.

Dysfunction of the Microbiome

The human gastrointestinal tract has in excess of 100 trillion microscopic organisms and archaea, which together make up the gut microbiota. The measure of microbes in the human gut outnumbers regular human cells by a factor of 10. As such, the human gut microbiota co-advanced with humans to accomplish a harmonious relationship prompting physiological homeostasis. This is a clear example of a symbiotic relationship.

When the gut is out of whack, the body's overall conditioning pays the price. The reason for this is that the microbiota helps digest food and absorb nutrition. When this process does not take place, the body becomes depleted of valuable nutrients. Needless to say, the body needs these little critters in order to fully gain the nutrition it needs.

Dysfunctions and deficiencies in the gut create a condition in which the body cannot fully receive the nutrition it needs. And while we have established that this is partly due to physiological factors which may influence the digestive system, the fact of the matter is that the vagus nerve also plays a critical role insofar as ensuring proper functioning of the body. When the vagus nerve is not at optimal levels, it is quite conceivable that the digestive tract will not be at its best either. The end result is any number of conditions that can arise from improper nutrition.

For example, improper nutrition may result in vitamin deficiency. Deficiency of the B-vitamins may lead to pernicious anemia, nervous system dysfunction and chronic pain. As you can see, it is a feedback loop that fuels itself. That is why it is of the utmost importance to consider gut health as much as possible.

In general, promoting gut health may imply a mix of nutrition such as consuming probiotics such as those found in yogurt. But on the whole, a healthy vagus nerve can go a long way toward setting up a healthy environment for gut health. The most important thing to keep in mind is that the body is an interconnected network meaning that one component cannot fail in isolation. So, if one system falters, the rest of the body will also be affected accordingly.

Cardiac dysfunction

Since the vagus nerve is associated with essential biological functions, the breakdown of this nerve can produce altered heart rhythm. In particular, bradycardia (a slowdown of the heart rate) and tachycardia (an increase in heart rate) may result.

This specific point is completely in concordance with vagus nerve function as this vagus nerve regulates cardiac function. What this entails is that any failure to regulate the heart properly will lead to the conditions mentioned above. Indeed, any potential cardiac failure may result in grave consequences such as a heart attack which can be fatal.

Beyond that, cardiac dysfunction may not necessarily be so serious. But it can be serious enough to leave the sufferer with a significant alteration of their lifestyle. For instance, they may have difficulty engaging in physical activity or may experience chronic fatigue. These symptoms are hardly pleasant and represent a detriment to the quality of life in an individual.

When physiological causes for cardiac problems are discarded, the individual ought to seek proper treatment in order to help correct any dysfunction in their nervous system. This generally implies a reduction of stress and a combination of proper nutrition and relaxation. As you can see, it is the same formula that comes up time and again. Hence, it is important to consider the vital importance that getting away from stressors has on a person's overall health and wellbeing.

Ultimately, maintaining proper cardiac health is a combination of factors that depend largely on proper nervous system management. By now, we have made this point repeatedly. Thus, we sincerely hope that you have already begun to think about ways in which you can begin removing stressors from your life and finding the means to improve your nutrition, exercise and relaxation habits.

Hepatic Dysfunction

Hepatic dysfunction, that is liver dysfunction, may also be traced back to the vagus nerve. While there are clear lifestyle issues that affect liver health, the vagus nerve and its dysfunctions may also play a key role in leading the liver to suffer from abnormal function.

Causes leading to improper liver function are excessive alcohol consumption, increased use of certain prescription medication, a viral infection such as hepatitis and unhealthy eating habits. In such cases, the liver becomes "gunked up". This contamination of the hepatic tissue can lead to further issues starting with digestive problems and moving on to more severe issues such as liver failure.

However, liver dysfunction may also be associated with the vagus nerve. When the vagus nerve is unable to regulate proper digestion, the entire digestive system becomes affected. One of the most common conditions is known as "fatty liver". This condition implies a liver that is so contaminated that it is no longer able to filter any of the substances that are consumed by the body. In that regard, the body progressively becomes intoxicated until it reaches a point where one, or several, organs also begin to show signs of failure. The end result may be the body going into shock. While that may seem extreme, the fact of the matter is that the liver is one of the most important organs in the body. That is why great care needs to be taken to ensure proper hepatic health.

Chronic Stress

We have widely discussed chronic stress throughout this book and its detrimental effect on the nervous system. However, it should be pointed out that chronic stress is just another feedback loop that fuels the feelings of illness and overload that affected the nervous system in the first place. As such, it is a never-ending cycle that leaves the person drained both emotionally and physically. In some cases, chronic stress is one of the leftover byproducts of burnout. Some folks never fully recover from burnout and therefore have to be increasingly careful to avoid falling into the same pattern again.

ADHD and Hyperactivity

ADHD is a neurodevelopmental disorder, which can influence various regions of the brain. It is not an indication of a lack of intelligence or even disability. With proper care and treatment, those with ADHD can effectively overcome the difficulties posed by ADHD. It is highly common in children though it also affects adults.

Folks with ADHD experience:

- Social anxiety
- Difficulty following instructions
- Negligence – experiencing issues concentrating, overlooking guidelines, undertaking one task and then moving onto the next without finishing anything
- Impulsivity – talking over others, having a short attention span, being clumsy
- Sleeping difficulties
- Hyperactivity – consistent eagerness and restlessness
- Inability to carry out complex cognitive tasks due to a lack of concentration and focus

A person coping with ADHD may experience some, or all, of the following:

- Difficulty following rules
- Following through on tasks
- Experience difficulty while playing with other children of the same age group
- experience issues sorting out tasks and exercises
- Being withdrawn as a means of keeping a safe distance between themselves and other children
- A lack of focus and attention to detail especially in schoolwork and other related tasks
- Generally losing things or forgetting where they had been placed.
- Apparent sloppiness and disinterest in neatness
- Appearing not to listen when spoken to directly
- Not begin able to complete tasks such as homework or assigned tasks such as taking care of household chores

There is no conclusive evidence as to the precise reason for ADHD. The main hypothesis is that ADHD is an acquired neurodevelopment disorder. Possible breakdown of the vagus nerve may lead the child to develop inadequately thus leading to the condition. Other contributing factors may include:

- Drugs – consumption of nicotine, alcohol or drugs during pregnancy
- Lead (and other heavy metals) – persistent presence of low degrees of lead may impact conduct and brain science
- Neurophysiology – which incorporates differences in biological systems, electrochemical action in the brain and even gut health

- Absence of early connection – if an infant does not bond with their parent or guardian, or has traumatic experiences identified with connection, this may add to their mindlessness and hyperactivity.
- Hereditary qualities – some examination recommends conceivable quality changes which might be present

A person with post-traumatic stress disorder may have symptoms resembling ADHD, however, it will require different treatment.

Chronic Fatigue Syndrome

Chronic fatigue syndrome (CFS), otherwise called myalgic encephalomyelitis (ME), is an ailment that influences an individual's nervous system (usually called a 'neurological disease'). It can happen at any age and can influence children just like grown-ups.

The term 'myalgic encephalomyelitis' refers to pain in the muscles, and aggravation in the brain and spinal cord. ME/CFS is a disconcerting sickness to which a conclusive origin has not yet been determined. For certain individuals, the condition might be suddenly activated by a viral disease, poisonous agent, sedative, inoculation, gastroenteritis or injury. In other individuals, ME/CFS may grow gradually over months or years.

Around 30 percent of individuals with ME/CFS will have subtle symptoms. Many of these individuals will have the chance to recover rather quickly through a conventional course of treatment. Around 50 percent will have a moderate to a serious case of ME/CFS and not have the option to bounce back quite so quickly. Another 20 percent will encounter serious ME/CFS and need to remain at home or on bedrest until treatment begins to take effect.

There are numerous subtypes within the range of ME/CFS, which implies that a management plan must be created for every individual with the condition. Applying a specific treatment for one subtype can be harming to another subtype. An individual management plan must be produced for every individual with ME/CFS.

Since ME/CFS is an extremely intricate, multi-system, chronic disease, numerous different side effects will happen and should be available for determination. These include:

- Sleeping disorders
- Palpitations, increased pulse or shortness of breath
- Sensitivity to light, smells, contact, sound, food, synthetic compounds, and meds
- Pain or throbbing in the muscles, joints or head
- Inability to adapt to temperature changes

- Gastrointestinal distress, for example, sickness, blockage, bloating or diarrhea
- Issues with cognitive tasks such as concentrating, bad memory, blurry vision, awkwardness, muscle spasms which can also be termed as 'neurocognitive issues'
- Urinary incontinence
- Sore throat, delicate lymph hubs and influenza-like symptoms
- A drop in circulation, dizziness or pale skin
- Sudden fluctuations in weight be it gain or loss

An individual's manifestations will vary over brief timeframes, even from hour to hour.

Chronic fatigue is generally traced back to nervous system overload. In which case, treatment of the vagus nerve may help to alleviate these symptoms or completely reverse them. Therefore, it is definitely a good idea to double-check if there has been any damage to the vagus nerve.

Sleep Issues and Circadian Rhythm Disruption

There are several biological and environmental factors that trigger the brain and cause good or bad sleep. Thus, there are two vital concepts in the human body that trigger the brain and influence a good or bad sleeping experience. Temperature and metabolism influence the level of brain activity since an increase in any of the two leads to an increase in brain activity. Dreams usually occur in the last third of an individual's sleep when brain activity is at its highest. This stage of sleep is known as the Rapid-Eye Movement stage where, depending on their body activity, an individual can experience a bad or good dream.

Foods that rapidly increase the body's metabolism, such as certain condiments and caffeine elevate body temperature and metabolism. In turn, there is an increase in the average brain activity where the individual will take a longer time to move from being fully awake to fast asleep and vice versa. In a similar fashion, any food that adds to the sugar level of the blood, such as sugary foods, increases body temperature and metabolism thereby influencing bad sleep. The increase in the activity of the brain is a consequence of the increase in brain waves.

There are other activities that also trigger brain wave activity causing good or bad quality of sleep. There have been several arguments about the definite influence of sleeping positions in determining the overall quality of sleep. There is evidence to show that poor body positioning and discomfort trigger the brain to produce nightmares and poor sleep. The positioning of the body calls the attention of the brain because of the constant communication it relays with the central nervous system.

For instance, sleeping on the stomach can have significant sway in causing bad sleep in an individual. This is because of the discomfort and strain it places on other body organs and the consequential brain activity through nerve connections. This is why sleeping on your stomach can be uncomfortable since it is plainly uncomfortable and distressing. This is similar to other poor sleeping positions such as sitting upright or having the neck raised too high. Poor body positioning triggers more brain wave activity causing a bad quality of sleep and a lack of rest upon waking.

With that in mind, an overactive nervous system can lead to increased brain wave activity throughout the course of a night's sleep, that is assuming that the individual can get to sleep. This is important to keep in mind as having trouble falling asleep is one of the most common issues that afflict people who are going through issues related to the vagus nerve. In short, addressing any potential issues in the nervous system can go a very long way toward improving sleep quality.

Antisocial Behavior and Lack of Social Interaction

Personality disorders are mental health conditions that influence how somebody thinks, sees, feels or identifies with others. An antisocial personality disorder is an especially testing sort of personality disorder portrayed by hasty, flighty and regularly inappropriate conduct. An individual with an antisocial personality disorder will commonly be manipulative, misleading and neglectful. Moreover, they tend not to take other individuals' feelings into account. Like different sorts of personality disorders, an antisocial personality disorder may range from mild inappropriate social interactions to intermittent improper conduct to overstepping the law and carrying out criminal actions.

Indicators of antisocial behavior include:

- The need to blame others for their shortcomings as opposed to taking personal responsibility
- Lack of concern, lament or regret about other individuals' distress

- Display lack of concern for ordinary social conduct
- Violating the law on a consistent basis
- Experience issues with forming long-term commitment and relationships
- Not being able to control their emotions
- Abuse, control or damage the privileges of others
- Reprimand others for issues in their lives

An individual with antisocial character disorder will have a past filled with lead disorder during youth, for example, skipping school (not going to class), wrongdoing (for instance, carrying out violations or substance abuse), and other troublesome and forceful practices.

PART III: THE MIND BODY CONNECTION

Chapter 7: The Physical and Emotional Connection Between the Mind and the Body

In ancient Greece, three specialists would see a patient in tandem. They were the "knife" specialist, the "herb" specialist, and the "language" specialist. The individuals who "designed" medication comprehended there was an association between the mind and body and functioned in a similar manner. Our cutting-edge Western doctors (specialists, physicians, and pharmacists) will only occasionally talk with one another regarding the specific course of treatment for a patient.

There is expanding proof the ancient Greeks were correct: our considerations, feelings, and states of mind can influence how our organism works. Also, what we do with our physical bodies can influence our psychological state. Indeed, until around 300 years ago, most conventional medical treatments regarded the mind and body only in a general sense. It was not until the seventeenth century that Western societies started to consider the possibility of the mind playing a role in physical maladies. Analysts started going back to the mind-body association in the late twentieth century, and from that point forward, there has been a noteworthy increase in the amount of information that evidences how our bodies and minds share a common linguistic framework as they are always speaking to each other.

Prolonged exposure to stress can emerge from events such as worry about a friend or family member's wellbeing and health, living in perilous conditions, financial considerations, unrealistic demands in the workplace, and so on. The experience of prolonged periods of stress causes an increase in heart rate, inappropriate breathing, muscle pain and discomfort, and circulatory issues, among many of the physical ailments we have discussed. Most side effects of incessant stress are physical such as migraines, stomachaches, muscle pain, sleep problems, chest pain, weakness, changes in sex drive among others. We have also explored the mental and emotional issues that arise such as anxiety, depression, and even antisocial behavior. Stress likewise causes increased production of the cortisol hormone which analysts have connected to medical issues such as weight gain, insulin resistance, and even cognitive decline.

Perhaps the most evident impact of incessant stress, which we frequently consider as an illness itself, is anxiety. Since our bodies are intended to deal with smaller doses of mental and emotional stress, it is vital for us to remain focused on our surroundings in order to deal with any situations that may arise at any given point. In any case, if we are not prepared to deal with prolonged stress, we may face a considerable uphill battle when looking to maintain proper mind-body balance.

It is crucial that we perceive the association between our bodies and psyches if we intend to feel our best. If you happen to feel anything less than your absolute vest, you might want to visit your primary care physician to check nutrient levels and screen for thyroid or gastrointestinal issues. Specialists could consider persistent stress as a risk to wellbeing and urge patients to talk with a licensed therapist when needed.

With that in mind, physicians need to work in tandem with therapists in order to uncover the causes of inexplicable illnesses that may be afflicting a patient. This is often the case when a battery of tests has been run and there are no discernible causes that can explain the ailments of the patient. In short, achieving full health and wellbeing is not just a matter of seeing your doctor and taking meds, it is also a matter of digging a bit deeper into your overall psychological and emotional state.

One of the most extraordinary concepts on how constant stress can influence the body is called "broken heart disorder." The experience of stress, because of a broken relationship, or even divorce, can cause significant amounts of stress for prolonged periods of time to a point where the individual may end up completely exhausted, both physically and emotionally. Indeed, prolonged exposure to such circumstances may prompt cardiovascular breakdown and even cognitive decline. The New England Journal of Medicine published a study on hormones such as adrenaline, noradrenaline, and cortisol discharged in the body, in abnormally high amounts, as a result of prolonged stress or anguish, in which the guilty party was identified as broken heart disorder. Specialists discovered treating this sort of cardiovascular breakdown with customary pharmacology would not be viable, though psychotherapy focusing on managing feelings and expectations helped alleviate the worst parts of the symptoms.

Based on the previous discussion, we can see how stress is an incredibly powerful force that can impact a person in a myriad of ways. In fact, most of the physical ailments that a person can manifest may be traced, one way or another, to emotional and psychological issues. These issues may have their roots in childhood, or they may be unresolved issues that have lingered and subsequently festered over time. The fact of the matter is that these physical manifestations are the living embodiment of the mind-body connection. Hence, attempting to ignore this relationship is a futile task. We must acknowledge the fact that the connection that exists between both aspects of the human condition make it crucial to develop a working knowledge of this connection.

Given the fact that the nervous system is connected to the brain, which is believed to the be organ closest related to thought and emotion, we can clearly see the connection between our feelings and our emotions and how the body can begin to express the manifestation of these feelings. This is a clear indication that there is a direct causal link between what the mind feels and what the body manifests at various levels. As such, there is no doubt that we cannot ignore the role the mind plays in overall health and wellness any longer.

However, most physicians will first attempt to discover the underlying physical causes of illness. After all, physicians are trained to do so. But often, physicians ignore the role that the mind plays in maintaining health or breaking it down. And just like the mind can cause illness, the mind can also heal. This is a very important assumption to keep in mind as the mind-body connection is indisputable. The body of research in this area is consistently growing. As a result, we cannot ignore that there is a divide between the mind and the body. In fact, the time has come for us to embrace the fact that our thoughts are just as likely to heal us as they are to hurt us.

With that in mind, it's worth digging deeper into the connections among other body systems and the mind. For instance, the connection between the mind and the gut, while often overlooked, are clear and coherent. When the mind is free of stress, the gut reacts accordingly, and vice versa. Yet, it is far more often that the mind affects the gut than the other way around. When the gut is ill, that affects the rest of the body. Consequently, the body enters a negative feedback loop in which it is unable to rid itself of the persistent ill effects of being sick. Rather, it enters a cycle in which it only fuels the patterns that are causing it to be sick in the first place. This is why we need to address this issue in closer detail.

Chapter 8: How the Mind Talks to the Gut

Ever "gone with your gut" when settling on a choice?

You are most likely accepting a sign from your gastrointestinal tract, which discusses, literally, with your brain. Constant digestive distress has been down to reduce cognitive ability and generate positive feelings. When we become debilitated with conditions like intestinal infection, our brains become reworked through a procedure called neuroplasticity, which changes the associations between the nerve signals among the various interconnect systems.

Stress can impact the sort of microscopic organisms possessing the gut, making our gut configuration less favorable and progressively allowing hurtful microbes to take a foothold. It can likewise build irritation in the gut and break down immunity to contamination and even allergies to certain foodstuffs.

The brain and gut address each other through a system of neural, hormonal and immunological messages on a consistent basis. In any case, this solid correspondence can be exasperating when we are under stress or experience constant digestive distress in the digestive system.

Due to the amount of nerve endings and transmitters that exist in the gut, it is called the "second brain". There is good reason to make this claim as the amount of information that is processed in the gut enables the body to repair itself, absorb nutrients and provide the brain with the necessary elements it requires for the overall functioning of the body's various biological systems.

As such, this ongoing dialogue between the brain and the gut means that there is a direct link between the CNS and the digestive system. Moreover, if we consider the fact that the brain is the main processing center where the mind manifests itself, then there is no doubt that the link between the mind and the gut is very much real.

This brings us back to the point about the mind being able to both make the body ill and heal it. This proposition picks up significant steam when considering the existence of so-called psychosomatic illnesses. These illnesses have their roots in psychological and emotional causes as opposed to purely physiological ones. When these causes are explored, usually after deep periods of introspection, a root cause may be identified. When the root cause is identified, the psychological burden can begin to be lifted off the nervous system and eventually dissipate the stress and anxiety that may be accompanying the individual everywhere they go.

Upon closer examination, this causal link between mind, feelings, and gut truly gives credence to the notion that there is such a thing as "gut feelings". While some may argue that gut feelings are a figurative way of explaining the role of intuition in the life of humans, it is certainly worth examining at a closer level. Gut feelings are often associated as unconscious choices that individuals make, not based on facts or evidence, but rather on assumptions and guesswork. The likelihood of being right on these hunches is, at best, 50/50. This idea is more the product of the law of probability more than any reasonable assertation. In truth, the fact that we, as humans, have the extraordinary ability to intuit things without rationally thinking them through is more the product of perception and clarity than any supernatural ability. Nevertheless, the gut does play a pivotal role in this endeavor as it serves as a secondary processing unit. And while the gut does not produce articulated thought in the same manner the brain does, it does provide enough data for the brain to arrive at a reasonable conclusion even if it doesn't seem perfectly understandable at the time.

So, the next time you experience a "gut feeling" ask yourself what's really on your mind. It could be that the feelings you are perceiving are more of a manifestation of underlying thoughts and even repressed feelings that have yet to surface at a reasonable moment. Therefore, your gut will tell you far more than you could have ever thought possible based solely on your intellectual processes.

Chapter 9: About Gut Feelings

What is Gut Instinct?

A large portion of us has encountered the feeling of knowing things before we know them, regardless of whether we cannot clarify how. You delay at a green light and miss getting hit by a speeding truck. You settle spontaneously to break your no-arranged meetings strategy and end up gathering your life accomplice. You suspect that you ought to put resources into a little online startup and it progresses toward becoming Google.

As indicated by numerous analysts, instinct is undeniably quite material. The natural right brain is quite often "perusing" your environment, in any event, when your cognizant left brain is generally locked in, the body can enlist this data while the cognizant personality remains willfully ignorant of what's happening.

So, as we have discussed earlier, does it mean that you can truly intuit things around you without consciously having to process them? Turns out you can, particularly if you figure out how to identify which signs to concentrate on — regardless of whether they are sweat-soaked palms, a strong feeling in the pit of your stomach, or an unexpected and incomprehensible conviction that something is going on. These may all be subconscious manifestations coming from your "second brain", but that somehow the "first brain" is unable to process consciously.

Another hypothesis purports you can actually feel chemical changes in your brain as they occur. This may explain why some folks can literally describe their thought process as it is happening. Others may be able to pick up on these processes but may be unable to articulate them in an intelligible manner. While this doesn't mean that these folks are somehow less intelligent, it does mean that others are more in tune with their feelings and how to express them in a more articulated manner.

This implies if something in the earth is even marginally perceptible — the speed of a moving toward the truck, the somewhat bizarre conduct of somebody at a gathering — your mind can somehow pick up the chemical changes in your brain which leads to that "abnormal" feeling. Regardless of whether you focus or not can have a significant effect. You may meet your future life partner — or meet your new boss. Those signs convey a great deal of significant data, so it is wise to hone these skills. In a way, this is more about perception of reality than anything else you could potentially do.

The advantages of tuning in to your senses go a long way past following through on life-or-passing choices. Living all the more naturally requests that you are at the time and that makes for an increasingly energetic life.

In any case, gut impulses are a long way from dependable. The brain's expertise based on fact and evidence can trigger doubts of new (however not hazardous) things or cause you to be particularly receptive to individuals who essentially help you to remember another person.

So, how would you pick which gut feelings to trust? It is a matter of "going along to get along" and finding some kind of harmony between gut intuition and normal reasoning. When you have seen a logical connection, you can draw on the sensible side of your personality to gauge your decisions and choose how best to follow up on them.

After all, there is no reason why you shouldn't trust your gut instincts unless you can be sure that they are wrong. Of course, there are plenty of stories out there of people who went against their better judgment and trusted their instincts. However, their stories are not nearly as common as those in which the protagonists happen to miss the mark by following their hunches.

Again, this point is not meant to discredit the merits of hunches and instincts. If anything, we should all be in tune with our feelings in such a way that we are able to recognize when something deeper inside of us is trying to tell us that something isn't quite right. Perhaps you get a sudden urge to do something that you normally wouldn't. All of those manifestations of intuition largely depend on what we are able to perceive long before it actually happens.

One contending theory is that when both the brain and the gut are in good health, they are both able to combine their processing power. This means that the sensory information that enters the body is processed by the brain with the aid of the gut. As a result, you are able to perceive situations before they happen thus giving credibility to the notion that you can intuit things without necessarily being aware of them.

Based on the previous premise, if your gut and brain both combine to process information which was not previously available, then it is safe to say that you "know" things before the brain is actually able to arrive to a logical conclusion. The truth is that you are generally able to rationalize the events that occurred after the fact, meaning that in hindsight, you are able to make sense of why your guess was right. In any event, you have the opportunity to dissect what happened and therefore come to a conclusion as to why you were right, or perhaps why you wrong.

At the end of the day, when you improve your gut health, you are giving your cognitive power a significant boost insofar as being able to combine the processing power that is within your body. When all systems are humming at the optimal capacity, you are then able to really make sense of the world around you even if you aren't always consciously aware of why things are the way they are.

Hence, don't be afraid to go on a hunch especially if it doesn't seem to contradict your better judgment right at once. Of course, it might be that you can find logical inconsistencies with the hunch once you drill down and look at the deficiencies in your thought patterns. But that doesn't mean that you should discard your feelings off hand. It could be that your body is trying to tell you something that you know at a deeper level but may be reluctant to accept at a more conscious level.

Chapter 10: How the Gut Talks to the Brain

The article "Digestive Distress: A Civilization Disorder" by Watson and Collins, provides intriguing insights into the prevalence of digestive disorders. The authors of the article focus on providing information about the differences that are present in women and men when contracting the disease. According to research from the authors, women display higher rates of infection than in men in several countries. The biological differences in the make-up of the body of a man and woman result in different effects on the digestive system. The authors highlight the fact that the disease is a significant disruption to civilization as it is responsible for several deaths. The community is slowly being disintegrated as a result of the prevalence of harmful diseases such as digestive disorders that are usually preventable. The article analyzes different causes of the disease and offers the insight of the authors as appropriate recommendations to follow.

The article also provides information about the different types of cancers responsible for a high number of deaths. The authors ensure that they provide appropriate information by referencing different scientific studies from institutions around the world. The findings of the authors are accurate and precise in describing the harmful consequence of digestive disorders in society. There is information about the awareness program in the United States that educates the population on the dangers of digestive diseases. There is a strong emphasis by the authors on insisting that women change their eating habits for the sake of preventing digestive disorders among other digestive disorders. The biological differences between both sets of the population mean that women need to exercise greater caution than their male counterparts in preventing the prevalence of the disease. The authors conclude by suggesting that digestive disorders have the potential of increasing its scope and harm in society if no appropriate control measures are implemented.

While there may be clear differences in the propensity to certain types of cancer according to gender, it is important to note that gut health and the broader digestive system can break down in equal proportion to men and women. As such, it is worth considering the following guidelines when looking to protect how the gut and brain communicate especially with the heightened risk of cancer among other potential illnesses.

Diet

The diet solutions of most people in society are perhaps the most significant cause of digestive issues. Poor nutrition, inadequate diets and the increase in pollutants in the body is accredited to diet as a cause of all sorts of digestive maladies in human beings. The body requires adequate nutrients and the right balance of food in order for all the organs to function properly. Any inadequacies result in the failure of some body organs and unfavorable biological reactions that may result in serious illness such as digestive disorders. The food in the modern world certainly does not help in allowing the population to retains high levels of health. A majority of the manufactured food products have a high amount of chemicals and other dangerous, unnatural substances that damage the body. Maintaining a healthy and strict diet is a difficult responsibility for most people living in the modern world with several alternative food products available to try.

Doctors and physicians around the world have let it be known that a majority of patients suffer as a result of their own actions. The high consumption of dangerous foods continuously results in bodily damage in the intestines. Some of these food products also prevent the body from carrying out essential functions, such as metabolism and the removal of waste. The accumulation of these harmful substances in the body causes massive cell and gene mutations. The colon is most vulnerable as it pays the primary responsibility of absorbing water for the body. The poor dieting regimes of most people in spite of them thinking that they are eating healthily result in digestive disorders. The dieting regimes of each individual require thorough scrutiny if digestive disorders are going to permanently disappear from the community. The digestive disorders awareness month in the United States aims at encouraging healthy diets to the population as a way of averting this disease in the community.

Fiber

Fiber plays an extremely important role in the digestion of food and nutrients in the human body. In terms of consumption, there are two different types of fiber than are accessible through nutrition. First, soluble fiber can be digested in the body through the normal process of digestion. Secondly, insoluble fiber is that which cannot be digested but instead passes through the gut. It is vital to note that fiber primarily comes from plants alone; it is not possible to acquire this essential nutrient from meat and other such sources. The absence of soluble fiber in the diet of an individual contributes greatly to the prevalence of digestive disorders in their lives. This is because this nutrient is responsible for reducing the levels of cholesterol in the blood, limiting the potential of an increase in body fat.

Individuals who consume high amounts of soluble fiber remain relatively healthier than those who consume high amounts of red meat and alcohol. Biologically, soluble fiber contributes directly to the digestion process as it allows for the easier absorption of nutrients in the body. The sources of soluble fiber include oats, barley, rye, fruits, root vegetables such as carrots and potatoes and golden linseeds. Insoluble fiber, however, cannot be digested and moves down the gut to help other foods move more easily in the digestive system. They are responsible for keeping the digestive system clean and healthy and contribute tremendously towards weight loss. Diets that have little or inadequate soluble and insoluble fiber are responsible for causing a high prevalence of digestive disorders in the human body. The credible sources of insoluble fiber that can help in reducing the chances of this cancer include bran, wholemeal bread, cereals, seeds, and nuts.

The Mouse Model

The research on the gnotobiotic mouse model shows that digestive disorders are preventable by relying on dietary fiber. Conflicting epidemiological findings suggest that dietary fiber does not protect against digestive disorders. Experiments that involved using mice, however, demonstrate that fiber is pivotal in the prevention of digestive disorders. In the experiment, scientists would monitor the digestion of fiber in the mice and analyze the effect of the hormones and proteins. In their findings, the gut microbiota is responsible for fermenting the fiber into short-chain fatty acids such as butyrate. The fatty acids would offer protection to the internal colon lining of the mice and limits the potential of the growth and expansion of abnormal cells. The butyrate accomplishes this by preventing the accumulation of β-catenin protein to hazardous levels. The breakdown of the fiber in the mice is an excellent example of the role that fiber plays in reducing the instances of digestive disorders.

Meat

Red meat is much more harmful than white meat in controlling digestive disorders. Scientific evidence shows that high consumption of red meats increases the chances of digestive disorders in individuals. Moderate consumption of this meat is instrumental in individuals who have never experienced the disease. The common sources of this diet include lamb, beef and liver, and it causes serious health problems in individuals when consumed in high amounts. The danger that these food options pose is also evident in processed meats such as bologna, hot dogs and lunch meat. White meats are better alternatives as diets and a source of nutrition because they do not have a high percentage of cholesterol than their counterparts. The continuous consumption of this option instead of red meat prevents the sudden gain of weight that is a common characteristic of red meat diets.

High cholesterol levels in the body encourage the release of insulin. This hormone directly contributes to the growth of cancerous cells in the colon by making conditions favorable for the mutant cells. The methods of cooking meat also reveal the flaws of this diet option in encouraging the prevalence of digestive disorders. Scientific evidence shows that cooking meat at very high heat temperatures can be hazardous for the digestive system. relationship is because the heat can create chemicals in the process of cooking that increase the chances of contracting digestive disorders. Broiling, frying or grilling attracts the mixture of the meat with various chemicals at high temperatures. The situation is worsened in the case of processed meats that already have preservative chemicals in them. Consuming meat that is prepared using these methods for long periods of time leaves the victim vulnerable to consuming pollutants and suffering from digestive disorders.

The lifestyle and dietary options of the community are going to be influential in determining the prevalence of digestive disorders. As long as there is a tendency to enjoy a life of opulence without careful regard for the health consequences will result in an increase in digestive disorders cases. Doctors and physicians from around the world are insisting on the importance of revolutionizing the feeding habits of all human communities. The reliance on foods that have high percentages of sugars and fats attracts the possibility of lifestyle diseases in the population and compromises the health of everybody.

Children in schools need to be given appropriate advice and adequate information on their lifestyle choices. It is possible to completely eliminate the threat caused by digestive disorders by ensuring everybody is aware of the importance of living a healthy lifestyle.

Starting this education in earnest from an early age will allow future generations to live much more healthy lives and experience higher life expectancy ratios. There is a possibility of eliminating digestive disorders in society, along with the other dangerous types of cancer responsible for millions of deaths across the globe. Education, awareness and proper dieting are the ways of guaranteeing a much healthier community.

How Communication Takes Places

When everything is humming along just fine, the neuroreceptors in the gut are free to communicate adequately with the rest of the body. In particular, the ongoing dialogue between the gut and the brain takes place through the vagus nerve. It is the vagus nerve that ends up facilitating this communicating since it mainly serves as a large highway for information to flow to and from. As a result, the brain is keenly aware of what's going in the gut and the gut is keenly aware of what the brain is attempting to communicate.

When this dialogue is fostered by proper nutrition and the removal of damaging foods, the gut is even able to repair itself. This also leads to the overall health of the nervous system and vice versa. In fact, we've talked so much about how negative feedback loops are created in the body. Now, in this particular case, we can focus on positive feedback since a healthy nervous system promotes a healthy gut while a healthy gut promotes a healthy nervous system. This interaction is a manner of give and take. In the end, the body is perfectly balanced with the rest of the biological systems.

At the end of the day, the body is able to tell the difference between foreign substances that might be potentially harmful and give the immune system a leg up. This is why you find that certain people are much healthier than others. After all, when you stop overloading your body, you are able to let it act freely. When it has the freedom to attack what it should be attacking, then you can truly focus on being healthy. Moreover, when you eliminate harmful foods from your diet, the body is no long tasked with helping the digestive system deal with harmful substances in food; the immune system and digestive tract are all focused on being ready to do their job.

So, this is why cleaning up your diet as much as possible is absolutely vital to ensuring that you have everything you need to make your life that much better. You can certainly improve your quality of life by improving your eating habits and fostering a positive communication link between your gut and brain.

Chapter 11: How to Improve Brain-Gut Health

A solid gut, which houses a fair microbiome, is increasingly impervious to the negative effects of inescapable stress. Omega-3 unsaturated fats, fat-dissolvable nutrients An and D, and adjusted probiotics would all be able to help recuperate the intestinal coating, lessen irritation, and give various exhibits of useful microorganisms. This makes your stomach related tract stronger to the destructive effects of stress.

Investigate What Your Digestive Symptoms Can Teach You

Your digestive system can be seen as an indicator of how you are adapting to life. Stomach related indications frequently give understanding into the base of what is causing your stress, enabling you to push toward recuperating. On the contrary, if you cannot detect any abnormalities, then you can be sure that you aren't suffering from any major conditions.

For instance, if you are inclined to obstruction you may investigate where in life you cannot give up. If you have constant acid reflux, you may take a gander at where you may feel you have been "scorched" or where you are clutching resentment or disdain. Investigating your stomach related indications from this figurative point of view can enable you to see your feelings, process them, and discharge them so you can more readily adapt to stress. Indeed, this is an approximation to the psychosomatic effects that mental anguish has on the body's physical manifestations.

Whenever you see a gut feeling or your digestive system is acting up, respect this shrewd system by focusing on what may go on in your life. When you figure out how to comprehend your feelings and reactions to stress and receive sound approaches to oversee stress, you can all the more adequately digest both nourishment and life.

Keep away from Negativity to Heal Your Gut

Negative considerations are an enormous supporter of stress in the current life. Figuring out how to perceive your considerations through care or other contemplation methods enables you to change your attitude. This diminishes ceaseless stress yet can likewise enable you to settle on more advantageous nourishment decisions that improve absorption. Uneasiness, despondency, and other uncertain feelings are regularly at the foundation of indulging and poor nourishment decisions that can further stress processing.

Energy and empathy improve the capacity of the vagus nerve, which is vital in the correspondence between the brain and stomach related system. Practices, for example, adoring benevolence contemplation can expand your confidence, which thusly balances the nervous system and decidedly influence processing. It definitely goes without saying that whenever you can positively charge yourself, you will be having a positive effect on your entire body. Your body feeds off your positive energy in the exact same manner your entire biological framework is affected by negative energy. As a result, you must make a point of cutting out as much negative energy as you can. Otherwise, you may find yourself contaminating your body with needless rubbish that may only lead you to further detriment. A wise choice is to focus on your loved ones and the experiences which leave you feeling better about life and yourself. It may be high time to do some house cleaning for the sake of better gut health.

PART IV: STIMULATING THE VAGUS NERVE

Chapter 12: The Benefits of Vagus Nerve Stimulation

Throughout this book, we have talked about the importance of caring for the vagus nerve. We have clearly established the reasons why the vagus nerve is so important and the negative consequences of ignoring its wellbeing. At this point, the time has come to discuss the ways in which the vagus nerve can better serve the body's overall wellbeing. In this chapter, we are going to focus on the benefits that you can derive from stimulating the vagus nerve in a positive manner.

Firstly, it should be noted that the key concept in vagus nerve stimulation is the reduction of stress on the nervous system. This begins with calming and soothing the CNS while allowing the PNS to do its job. When this occurs, a great deal of the stress and pressure on the vagus nerve is reduced. As a result, the vagus nerve can recover and eventually restore the proper balance in the entire body's systems.

A Natural Way to Stimulate the Vagus Nerve

The most common technique used to calm the nervous system is meditation. Now, meditation doesn't have to be a complex endeavor. In fact, most folks who are unfamiliar with meditation believe it to be some sort of mystical art that must be practiced atop a mountain.

The truth is that meditation can be practiced anywhere at any time. The key point to meditation is to free the mind from thought. This does not mean that the mind must be completely blank; that is virtually impossible What this means is that the mind must be free of those thoughts which cause it to fixate on negative aspects. For instance, if you are overly concerned about paying the rent at the end of the month, this fixation may lead you to lose sleep, eat poorly and become anxious at various points throughout the day. When you apply meditation to the mix, you can allow your mind the break the shackles of worry and even come up with solutions to the problems afflicting you.

The easiest way in which you can practice meditation is to take 5 or 10 minutes of your time and just close your eyes. When you attempt to relax, try deep breathing. This will allow enough air to enter your lungs. As your blood becomes rich in oxygen, the nervous system suddenly becomes energized by the rush of fresh air. If you happen to feel that you are becoming anxious, you can retreat to a "happy place". While that may should cheesy, it actually works. This tenet behind a happy place is that you are stimulating positive feelings. As a result, positive feelings become positive energy. When positive energy begins to permeate your body, you will be able to literally feel this vibe enveloping your body.

As you become more and more proficient with meditation, you will begin to see the following benefits:

1. Reduced anxiety

When you practice meditation, you often find that anxiety is reduced simply because you are able to shift your focus away from what is ailing you. Even if it is making a relentless assault on your conscious thought, you have the power to divert these negative thoughts into more positive means. For example, your meditation may consist of positive visualization in which you see yourself actually being successful at something. This visualization technique is so effective due to its simplicity. You don't need to do anything special; just breathe and imagine yourself achieving whatever you want to achieve.

2. Increased blow flow and circulation

Another benefit is the improvement of circulation in your body. When you are able to focus on diverting your mind from negative thought, the blood in your veins begins to flow more freely especially since the blood vessels begin to feel less constricted. This effect is often described as a warm feeling all over. This sensation of blood going through your veins is equal to having a strenuous workout. When you push yourself physically, your heart begins to pump blood quite forcefully. The end result is your circulation improving. The same effect can be achieved when the nervous system relaxes and focuses on regulating essential biological functions.

3. Decreased heart rate

If you find that your heart is racing all the time especially when you think about all of the things on your plate, your heart rate begins to pick up. On the flip side, if you are able to focus your attention on other, more positive thoughts, your mind then begins to shift the focus from stress and on positive energy. This gives your vagus nerve a much-deserved break to the point where it no longer pushes the heart to beat faster. Rather, the vagus nerve can focus on restoring the heart's proper rate. When this happens, you can literally feel your body begin to slow down. This, on top of proper circulation, will lead your cardiovascular system to achieve its optimal level of functioning.

4. Improved immune response

When the body is no longer overloaded with worry and concern, the immune system is able to take a step back a catch a breather. At this point, some folks claim that they get sick with a common illness like a cold or the flu. The fact of the matter is that when the immune system is not forced into overdrive, what it does it that it actually fights off bugs that might be in your system. However, your overexcited state may not allow you to actually feel sick. This is nothing more than a consequence of an excited state that keeps the individual going on pure adrenaline. When your immune system is able to take five, you will find that you no longer get sick as often, and when you do, your illness is not nearly a tough to deal with as it had otherwise been.

5. Better cognitive ability

Perhaps the biggest benefit of improving the vagus nerve is the overall boost to your cognitive abilities. When you manage to get worry and anxiety out of your system, you are able to free up valuable real estate in your brain so that you can dedicate it to the tasks that you actually need to get done. This is manifest in better grades in school, improved performance at work, or simply being able to focus more on the things which you normally do.

In addition to meditation, mindfulness is one of the best ways in which you can unlock the above-mentioned benefits. Mindfulness is a state in which you are living in the here and now. When you enter a mindful state, you are giving your mind the leeway it needs to think about the task at hand rather than worrying about whatever is on your mind. Sure, this may not solve the problem at hand, but it will at least you give some peace of mind while in the mindful state.

Chapter 13: Vagus Nerve Stimulation Techniques and Exercises

Microbiotic and probiotic manipulation is a new-found science that will be instrumental in the treatment of various diseases, particularly those that affect the Central Nervous System. The 'gut-brain axis' refers to the association between the gastrointestinal system and the central nervous system (CNS), which has been increasingly looked upon as a sort of symbiotic relationship in the body and is now seen as a possible avenue for treatment of CNS disorders. The gut-brain axis is an insightful approach towards solving health and medical problems associated with a breakdown in the Central Nervous System in the human body.

This approach has been discussed as a revolutionary approach towards treating different conditions that affect the Central Nervous System in the human body. Microbiotic and probiotic manipulation in the human body is important in treating and preventing multiple diseases that have long been associated with the nervous system. There is a clear link between gastrointestinal health and CNS disorders such as ASD that brings forth relevance to the manipulation process as a method of treatment. This method is gaining popularity among health care practitioners as they seek the most effective ways of addressing some of the problems experienced by their patients via the Central Nervous System.

The purpose of this form of treatment is to restore the neurological pathways in the central nervous system destroyed by disease. There is a rapidly increasing amount of evidence implicating host-microbe interactions at virtually all levels of complexity, ranging from direct cell-to-cell communication to extensive systemic signaling, and involving various organs and organ systems, including the central nervous system (CNS). This treatment approach is critical to getting the most appropriate method of implementing a relevant remedy for the central nervous system.

Self-healing through Yoga

Yoga exercises are ancient Indian practices that serve the critical purpose of 'uniting the body, mind, and spirit.' The essence of yoga exercises is to strike a perfect balance within the nervous system that puts the entire body at ease. Practicing yoga exercises on a constant basis is a good way of staying in shape and reducing stress, particularly in work environments where people spend significant portions of their time.

The yoga exercises prescribed are my personal favorite because I engage in them at least once a day. The exercises have become a tradition because they are effective ways of changing mood and feelings of exhaustion. When working behind a desk for several hours, energy levels wane and stress easily kicks in. Performing various stretches as prescribed in yoga for just a few minutes can work wonders by completely clearing the head.

STEP-BY-STEP process
1. Forward Bend

The first technique, the "Forward Bend", involves stretching the back and allowing the tension on the neck to disappear. The technique involves the individual first standing upright, then bending forward and allowing your knees to bend. The feet- hip-distance must remain reasonable and the individual should remain in this pose for six full breaths. Thereafter, fold the legs and hold down your head, shaking it first for six full breaths, and then nodding for six full breaths. The entire process should take no more than a few minutes, but it helps ensure that blood circulation is distributing an adequate amount of oxygen to the rest of the body.

2. Eagle Arms

Shoulder knots can be quite frustrating, particularly for those who spend most of their time hunched over a desk. The 'Eagle Arms' technique involves standing upright with the arms outward and parallel to the ground. Swing the arms, and then bend the elbows to the extent that the back of the hands can touch each other. Thereafter, hook the right arm over the left so that they are facing each other directly, remain in this position looking straight ahead and maintain the position of the elbows. Slowly pull the elbows apart as the shoulders remain relaxed, remaining in this position for five breaths then unwrap the arms and swing them together.

3. Band Stretch

The "Band Stretch" is another yoga exercise that involves completely laying down on the ground and stretching the legs. Begin by bending the left leg, with the left foot flat on the ground and then put your right foot on top of the left knee. Put your arms around the left thigh while pulling it towards you, stretching the hips on the right side. Remain in this position for a few breaths, and then switch up the process by starting over by bending the right leg to stretch the hips on the left side.

4. Square Breathing

"Square Breathing" is a straightforward yoga exercise that involves taking deep breaths as a remedy for clearing the mind and de-stressing. The biological process of breathing accounts for a significant part of brain activity because constant oxygen is needed for this vital organ. The technique must begin with the individual sitting upright and inhaling through the nose deeply and holding that breath. Thereafter, exhale through the nose, timing no more than five seconds on each occasion and allowing the air to move indiscriminately. Repeat the cycle a few more times as it supplies more oxygen to the brain and hastens the process of carbon dioxide exhalation, de-stressing the individual.

5. Heart Opener

The "Heart Opener" is another yoga exercise technique that is particularly effective for the chest region. While standing, reach the arms towards the back with the feet hip-distance apart, then hook the hands together at the base of the back. Slowly lift the hooked hands behind you, allowing them to stretch the shoulder blades as the body tilts and bends over. Remain in this position for about a minute as it reduces stress by stretching the back and allowing for effective blood circulation in the body.

6. Shoulder Stretch

The "Shoulder Stretch" is the last yoga technique that is applicable for a wide range of purposes. Interlock the fingers and raise the hands above the head facing upwards, ensuring the hands remain in line with the ears. While looking ahead, relax the shoulder blades and remain in this position for five full breaths, then allowing the arms to fall on the sides. Take deep breaths through the nose while conducting the stretch as it increases the rate at which oxygen is being absorbed by the blood and the vice-versa expulsion of carbon dioxide. This process reduces stress because it relaxes the shoulders and allows for the relaxation of the back.

The prescribed yoga stretches can be performed almost anywhere, even at work. The best time to perform these exercises is at the peak of activity when a break is needed. Taking some time off to conduct different body stretches helps to clear up the mind by boosting the circulation of oxygen in the body. This traditional Indian technique has been adopted by peoples from all over the world for its effectiveness in reducing stress. Yoga techniques are several in their types and sometimes depend on the physical fitness of the individual, but overall, they are particularly helpful. The breathing processes involved in yoga are the most essential aspect of the exercises because all the body parts work in tandem to reduce stress and instances of fatigue than an individual might experience.

A majority of the stretches are highly reliant on loosening the body and moving the limbs as freely as possible. Clothing must be taken into consideration when performing yoga exercises because tight jeans and skirts might not be appropriate for some of the stretches. Some of the stretches that involve completely laying on the ground must also be taken into consideration because they might be disruptive to the people in a work environment. The essence of yoga exercises is to reduce stress in the individual and restoring excellent oxygen circulation is a pivotal element of yoga exercises. The stretches become effective and successful to those who engage in it and find themselves stress-free if they develop a timetable and make it a routine in their daily lives.

Chapter 14: The Polyvagal Theory

Polyvagal theory clarifies three different pieces of our nervous system and their reactions to stressful circumstances. When we comprehend those three sections, we can perceive any reason why and how we respond to high measures of stress.

Polyvagal theory is an innovative approach that serves to stimulate the vagus nerve thereby unlocking its potential while repairing any damage that may have come to it. It is a captivating clarification of how our body handles stress, and how we can utilize different treatments it to revise the impact of injury.

Why is polyvagal theory significant?

For specialists, and psychology science lovers, too, understanding polyvagal theory can help with:

- Understanding significant mood swings
- Seeing how to peruse someone using body language
- Getting through physical injury and conditions such as PTSD
- Seeing how extraordinary stress prompts separation or even shutdown

We like to think about our feelings as ethereal, complex, and difficult to classify and identify.

In all actuality, feelings are reactions to an upgrade (inward or outer). Frequently they occur out of our mindfulness, particularly if we are distant, or incongruent, with our inward passionate life.

The nervous system is continually running out of sight, controlling our body's capacities so we can consider different things — like what sort of frozen yogurt we'd like to order, or how to get an "A" in school. The whole nervous system works with the brain and can assume control over our enthusiastic experience, regardless of whether we do not need it to.

Our basic want to remain alive is more essential to our body than even our capacity to consider remaining alive. That is the place the polyvagal theory comes in to play. In this next chapter, we are going to be taking a look at how you can put Polyvagal theory to the test.

Chapter 15: The Healing Power of Polyvagal Theory

The polyvagal theory depicts three neural circuits that underlie different methods for consulting with our condition. When we have a sense of security, we depend upon a neural circuit that advances social commitment practices. He calls this the social nervous system. This piece of the parasympathetic nervous system draws in neural structures that restrain our guarded systems. This depends upon the myelinated ventral vagus nerve which enables us to connect socially by looking, relaxing our voice tone, and communicating care with our face. Significantly, the social nervous system can encourage immobilization inside setting security to advance more noteworthy closeness or closeness.

At first, when we experience a risk, we may depend upon our social nervous system to determine the circumstance. We may connect for association or nearness with another to restore security. In any case, if this is fruitless or if the risk is progressively extraordinary, we will start to draw in the sympathetic nervous system initiation of battle or flight.

If we cannot resolve the compromising circumstance by battling or escaping then we will start to draw in an unmyelinated, developmentally more seasoned piece of the vagus nerve to endure. This is particularly the situation in circumstances such are reality compromising in which there will never be a way out. The dorsal vagal neural pathway is likewise part of the parasympathetic nervous system; in any case, this time immobilization turns into a guarded reaction. Ordinarily, this is alluded to as the "blackout" reaction. Some of the time, one can actually black out on the grounds that the dorsal vagal pathway diminishes blood stream to the brain. Shy of blacking out, this guarded pathway can prompt manifestations, for example, unsteadiness, queasiness, or exhaustion all side effects of separation.

Your physiology holds the recollections of injury as well as holds a significant key to recuperation. The Polyvagal theory guides us to another vital aspect for recuperating... your ability to connect with the social nervous system. You can encourage the strength of your social nervous system by creating careful attention to your body sensations, for example, your pulse or breath. This encourages you to identify your very own indications of stress and permits you to react immediately—before the stress feels overpowering or out of your control.

Consider the following;

- **Practice Attention Control.** Practice concentrating on specific signals in your condition that advise you that you are protected at this point. Check out your room. Notice the light sifting through a window, a bit of craftsmanship on the divider, or how it feels to peruse this article. You can likewise tune in to a most loved bit of music, grasp an article, or notice the quieting fragrance of a basic oil.

- **Self-Compassion.** Develop self-sympathy for your side effects. Perceive the physiological, substantial premise of side effects and why you can't just consider your method for your injury responses.

- **Create Somatic Awareness.** Learn to carefully follow unobtrusive changes in your body sensations and pulse. Identify your very own indications of stress. This will enable you to react immediately before the stress begins to feel overpowering or out of your control. We call this remaining in the window of resilience.

Conclusion

Thank you for making it through to the end of this volume on the *Vagus Nerve*. We hope it was informative and able to provide you with all of the tools you need to achieve your goals of improving your understanding of this important topic.

Please take the time to go over any part of this book which you feel is particularly important or relevant for you. Also, the information we have provided to help you improve your overall health and wellbeing. It is important for you to find a balance that can lead you to a better quality of life.

Indeed, the knowledge we have discussed in this book may be of benefit to you, or any one of your loved ones. So do take the time to get as much as you can out of this book. We are sure that you will not be disappointed in the results you can get from taking care of the vagus nerve. Plus, the information we have presented here will lead you to a better life, both physically and mentally.

We hope you will find plenty of benefits from the information we have distilled as a result of years and years of research and study.

Thank you once again for reading this book. See you at the next one!

COGNITIVE Behavioral THERAPY for Anxiety

CBT and Emotional Intelligence to get over Human Behavior Disorders. Set the Best Mindset to Control Fear and Depression. Lead your Life with Self-Discipline

By Albert Dales

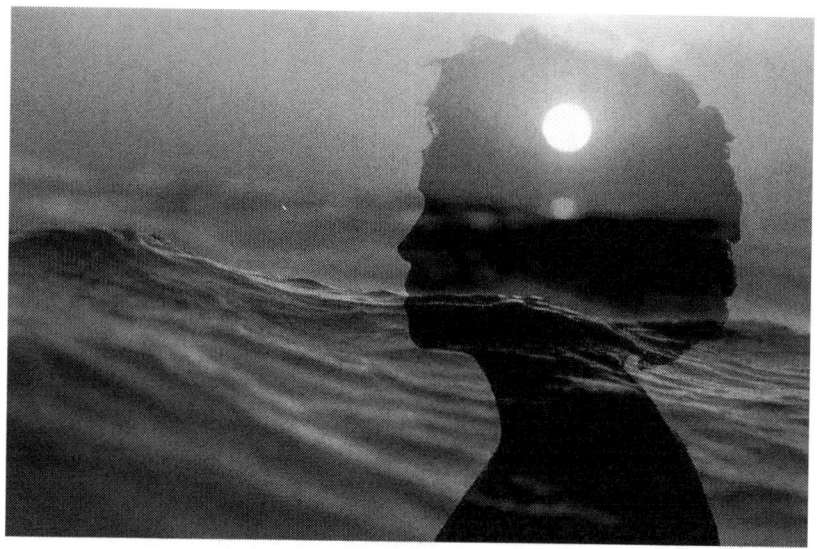

© **Copyright 2019 by Albert Dales - All rights reserved.**

The content contained within this book may not be reproduced, duplicated or transmitted without direct written permission from the author or the publisher.

Under no circumstances will any blame or legal responsibility be held against the publisher, or author, for any damages, reparation, or monetary loss due to the information contained within this book. Either directly or indirectly.

Legal Notice:

This book is copyright protected. This book is only for personal use. You cannot amend, distribute, sell, use, quote or paraphrase any part, or the content within this book, without the consent of the author or publisher.

Disclaimer Notice:

Please note the information contained within this document is for educational and entertainment purposes only. All effort has been executed to present accurate, up to date, and reliable, complete information. No warranties of any kind are declared or implied. Readers acknowledge that the author is not engaging in the rendering of legal, financial, medical or professional advice. The content within this book has been derived from various sources. Please consult a licensed professional before attempting any techniques outlined in this book.

By reading this document, the reader agrees that under no circumstances is the author responsible for any losses, direct or indirect, which are incurred as a result of the use of the information contained within this document, including, but not limited to, — errors, omissions, or inaccuracies.

Table of Contents

Introduction 73
Chapter 1: What Is Cognitive Behavioral Therapy (CBT)? 74
Cognitive Behavioral Therapy 75
How Does Cognitive Behavioral Therapy Work? 75
CBT and Self-Improvement 75
CBT Model 76
Chapter 2: Can CBT Help in the Management of Emotional Disorders? 77
How Does CBT Work? 77
Structure of CBT Sessions 78
Does CBT Work? 79
What Can CBT Help Improve? 79
How Does CBT Help with Anxiety? 79
How Does CBT Help with Depression? 80
Chapter 3: What Is Emotional Intelligence? 81
Emotional Intelligence Can Be Developed 82
Chapter 4: Defining Your Emotional Problem and Setting Goals 84
The Most Effective Method to Set SMART Goals 84
Specific 84
Why 85
Where 85
Quantifiable 85
Reachable 85
Significant 85
Time-bound 85
The Benefits of Goal Setting 86
Dopamine Boost 86
Important Experiences 86
Improved Performance 86
Creating Goals Can Make You Happier 87
The Downside of Goal Setting 87
Feeling of Failure 87
Depression and Anxiety 87
Chapter 5: Transforming Problems into Goals 88
Why Objectives are Superior to Issues 88
Objectives and Sub-Objectives 89
Chapter 6: Transforming Intention into Action 91
Understand Your Bias 91
Develop Your Own Leadership Vision Statement 92
Take an Interest in a Leadership Development Action Plan 92
Submit 92
Make the Next Logical Stride 92
Consider Yourself Accountable 93
Make a Move 93
Chapter 7: Identifying Solutions 94
Stage 1: Get Clarity 94
Stage 2: Don't Surrender! 95

Stage 3: Organize Yourself..........95
Stage 4: Set Your Intention..........95
Stage 5: Celebrate Your Progress!..........96

Chapter 8: Resolve Relationship Conflicts and Learn Better Ways to Communicate..........97

Step-by-Step Instructions to Establish New Habits..........98
  Be the Best You for Your Partner..........99
  Use Humor to Diffuse the Situation..........100
  Transform Conflict into Something Positive..........100
  Humor Is A Shortcut to Solving Relationship Problems..........100

Chapter 9: Overcome Emotional Trauma Related to Abuse or Violence..........101

What Are the Signs of Trauma?..........101
  Most Common Symptoms..........102
  Intense Stress Reactions..........102
  Post-Traumatic Stress Disorder (PTSD)..........103
What are the Signs of Trauma in Children and Youth?..........103
  Common Trauma Symptoms in Children and Youths..........103
  Step-by-Step Instructions to Deal with Trauma Symptoms..........104
  Tips for Supportive Family and Friends..........104
  Ways to Help Children Dealing with Trauma..........105
Effective Treatments for PTSD?..........106
  Cognitive Behavioral Therapy (CBT)..........106

Chapter 10: CBT Can Help in Mental Health Disorders 107

Anxiety..........107
  Reasonable, Realistic Thinking..........107
  Steps to Rational Thinking..........108
  Relaxation Strategies..........109
Depression..........110
Sleep Disorders..........113
  Concentrate on the Body..........113
  Quiet Your Mind..........113
  Sleep Apnea..........114
  CPAP Therapy..........114
Description of Sleeping Disorders..........114
  REM Sleep Behavior Disorder..........115
  Chronic Insomnia..........115
  Transient or Short-Term Insomnia..........115
  Normal Treatment Types for Insomnia..........115
Restless Legs Syndrome..........115
  Basic Treatment Types for Restless Legs Syndrome..........116
Narcolepsy..........116
  General Course of Treatment for Narcolepsy..........116
Substance Use Disorders..........116
  Managing Dependence and Addiction..........116

Chapter 11: Identifying Unhelpful Behaviors..........121
Chapter 12: Develop A Positive Mindset..........124
Chapter 13: Develop Self-Discipline..........129
Chapter 14: Improve Self-Esteem..........131
Chapter 15: Develop Self-Acceptance with Self Talk..........134

Why is Self-Acceptance So Difficult?..........134
Why Self-Acceptance is Important..........134

What Is True Self-Love?...135
Self-Love is Transparent..135
How Do You Comprehend Self-Love? 135
Self-Love Techniques 136
Chapter 16: Stop Overthinking; Change Negative Thinking 138
What is Overthinking?...138
Chapter 17: Take Care of Yourself and Your Environment 141
6 Reasons to Take Care of Your Environment 141
Chapter 18: Staying Focused on Your Goals 144
Make a Dream Board..144
Create and List Goals 144
Make Plans..145
Learning the Power of "No"..145
Tracking Your Outcomes 145
Focus on 1 to 4 Objectives 146
Conclusion... 147

Introduction

Congratulations on purchasing *Cognitive Behavioral Therapy for Anxiety* and thank you for doing so. The following chapters will discuss the most effective way you can use Cognitive Behavioral Therapy (CBT) to improve your health and wellbeing in order to tackle both common and complex disorders.

Dealing with anxiety can be an incredibly difficult situation that only those who have been through it can understand. If you, or a loved one, have been through this, then you can attest to the challenge that it poses. Most importantly, you need to find the means to deal with it in an effective manner.

That is where this book comes in.

We have produced a collection of both theory and practice which will help you understand and address the effects that anxiety has on your life. But more than just understanding what anxiety is, we seek to address the root cause. In doing so, you can find a great deal of alternatives in dealing with it.

This book isn't about finding a magical cure.

This book is about building the life that you want. It is about making the most of your opportunity to achieve your goals and create the life that you seek to achieve. If anxiety is getting in the way, then we are going to take the time to analyze it and find effective ways of getting rid of it.

Ultimately, you may not be able to let of it altogether. But you will find that understanding the onset of symptoms is a great way of managing them. Eventually, you will learn to control it so that anxiety will never run your life ever again. You will become the master of your own domain.

You are surely eager to get started. So, let's find out how we can get a grip on anxiety once and for all!

Chapter 1: What Is Cognitive Behavioral Therapy (CBT)?

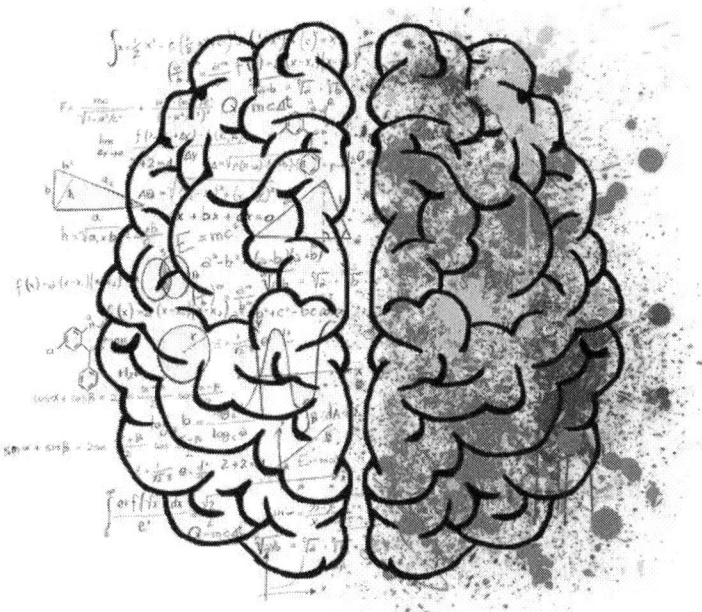

Cognitive Behavior Therapy (CBT) is a psychotherapy that has been demonstrated to be successful in more than 2,000 research works. It is an of delicate, organized, present-focused psychotherapy that enables people to identify objectives that are most critical to them and overcome obstacles that currently make meeting those objectives difficult. CBT enables individuals to show signs of improvement in multiple aspects of their lives and remain healthier overall.

CBT is derived from the cognitive model. This means that the way that you perceive certain circumstances is associated more strongly with your response to that circumstance rather than the actual circumstance itself.

One significant aspect of CBT is helping clients make sense of what they most need from life and advance toward accomplishing their vision. They learn skills to change their thinking and behaviors that contribute to the development of their vision.

CBT utilizes an assortment of cognitive and behavioral procedures, but it isn't characterized by the utilization of the procedures. We do a lot of thinking in a critical manner and we can change the way we think and behave from numerous psychotherapeutic modalities, including persuasive behavior therapy, acknowledgment and responsibility therapy, Gestalt Therapy, Person-Centered Therapy, goal-centered therapy, constructive brain science, relational psychotherapy, and with regards to character issues, psychodynamic psychotherapy.

Cognitive Behavioral Therapy

CBT is an organized, time-constrained, problem-centered, and objective-focused type of psychotherapy. CBT encourages you to be able to figure out how to identify, question, and change how they contemplate things and how it is able to take place in their mind. It also helps you identify your frame of mind and beliefs which will help you to understand what you need to change them.

Cognitive behavioral therapy is a psycho-social intervention theory that seeks to improve your mental health. It focuses on changing and challenging unhelpful distortions and behaviors that you have. It also seeks to help you improve your emotional regulation along with developing personal coping strategies that will target solving current problems.

CBT centers around the present time and place—on the issues that surface in everyday life. CBT causes individuals to analyze how they perceive what's going on around them and how these discernments influence the way they feel.

How Does Cognitive Behavioral Therapy Work?

In CBT, clients figure out how to identify, question, and change the thoughts, feelings, and behaviors that the client and therapist have identified are acting as everyday obstacles in the journey to achieving their life goals.

By observing and recording thoughts during upsetting circumstances, individuals discover that how they think can contribute to negative experiences, such as depression and anxiety. CBT decreases these issues by encouraging clients to:

- Consider their thoughts about what is happening to be subjective and able to be adjusted rather than absolute truths
- Identify irrationalities in their reasoning
- Consider challenging circumstances from different points of view

CBT and Self-Improvement

There are numerous self-improvement guides and sites dependent on cognitive-behavioral standards. Proof demonstrates that these assets are progressively valuable when the individual likewise gets support from a therapist, particularly if the person is suffering from low self-esteem and low motivation.

CBT Model

The CBT model is based on a two-path connection between thoughts and behaviors. Each can impact the other.

There are three degrees of cognizance:

Cognizant thoughts:

Rational thoughts and decisions that are made with full mindfulness.

Programmed thoughts:

Programmed thoughts can be defined as thoughts that stream quickly, with the goal that you may not be completely mindful of them. This may mean you can't check them for accuracy or importance. In an individual with a psychological issue, these thoughts may not be coherent at all.

Patterns of Thought:

Patterns are identified by examining core beliefs and individual guidelines for handling problems. These core beliefs and personal rules we have set for ourselves are molded by our life experiences, especially those during childhood when we are most vulnerable and impressionable.

Chapter 2: Can CBT Help in the Management of Emotional Disorders?

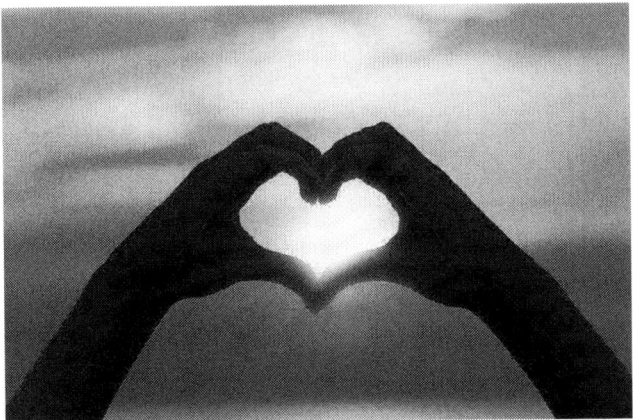

Cognitive Behavioral Therapy (CBT) is a form of talk therapy that can help individuals with emotional disorders gain the skills they need. At the point when you start CBT, you and your therapist will collaborate to identify your individual issues and concerns. You'll additionally figure out how to incorporate key strategies in light of these issues.

CBT depends on the understanding that our challenging encounters are straightforwardly identified with our thoughts, beliefs, and activities and because of this, it is conceivable to change the way we react to these challenging encounters by analyzing and modifying our thoughts and behaviors.

The span of CBT treatment shifts, commonly extending from six sessions to a much longer than that depending on your individual needs. You will usually meet with your therapist once every week.

After some time, CBT will enable you to increase your awareness of:

- How you can combine thoughtful strategies and consistent practices to improve your emotional well-being
- Your exaggerated reasoning and behaviors and how to change them
- The effect your beliefs and actions have on your general psychological well-being

How Does CBT Work?

Together with your therapist, you will work cooperatively to identify which of your own instances of reasoning and behavior add to negative states of mind. CBT offers specific procedures to inspect and modify these unhelpful thoughts and beliefs. These unhelpful thoughts are known as cognitive distortions, and they are directly challenged by practices within CBT. These practices eventually contribute to an overall process of cognitive restructuring.

You will also learn behavioral strategies that help contribute to your desire to change your thoughts and reach your goals. There are numerous CBT methods, including:

Relaxation preparing: An assortment of procedures used to quiet the sensory system. Models incorporate breathing activities, improved self-care abilities, and progressive muscle relaxation.

Anxiety and avoidance hierarchy worksheet: An instrument used to survey anxiety levels about specific circumstances.

Guided imagery:
- Using words, music, or pictures to evoke positive and relaxing envisioned situations.
- *Objective critical thinking:* A six-step procedure to identifying the best answer for an obviously characterized issue in the wake of thinking about significant choices.

Subjectivity of Perception:

- Consider how others may perceive a specific circumstance differently.

These are only a couple of ways to successfully engage in CBT. You and your therapist will decide the correct one based on your needs.

Structure of CBT Sessions

A typical session of CBT starts with a careful examination of your state of mind and anything you might be struggling with to begin to make connections. Your therapist may utilize an assigned agenda based upon what route they decide to take in treating you.

Next, you share any issues you're dealing with right now or have dealt with recently (often in the past 30 days) and how you believe these issues are contributing to your overall wellbeing. You will utilize that data to organize a goal for that particular therapy session.

During the session, you and your therapist will survey past sessions and the time between sessions. You'll examine how you used your newfound skills and consider the possibility that using these skills impacted your state of mind in that moment or during that week.

Your therapist will function as a mentor or coach to enable you to compartmentalize the present issue you've identified so you can learn about and apply a CBT skill or method to address that issue.

Finally, every session normally finishes with an arrangement for you to practice a CBT strategy or ability on your own after the session, and you will report how it went at the following session. This commonly incorporates homework-style exercises, such as being mindful of your behaviors or potentially thoughts in a diary or application specifically worked for CBT.

Does CBT Work?

Studies have seen CBT as powerful as an independent treatment for:

- Anxiety and depression (which often co-exist and are interrelated)
- Tics
- Marginal character issue
- Substance abuse (aside from a narcotic-use issue which requires more intense, substance-focused treatment due to the severity of risks that exist within this specific addiction.)
- Post-Traumatic Stress Disorder (PTSD)
- Health and dietary issues

Frequently, therapists will recommend returning for an "adjustment," should concerning indications reappear any time after a full course of treatment is finished.

What Can CBT Help Improve?

- CBT has proven to be successful at improving results for a range of psychological well-being difficulties, including anxiety and depression.

How Does CBT Help with Anxiety?

Research demonstrates that CBT is the best psychotherapy for treating anxiety issues. Using CBT requires identifying unhelpful behaviors and perspectives and replacing them with increasingly versatile thoughts and behaviors that can reduce and ultimately destroy anxiety.

One of the most well-known standards of CBT for anxiety is that moving toward the things that cause anxiety, as opposed to maintaining a strategic distance from them, can really help calm anxiety symptoms over the long haul. During the time spent confronting anxiety, CBT inspects specific thoughts identified with anxiety and replaces them with increasingly supportive and reality-based thoughts.

CBT additionally involves the learning and practicing of relaxation skills--for example, progressive muscle relaxation--to quiet the body and brain and prepare them for the changes you seek to make.

How Does CBT Help with Depression?

CBT treats the thoughts and behaviors that have prompted your depression, and those that keep contributing to a discouraged state of mind and beliefs based on low self-esteem. For instance, if you've been in your house for various days, a CBT system called "behavioral initiation" may urge you to go out and take a walk – basically forcing you to engage in rhythmic movement.

You may attempt to likewise identify pessimistic ideas you hold about yourself, such as comparing yourself to others constantly resulting in you feeling poorly about yourself. A CBT therapist will assist you in identifying the negative thoughts and beliefs that are normal in individuals with depression and work with you to identify elective thoughts that are progressively useful or versatile.

Changing even one behavior or thought can have significant influences on one's state of mind and can help one rise above negative thinking, self-doubt, and pessimistic views of the world and others.

Chapter 3: What Is Emotional Intelligence?

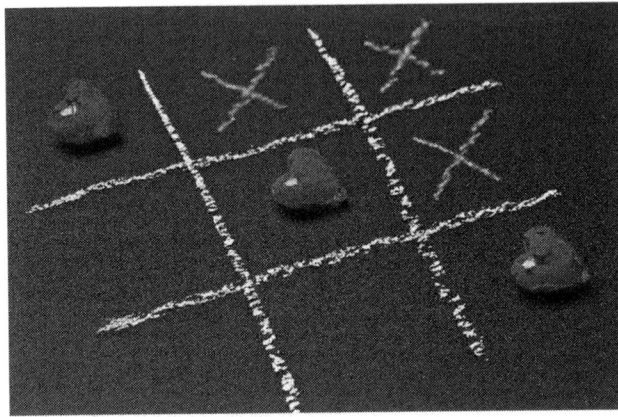

Emotional intelligence is the "something" in every one of us that is somewhat impalpable. It influences how we oversee behavior, explore social complexities, and settle on choices that accomplish positive outcomes. Emotional intelligence is comprised of four main abilities that can be divided into two essential skills: individual capability and social fitness.

At the point when emotional intelligence originally appeared and became popular in 1995, it acted for many as the missing connection in an impossible-to-miss discovery: individuals with normal IQs beat those with the most noteworthy IQs 70% of the time. This irregularity tossed a gigantic wrench into what numerous individuals had constantly accepted as the sole predictor of intelligence and accomplishment—IQ. Many years of research currently point to emotional intelligence as the basic factor that sets star entertainers and other celebrities apart from the remainder of the population.

- **Individual ability** is comprised of your mindfulness and self-administration skills, which focus more on you independently than on your communications with other individuals. Individual skills are your capacity to remain mindful of your feelings and deal with your behaviors and tendencies.
- **Social fitness** is comprised of your social mindfulness and relationship to personal executive functioning skills; social skills are your capacity to comprehend other individuals' dispositions, behavior, and intentions, so as to improve the nature of your connections.
- **Mindfulness** is your capacity to identify or name your feelings and remain mindful of them as they occur.
- **Self-Management** is your capacity to utilize consciousness of your feelings to remain adaptable and direct your behavior accordingly.
- **Relationship Management** is your capacity to utilize mindfulness of your own feelings and the feelings of others to perceive your connections properly and thus, engage in them accordingly.

- **Social Awareness** is your capacity to precisely read and tune into the feelings of other individuals in order to understand what is happening around you.

Emotional Intelligence Can Be Developed

The correspondence between your "emotional mind" and your "thinking mind" is the core of emotional intelligence; how well and how often they interact with each other will determine your emotional intelligence. The pathway for emotional intelligence begins in the brain, at the spinal cord. The stimuli you receive from all life experiences enter here and must venture out to the front of your brain before you can begin to understand your experience. Nevertheless, first, they travel through the limbic framework, where feelings are created. According to this natural order, we have an emotional response to situations before our thoughts and beliefs can lock-in. Emotional intelligence requires viable correspondence between the emotional and reasoning focuses of the brain.

"Plasticity" is the term nervous system therapists use to depict the brain's capacity to change. Your mind develops new associations as you adapt to new skills. The change is slow as your synapses begin to grow and new connections are formed, but it is worth it, and it is possible.

Utilizing methodologies to expand your emotional intelligence permits the billions of minuscule neurons covering the path between the balanced and emotional focuses of your mind to branch off little "arms" (much like a tree) to connect with different cells. A solitary cell can form 15,000 associations with its neighbor cells. This chain response of development guarantees that it is simpler to kick this new behavior without hesitation later on. When you train your brain by consistently utilizing new emotional intelligence systems, genuinely wise behaviors become habits.

How much of an effect does emotional intelligence have on your expert achievement? The short answer is: a ton! It's a ground-breaking approach to center your energy one way with a huge outcome. Emotional intelligence is the most grounded indicator of success, defining achievement in a wide range of ways.

Your emotional intelligence is the establishment of a large group of basic skills; it impacts nearly everything you say and do every day.

Over time, we have discovered that the most successful aspect of top entertainers is likewise high emotional intelligence. On the other hand, only a couple of basic or non-famous entertainers are high in emotional intelligence. You can be a top entertainer but without emotional intelligence, your chances of becoming successful are slim.

Normally, individuals with a high level of emotional intelligence get more cash-flow. This individual will, on average, earn $30,000 more every year than individuals with a low level of emotional intelligence. The connection between emotional intelligence and profit is immediate to such an extent that each point increment in measured emotional intelligence adds $1,200 to a yearly pay. These discoveries remain constant for individuals in all businesses, at all levels, in every region of the world. We have not yet discovered a single job where performance and pay are not related to the emotional intelligence of the employers and employees.

Chapter 4: Defining Your Emotional Problem and Setting Goals

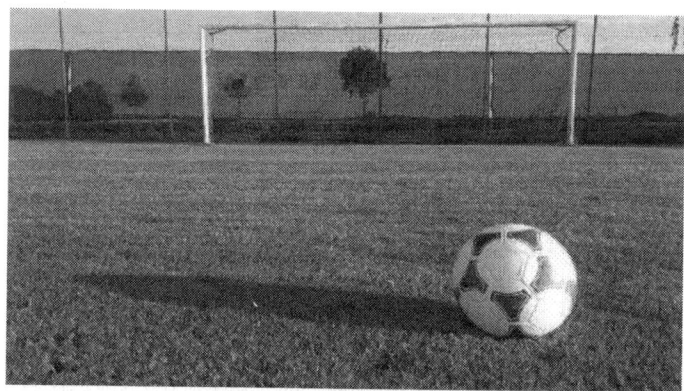

One challenge with an objective goal setting is that it conflicts with how your mind normally functions. Past research demonstrates that your brain naturally needs to organize and pick routine over curiosity each time alone. Bodes well – its top employment is consistently to protect you. When attempting to change a behavior, brain circuits for constant and objective-coordinated activity fight it out in your mind for control. Hence why any objectives that require radical behavioral or thinking changes will be met with opposition at first.

Additionally, your brain is wired to look for remunerations and keep away from agony, distress, and fear. Nevertheless, that doesn't imply that the more agreeable way is to your greatest advantage. It just implies that your mind has a natural inclination toward it. Truth be told, these inclinations are "demotivators" and leave you with the craving to return back to the wellbeing of your routine behavior and thought designs. In any case, with cognizant exertion, you can abrogate these feelings and change your mind and behavior.

The Most Effective Method to Set SMART Goals

An effective objective-setting practice is to choose what you need to accomplish and after that record a "brilliant" objective. Keen objectives are characterized as:

Specific

A specific objective should respond to these five inquiries:

- What precisely would I like to accomplish?

Why
- Specific reasons for or advantages of achieving the objective.

Where
- Identify an area.

Which limitations or cutoff points are critical to consider?

Quantifiable

A quantifiable objective will reply:

- What amount or what number of?
- In what capacity will I know when it is cultivated?

Reachable

A feasible objective will respond to the inquiry:

- In what manner can this objective be cultivated?

Significant

An important objective will answer yes to these questions:
- Does this appear to be beneficial?
- Is this the perfect time?
- Does this match our different endeavors/needs?

Time-bound

- Goals that can be achieved within a set timeframe.

A time-bound objective will reply:
- When must I be done?
- What would I be able to do half a year from now?
- What would I be able to do a month and a half from now?
- What would I be able to do today?

The following stage, where numerous objective setters miss the mark, is to list the steps you have to take, and after that, begin to take those steps.

Inquiries to consider include:

- Who can enable me to accomplish my objective?
- What exercises do I have to finish to accomplish my objective and in what time period?
- What assets do I need?

Furthermore, you will need to locate a strong friend or support system to enable you to remain on track with your objective. You should meet up regularly to identify and discuss issues to help with remaining focused on the objective.

The Benefits of Goal Setting

Dopamine Boost

At the point when you need something and get it, regardless of whether it's a reward, piece of candy, or instant message — your mind gives you a dose of dopamine. Dopamine is frequently called the "good vibe" synapse.

According to this neuroscience, it's conceivable to maintain and increase dopamine levels by defining little objectives and achieving them. For example, your brain gets a spike in dopamine if you believe in yourself and your abilities and go out and succeed in something that you did not believe you would be able to succeed, or that others perhaps doubted you would accomplish. This is one explanation as to why individuals like daily agendas. It feels great to accomplish goals you have set for yourself in part because it causes a spike in dopamine. Each time your brain gets a hit of dopamine, it urges you to repeat the preceding behavior.

You'll keep the dopamine streaming if you separate objectives into smaller, more easily attainable steps. For instance, if you need to practice three times each week, scratch-off every accomplishment with a marker on a schedule so your mind sees and registers the achievement. If you need to write a book, make an objective to write for 10 minutes consistently and reward yourself when you do.

Important Experiences

Defining objectives can provide you with important learning experiences that will improve your psychological wellness as well as your life by and large. The training can show you significant exercises related to numerous things from autonomy, versatility, and rivalry to absolution and benevolence. These abilities are known to be significant supporters of your emotional well-being and happiness.

Simply put, defining objectives can enable you to develop and grow as an individual. Probably the greatest fulfillment in life is seeing your life advance in a positive, healthier, more beneficial direction. Along these lines, moving in the direction of and accomplishing objectives can give your confidence a boost, which can improve your general psychological well-being and overall life fulfillment.

Individuals who set objectives are more joyful and increasingly productive, yet in order to reap these benefits, your objectives must be the correct sort of objectives.

Improved Performance

Research demonstrates that defining objectives can expand execution when:

- Rewards--for example, cash--are given for objective achievement
- The objectives are specific and adequately challenging

- Constructive criticism is given to show progress in connection to the objective
- Appointed objectives are reasonable and settled upon by the person
- The subjects have adequate capacity to achieve set objectives

Creating Goals Can Make You Happier

- One examination had individuals take an interest in three short, one-hour objective-setting and planning sessions on the web. The therapists at that point compared these individuals with control groups that did not engage in the sessions. The outcomes revealed a causal connection between objective-setting and happiness and fulfillment.

The Downside of Goal Setting

Feeling of Failure

Accomplishing an objective feels incredible, creates a feeling of achievement in us, and sends your cheerful neurochemicals straight through your brain to make you feel good overall. On the other hand, though, not meeting an objective or getting off track incidentally feels quite lousy. At the point when somebody doesn't hit their objective mark, it can prompt self-analysis, and thus a feeling of disappointment. Nevertheless, numerous successful individuals reveal to us that disappointment is a normal and important part of progress.

Depression and Anxiety

Not all objectives are made equally. Objectives with no specific purpose can even be terrible for your psychological wellness. If an objective is excessively dubious, it's harder to reach, and you don't have the simplest idea when or if you've even arrived at your goal. One investigation found that general, unclear, and vague objectives made discouraged individuals feel increasingly discouraged.

Defining objectives can increase anxiety. One investigation found that as you would expect, anxiety increased with objective difficulty and self-assurance diminished.

Chapter 5: Transforming Problems into Goals

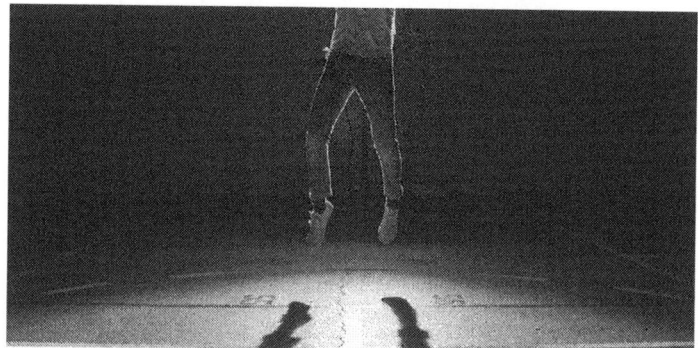

With regards to inventive critical thinking, which is progressively successful? Concentrating on the current issue, or on defining objectives for what we'd like to achieve?

If you stop and consider it, individuals all the more regularly use innovativeness to discover a method for accomplishing an objective rather than to tackle an issue. Someone who writes books, for example, wouldn't consider that they may have an issue with writing bad books. Instead, they would be focused on having their goal of writing another book. Another example is within the realm of business. A business may not need items at all in order to succeed, but their executives may feel they should so that they can liven up the business and take it to the next level.

In addition, any issue can be repeated as an objective. Sales are down? Your objective, at that point, is increment sales. Your production line is wasteful? At that point, you need to improve the productivity of your production line.

Why Objectives are Superior to Issues

All the more critically, I accept that there are significant favorable circumstances to utilizing "objective" as the point of the inventiveness procedure. Right off the bat, interpreting an issue (if you are beginning from an issue) as an objective urges you to scrutinize the issue. This, in my experience, is the place a great many people mess up when attempting to take care of issues. They promptly attempt to fix the issue and neglect to attempt to understand the issue appropriately first.

Creating objective explanations from issues makes you consider the issue and what part of it you really wish to unravel. If you state, "We have to build sales," a great many people will promptly answer, "Obviously you do. Each business does! What would you like to do? Improve your business procedures? Improve your product or service marketing? Make your item increasingly alluring?"

With these inquiries, you may understand that you will likely create more leads for your business group. Or, on the other hand, you may understand that your items are seen as outdated by the young people you are attempting to sell to, so you have to make your items increasingly current and 'attractive'. Simply put, these two objectives are incredibly different; however, either or both could be objectives you have to take a stab at so as to accomplish your overall objective of selling more.

What's more, I accept that utilizing imagination to accomplish an objective is more positive and inspiring than utilizing it to take care of an issue. Of course, it is basically something very similar. Be that as it may, which challenge do you figure a great many people would discover all the more fascinating?

"Our line of young ladies' shoes is obsolete, and sales are falling. How might we fix this?"

– or –

"How about we make our line of young ladies' shoes more stylish and attractive! How might we do this?"

Objectives and Sub-Objectives

Working with objectives rather than with issues also makes it simpler to turn enormous, daunting objectives into smaller, sub-objectives. This can be significant as well. I find that when individuals come to me with issues that need to be understood better, these issues are the consequence of different issues, every one of which should be tended to. In any case, the idea of core issues and sub-issues appears to be odd. More regrettably, it appears to be discouraging!

All things considered, I accept that if we plan to concentrate innovativeness on achieving expressed objectives, we will get rewarding outcomes. What do you think? What is your experience?

In conventional medicinal language, patients present themselves with a "great injustice" which makes therapists sound like they are working in advertising. It additionally makes our patients sound like a load of complainers. Another way medical professionals are instructed to conceptualize patients' purposes behind their visits is the "issue list." For individuals with convoluted lives or long ranges of time between their therapeutic visits, that rundown can be long and feared by doctors.

It can appear to be a shopping list for a large family. Any wise customer realizes that it's ideal to consider to be thorough and to take time to plan your visit to the supermarket. You would burn through a great deal of time and do significantly more aimless strolling through grocery store aisles if you did not plan your trip and instead just went to take a look at everything and decide there what to get.

At the point when patients don't present all of their problems in advance, their primary care physicians can end up being shocked by concealed information that comes to the service after so much time was already spent with this patient. Even the most thorough assessments do not always show everything that is going on with a patient.

You can assist your primary care physician with learning about you and helping you by introducing every one of your worries when booking your appointment and toward the beginning of each visit. This will guarantee that the therapist is better prepared to deal with your worries.

There are times in our lives when we are overwhelmed with our circumstances or simply feeling depressed. There are patients in these states, and it's difficult for them to realize where to start. They have no idea what they want or need. In these circumstances, it very well may be useful to ask, "What are your objectives?" For instance, "How might you want to feel? Where might you want to be?"

If you are discontent with a relationship or work circumstances, we can ask, "How might I improve them?" It's imperative to invest some energy transforming our issues into objectives. It can carry trust and a positive point of view to a difficult circumstance. It can engage us when we have felt powerless. Picturing your objectives is the initial phase in a dynamic arrangement towards better well-being and happiness.

Chapter 6: Transforming Intention into Action

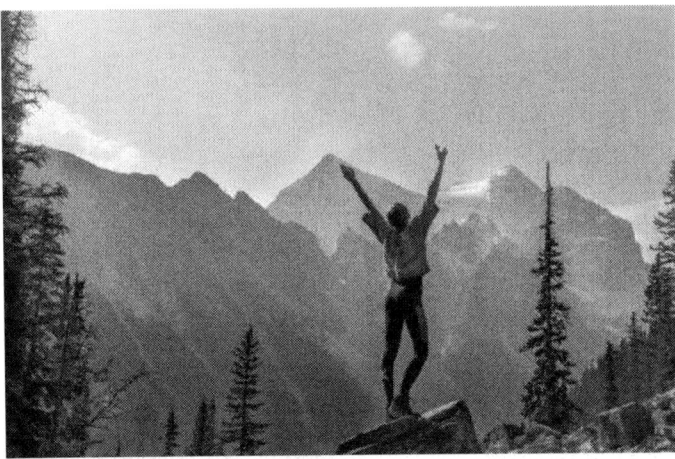

When taking a look at how pioneers rate themselves compared to how others assess them, leaders in the lowest quartile often assess themselves at a higher level than others who have assessed them. Interestingly, the most effective leaders, all things considered, assess themselves at a lower point by a margin of 70% most of the time.

You consistently attempt the most popular diet at any point in time, yet you can never seem to stay in shape. You purchase a rec center enrollment each New Year, yet never make it to the rec center. Understudies mean to get extraordinary evaluations, however, organize different exercises over contemplating and going to classes. Individuals expect to resign affluent, however, don't take the predictable activities important to manufacture riches. You plan to land on schedule but are interminably late to everything in any case.

Being an extraordinary pioneer originates from taking a stab at significant changes and developing updated value systems. Making change is never easy, and under certain circumstances, it can be tough. Yet, extraordinary pioneers figure out how to love being awkward. Growing new beliefs takes responsibility and diligent work until the correct beliefs are solidly settled in into our day by day activities.

The accompanying tips will assist you with turning to transform intention into action without hesitation.

Understand Your Bias

Strangely enough, individuals will, in general, assess themselves based on their goals, yet judge other individuals based on their deeds. It's a normal human reaction to do so. We judge others before we understand their intentions, thus resulting in biases. Rather than judging other people, focus on your own actions and intentions behind those actions. Start by reflecting on the moves you have made which have contributed to the achievement of your goals.

Develop Your Own Leadership Vision Statement

Your own leadership vision statement is the manner in which you wish to be perceived in a leadership role. From multiple points of view, your own leadership vision functions as a preset leadership declaration. Another way of going about developing your vision is to imagine what people would say about you at your funeral. As such, what would you like people to say about you? The answer to this question will help guide your endeavors in such a way that your vision will take shape.

Take an Interest in a Leadership Development Action Plan

One of the best ways in which you can assess your leadership skills and performance is to elicit a group of collaborators to determine how they judge your vision and leadership skills within a real-world context. If this assessment determines that your vision is on par with their expectations, then you can feel satisfied. Otherwise, you may need to determine in which ways you need to improve. Extraordinary pioneers acknowledge productive input and set objectives to take their leadership abilities to a much more significant echelon.

When you set your goals, it isn't enough to simply have good intentions. Everything you do in your day to day life ought to be lined up with the goals that you are looking to achieve. Sure, the first step toward making a successful transition is to have clear goals and objectives. But at the end of the day, there is not much that you can achieve unless you actively pursue your goals. If it were enough to set clear goals and objectives without the need for execution, then the world would be filled with exceptional leaders. This is why it is of the utmost importance to follow through as much as you can.

Submit

Responsibility is built up every day; each of our choices contributes to or takes away from our personal responsibilities. As of now, have you made the pledge to turn your goal into a reality?

Make the Next Logical Stride

The best aims frequently become mixed up in an ocean of stalling. As Christopher Parker stated, "Dawdling resembles a charge card. It's a great deal of fun until you get the bill." That is why procrastination, that is, putting things off for later is one of the biggest obstacles that you will have to overcome. You can't expect to be successful at every turn without putting in the requisite hard work. Moreover, focused work is essential if you are keen on making the most of your talents and efforts.

Consider Yourself Accountable

Consider yourself responsible for completing the activities you've focused on. Set aside the effort to reflect hourly, every day, week after week, month to month, or year to year the moves you're making to transform your goals and objectives into the real thing.

Make a Move

There are inspiring folks all around us who have incredible goals, dreams, and hopes for the future. However, good intentions are simply not enough. By being wishful without any effort, you will have a hard time parlaying that into a successful outcome. So, try your best to resolve to make things happen as much as possible.

Chapter 7: Identifying Solutions

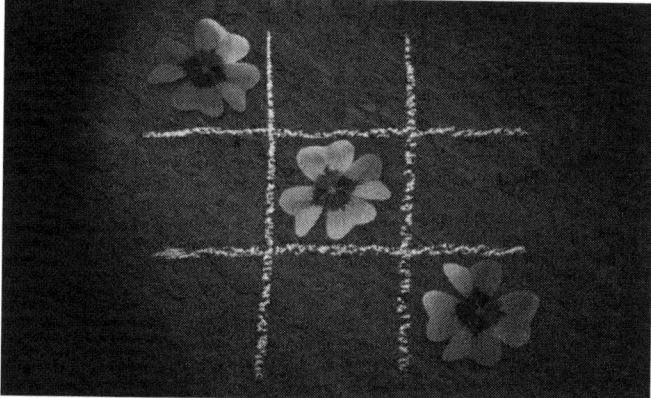

As you may definitely know, finishing a goal or a thought can end up being much harder than we had recently envisioned. As the underlying energy of a thought or objective wear off and the questions and 'what ifs' start to sneak in, what from the outset appeared to be a generally excellent expectation, all of a sudden turn into a task we would prefer to disregard. That is before another well-meaning goal tags along. Just envision the amount we could do with our lives if we oversaw our expectations as far as possible. Think about the degrees of enormity we could reach and the power we would appreciate! At this point, you could have turned into an acclaimed writer, be getting a charge out of that late spring house in the nursery, traversing India or be CEO of a multi-million-pound business.

Do you frequently wind up speaking groggily about what's to come? Fantasizing or discussing 'the day' when you will at least get around to composing your first novel or will go into business, or even get around to beginning that diet? We are for the most part liable for it. Regardless of the amount we plan and discussion about what we expect to do or accomplish, we never appear to get any more remote than our expectations, regardless of how great they may initially appear.

Be that as it may, it's not very late! This could in any case all be valid for you! If you are blameworthy of not staying with your honest goals, at that point read on, for the five stages that you have to transform your well-meaning goals into positive activity.

Stage 1: Get Clarity

- Since you have set your goal, it's now a great opportunity to come up with a strategy!
- There is no point rushing into something aimlessly, regardless of how anxious you might be to achieve your goal. Success is about planning and the clearness of your vision. This can give you the advantage of clarity to look forward and choose what you will need to do to transform your goal into a triumph.

- Before you can make a move, setting up the means that you should take to arrive at your objective can be fundamental for your long-haul triumph. Along these lines, get clear on your vision. See yourself toward the end goal! At that point rationally go through what the voyage there will resemble, to perceive what activity you should take in transit.

Activity Needed: Write down five steps you take to help you towards accomplishing your objective.

Stage 2: Don't Surrender!

- Sooner or later, you may be enticed to quit attempting. It may be on the grounds that you hold the belief that you are not arriving at your objective quickly enough since you are worn out or even in light of the fact that you think you have done sufficient. As of now, it is significant that you prop up regardless. Have you known about the revitalizing burst of energy ideas? It is a marvel in separation running when a competitor who is too worn out to even consider continuing all of a sudden finds the solidarity to proceed. All things considered; you can likewise get a revitalizing burst of energy when attempting to accomplish something. Simply sit tight for it and don't surrender. To help get a revitalizing burst of energy give centering a shot your objective and envision the amount you would then be able to make the most of your triumph.

Stage 3: Organize Yourself

- Without association and the fundamental devices, you may require, you could be putting yourself at a genuine inconvenience, thwarting your odds of arriving at your objective.
- Regardless of how solid our aims might be, if we don't encircle ourselves with the apparatuses and condition that we have to achieve our objectives, at that point, even the most unshakable of individuals may feel slanted to surrender. We ought to act naturally spurring in each perspective we can!
- To start with, so as to improve sorted out, attempt and plan ahead by considering what you may need to make arriving at your objective that tad simpler. For instance, if you will probably get in shape, you could prepare and watch that you have the accompanying; healthful plans, the right exercise center wear, pre-arranged shopping records, and a morning plan, to guarantee that you allow for breakfast.

Activity Needed: Take activity today! It was hesitation that kept you from overseeing your aims as far as possible in any case; in this way, cause a rundown of what you can do today to guarantee that nothing prevents you from defining off towards your objective tomorrow.

Stage 4: Set Your Intention

- Once in a while, the explanation we can't stay with a goal is that we have such a large number of! So as opposed to overpowering yourself with various thoughts and points, why not choose one specific objective?
- Setting a portion of your different objectives aside for later may feel somewhat disappointing, particularly when you so frantically need to prevail at them all. Be that as it may, it is imperative to recall that while you were attempting to clutch these aims, you were really prevailing at none of them.
- Take a stab at adhering to one objective for some time and see what improvement you start to make. You can generally toss another in with the general mishmash sometime in the future!

Activity Needed: Set your sights on one objective as it were. Use dream sheets and visual tokens of your objective to keep you concentrated on what it is that you need to accomplish. Furthermore, have faith in what you need to pull in.

Stage 5: Celebrate Your Progress!

- Inspiration is critical when you are hoping to accomplish something, regardless of how enormous or little. Arriving at any objective requires diligent work and serious persistence, and if you don't reward yourself routinely or recognize your triumphs, you can immediately end up unsatisfied and lose your motivation.
- Regardless of what your goal is, whether it is to lose weight, set out on another vacation, make sure you monitor your progress. Each time you hit an objective-- for example, arriving at a specific weight or amount in your savings, celebrate what you have accomplished! Treat yourself to something nice or have a little shopping spree on something that you will need once you've arrived at your objective; for example, a nice dress or a traveler's backpack.

Activity Needed: Be sure to record the majority of your progress in a diary or on a calendar. Honor your achievements. What's more, when you contact them, salute yourself with a merited reward!

At the point when you take one goal, center around it, make a game plan and persuade yourself however much as could reasonably be expected. At that point when your next well-meaning goal goes along, you can feel certain, realizing that this time you can be overseeing it as far as possible.

Chapter 8: Resolve Relationship Conflicts and Learn Better Ways to Communicate

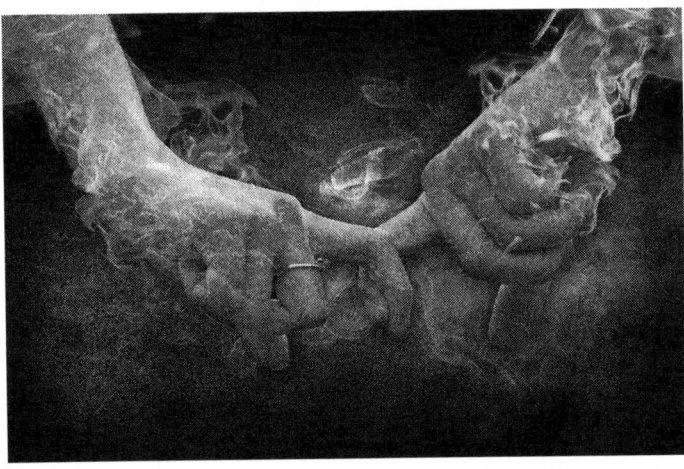

Break the example of a threatening vibe and give the contention positive energy. Try not to get guarded; don't pound your point; don't attempt to win. For what reason would you need your partner, the individual you cherish, to lose?

A contention with your partner can make you feel assaulted or compromised, powerless and frail, and this can make you backlash and retreat. At the point when things your partner does upsets you and you feel that you're under attack, you're more averse to react usefully and bound to fall back on old reserves like "the silent treatment" that, at last, accomplish more damage than anything else. This will in the long run reason your relationship to separate totally.

Clashes are open doors for you and your partners to adjust on esteems and results. They are opportunities to comprehend, acknowledge, and grasp differences. Put yourself in your partner's place and attempt to get their experience. These encounters and feelings can be awkward, yet if we generally decide on solace then we can never develop.

If anybody inquired as to whether you realized how to determine strife, you'd likely state truly, and if they asked you whether the quiet treatment was a brilliant method to manage struggle, you'd more likely than not state no. You know not to turn to these senseless strategies, however, if you're harmed enough, you do it in any case. Why? Why fall back on negative examples as opposed to attempting to really fix the correspondence issues close by?

If you wind up in a retaliatory winding, a great strategy is to utilize silliness to break the example; make the contention ludicrous.

Funniness is an easy route to tackling relationship issues. It can discharge strain and enable you and your partner to concentrate on what you both need instead of on what you both don't need.

What do you need? What would it be a good idea for you to concentrate on? Make sure to acknowledge, instead of diminishing. Every one of our partners gets things done or have beliefs, that irritate us. Concentrate rather on what they bring to the table, how they affect you and the characteristics that you adore. You'll see that you'll before long begin to miss even the things that used to make you insane, in light of the fact that they are a piece of that entire individual, your partner, whom you revere.

Use strife as a chance to re-adjust your qualities and objectives, to infuse enthusiasm and energy into your relationship. Keep in mind the two couples at the bistro? The fruitful couple, who put energy into seeing each other's needs, reaffirmed their help for each other. She supported his need to leave at a specific hour and he upheld her need to associate with friends. They additionally made a fun round of it as a tradeoff, promising to return home early enough to get to know each other.

Tune in to your partner, comprehend what they're stating and why they feel the manner in which they do. Speak the truth about your own inclination and feelings. Be your legitimate self, since strife is a chance to really associate with your partner.

Struggle is additionally a chance to get familiar with your partner and adore them on a significantly more profound level. It's a chance to add energy and to take your relationship to the following level. Figure out how to consider Cassius to advance to something better, as opposed to as motivations to withdraw. Whenever you wind up contradicting your partner and considering how to spare your relationship, see the world positive in the circumstance as opposed to the antagonism, and effectively choose to move in the direction of an increasingly steady future together. Together.

Step-by-Step Instructions to Establish New Habits

You should need to be useful to get it going, particularly if you have to beat your very own hurt emotions to make sense of how to fix your relationship. You may have an awesome store of learning, skills, and apparatuses, however, if you do not have the expectation to utilize them, the fact of the matter is debatable.

We have a belief of fighting back and reacting to a threatening vibe with a greater antagonistic vibe, which makes an endless loop that amplifies and raises the cynicism of a contention. This is known as the retaliatory winding, and it can make a relationship wilt and, in the end, end. You're utilizing negative beliefs to self-harm.

What causes this? A contention winds up unsafe when you're centered around safeguarding yourself from assault instead of taking care of the issue that would enable the relationship to defeat the obstruction. By concentrating on your agony and enduring, you are guaranteeing you'll encounter business as usual, on the grounds that you're neglecting to put your energy toward the one thing that will forestall the torment and enduring: discovering answers for help you figure out how to spare your relationship.

Be that as it may, our center decides our course. If we would prefer not to hit the post, we have to concentrate on what we need: steer the vehicle toward either side of the shaft. By changing our center, we can change the outcome. The exercise applies to your relationship. If you center around where you don't need your relationship to wind up, battling and giving annoyance a chance to work over, you'll get yourself where you would prefer not to be – either in a difficult, unfulfilling relationship or isolated from your partner by and large. If you center around settling struggle and developing together, you'll be centered around the results that you need, and you'll accomplish them. That is, imagine yourself discussing great with your partner. You two are satisfied and content with each other and have the devices you have to make a beautiful, energetic, durable relationship. Where the center goes, energy streams.

By exchanging viewpoints and center, you can divert a contention from something awful into a chance to take your relationship to the following level. This requests the goal, which you set early and practice at the time. You figure out how to react not with heightening, however with valuable advances that shore up the establishment of your relationship.

Be the Best You for Your Partner

Do you wind up asking, "How might I spare my relationship?" Use strife as a chance to re-adjust your qualities and objectives, to infuse enthusiasm and energy into your relationship. Keep in mind the two couples at the bistro? The effective couple, who put energy into seeing each other's needs, reaffirmed their help for each other – she upheld his need to leave at a specific hour and he supported her need to associate with friends. They spoke with one another, evaluated each other's needs and made it a fun issue to fathom as opposed to letting something minor transform into a significant contention. They likewise made a fun round of it as a tradeoff, promising to return home early enough to get to know one another.

Tune in to your partner, comprehend what they're stating and why they feel the manner in which they do. Speak the truth about your very own feelings and feelings. Be your bona fide self, since strife shouldn't be seen as the finish of a generally extraordinary relationship; see the struggle as a chance to genuinely interface with your partner.

Rather than review struggle as a risk to the relationship you share with your partner, see it as a productive instrument. Strife is likewise a chance to get familiar with your partner and adore them on a considerably more profound level. It's a chance to add energy and to take your relationship to the following level. Figure out how to consider making the change to something better, as opposed to as motivations to withdraw. Whenever you end up contradicting your partner and considering how to spare your relationship, see the positive in the circumstance instead of the negative, and effectively choose to move in the direction of an increasingly steady future together.

Use Humor to Diffuse the Situation

If you wind up in a retaliatory winding, a great strategy is to utilize silliness to break the example. If you feel a contention raising, pause for a minute to crash it. Sing a tune that makes your partner giggle. Make the contention crazy.

Transform Conflict into Something Positive

Break the example of a threatening vibe and give the contention positive energy. Try not to get guarded; don't pound your point; don't attempt to win. For what reason would you need your partner, the individual you cherish, to lose? At the point when you acknowledge that there are no washouts in adoration and that you need to win together, you can get down to concentrating on relinquishing insignificant contentions and grasping solid correspondence.

Clashes are open doors for you and your partners to adjust on esteems and results. They are opportunities to comprehend, acknowledge, and grasp differences. Put yourself in your partner's place and try to get their experience; this is the manner in which you figure out how to spare your relationship. These encounters and feelings can be awkward, however, if we generally settle on solace then we can never develop.

Humor Is A Shortcut to Solving Relationship Problems

It can discharge pressure and enable you and your partner to concentrate on what you both need cherishing, upbeat relationship. As opposed to what you both don't need, another inconsequential contention.

When you're figuring out how to fix your relationship, there are a couple of inquiries you have to pose to yourself: What do you need? What would it be a good idea for you to concentrate on? Make sure to acknowledge, as opposed to reducing. Every one of our partners gets things done or have beliefs, that disturb us, in light of the fact that no person is flawless. Rather than dwelling on their negative attributes or unfortunate beliefs, center rather around what they bring to the table, how they affect you and the characteristics that you cherish. You'll see that you'll before long begin to miss even the things that used to make you insane, on the grounds that they are a piece of that entire individual, your partner, whom you venerate.

Chapter 9: Overcome Emotional Trauma Related to Abuse or Violence

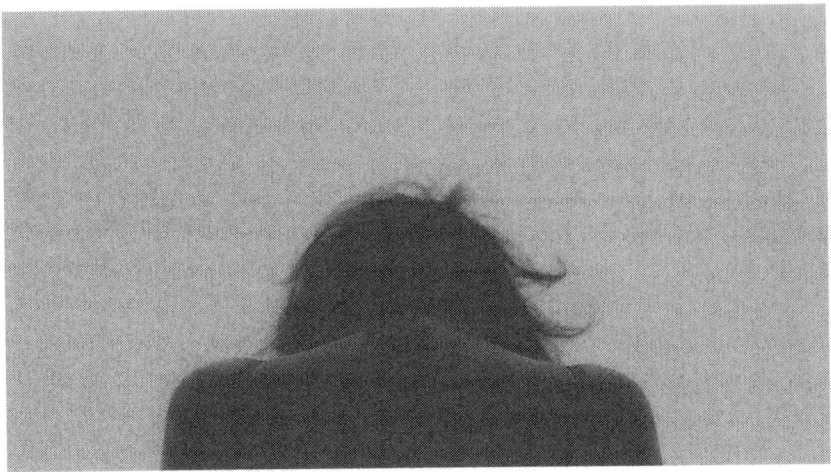

Following a profoundly upsetting or disturbing occasion or injury, it isn't abnormal to feel stressed and overwhelmed. Horrible accidents involve witnessing or experiencing real or imagined death, serious harm to oneself or others, or anything that otherwise causes shifts to one's perception of themselves and others. Examples include violent interpersonal attacks (for example sexual or physical assault, robbery, mugging), abuse, and serious car accidents.

Reactions to traumas might be exemplified by an intense stress response, which is a brief condition that we are in following a horrendous accident. The side effects start close to the horrendous mishap and can vanish inside hours, days, or weeks.

When a person goes through a particularly traumatic experience, they may end up developing a condition known as Post-traumatic Stress Disorder (PTSD). This condition is common in people that have gone through a horrendous experience such as a terrible car accident or soldiers who are exposed to prolonged exposure to stress during combat operations. It is not easy to recover from PTSD as there may be a need for a combination of medication and therapy. In addition, recovery time depends on the severity of the case, the type of trauma and the individual's own mindset. In short, PTSD is a difficult condition to deal with but not impossible to treat.

What Are the Signs of Trauma?

Trauma can easily fly under the radar. This means that it may not have overt manifestations. As such, the sufferer may not lash out in any evident manner. Rather, they may exhibit signs such as being quiet, withdrawn and have difficulty socializing.

So, it is important to take a look at the most common symptoms of trauma.

Most Common Symptoms

1. Being effectively frightened by boisterous clamors or abrupt developments.
2. Tension or fear of risk to self or friends and family, being separated from everyone else, being in other terrifying circumstances, having a comparable occasion happen once more.
3. Flashbacks where pictures of the horrendous accident come into your psyche all of a sudden for no obvious explanation, or where you rationally re-experience the occasion.
4. Physical indications, for example, tense muscles, trembling or shaking, sickness, migraines, perspiring, and tiredness.
5. Distraction with pondering the injury.
6. Absence of enthusiasm for normal exercises, including loss of hunger or enthusiasm for sex.
7. Feelings of isolation, bad luck, and intense loneliness.
8. Problems with sleep such as nightmares, flashbacks or being unable to fall asleep due to constant thoughts pertaining to the traumatic event.
9. Shirking of circumstances or thoughts that help you to remember the horrendous accident.
10. Issues with speculation, focus, or recollecting things (particularly parts of the awful mishap).
11. Self-blame and second-guessing are also common. The sufferer replays in their mind, over and over, about how they could have done things differently in order to avoid the outcome. This may also be punctuated by feelings of guilt.
12. Outrage or peevishness at what has occurred, at the pointlessness, all things considered, at what made the occasion occur, regularly asking "Why me?"
13. Not every person will encounter these responses or experience these responses to a similar degree. There may likewise be different responses to add to the rundown. Notwithstanding, as a rule, these side effects will vanish after a generally brief timeframe.

Intense Stress Reactions

1. An underlying condition of dissociation
2. Being unsettled, or jumpy
3. Discontinuing normal activities (e.g., from work to social circumstances)
4. Tension manifests in the body (e.g., muscle tightness, headaches, stomach aches, inability to sleep)
5. Thinking about what occurred most of the time
6. Feeling disorientated or confused
7. Feeling discouraged or depressed
8. Difficulty remembering important details of the stressful event

Post-Traumatic Stress Disorder (PTSD)

1. PTSD, for the most part, creates inside 3-6 months of the awful mishap and includes the accompanying:
2. It is common for the individual to relive the events. Sudden flashbacks are common while specific reminders may trigger memories of the event.
3. Bad dreams about the injury and upset sleep
4. Staying away from things, thoughts and emotions that help you to remember the horrendous accident
5. Difficulty recollecting significant parts of the injury.
6. Withdrawal from your loved ones
7. No enthusiasm for ordinary exercises
8. Indication of expanded excitement and nervousness
9. Serious excitement and nervousness when looked with tokens of injury
10. Having discouraged or crabby mind-set (and blowing up effectively)
11. Difficulty focusing on and recollecting different things
12. Having discouraged or crabby mind-set (and blowing up effectively)
13. PTSD can be a debilitating condition in terms of social interaction. It can severely limit a person's ability to interact socially thereby affecting their ability to connect with others at a personal level.

What are the Signs of Trauma in Children and Youth?

Children and youth may likewise encounter mental responses to an awful trauma. They respond to frightening occasions from various perspectives, and there is no run of the mill or typical response. Younger kids, specifically, may think that it's difficult to understand what has happened to themselves, their friends, or their family. They may distract themselves or reenact the traumatic incident during play (e.g. playing with firetrucks constantly after surviving a serious house fire).

Like adults, they will experience seriously distressing emotions. On the other hand, unlike most speaking adults, they will be unable to verbally reveal to their true feelings. On the contrary, they are prone to express themselves through their behavior in such cases. In the event that a traumatic event occurs to a loved one, all family members will feel the same impact. This entails the entire family's involvement so they can rally around the affected member and provide them with the love and support they need.

Common Trauma Symptoms in Children and Youths

1. Being scared or anxious, particularly around nighttime or when away from caregivers
2. Being more submissive or obedient than typically expected

3. Your kid may demonstrate 'immature' behavior
4. Your children may have bad dreams and experience difficulty sleeping
5. Wetting the bed
6. Having a throbbing pain somewhere in the body
7. Your child might be more deceitful or sneaky than usual
8. Your child might be more irritated than usual
9. You may observe behavior intended to get attention such as temper tantrums over seemingly unimportant things.
10. You may observe a decline in school performance as compared to before the traumatic incident occurred

These issues are, for the most part, normal responses to abnormal circumstances that have impacted the family in a significant way. Thus, it's crucial to avoid harsh reactions such as punishing the child for their behavior.

Step-by-Step Instructions to Deal with Trauma Symptoms

1. Safety is one of the main concerns. If you find that symptoms are progressing significantly, finding a safe place is important in order to avoid any potential harm.
2. Talking to someone you can trust about your feelings is essential.
3. Conversing with loved ones may likewise be great. Getting love and understanding from your loved ones is necessary to eventually confront your issues.
4. Learn to identify your feelings. But keep in mind that many of them are normal for anyone who has been through anything like it.
5. Remember that healing takes time. And while the incident may have occurred in a short period of time, your recovery will take time. Don't get ahead of yourself. Rather, be patient and don't push yourself more than you need to.
6. Acknowledge the fact that it might require some investment to change.
7. Invest energy accomplishing decent things – relaxation, taking strolls, seeing new and wonderful places, and spending time with friends. Make it a point to enjoy the good things in life every day.
8. It is absolutely necessary that you go up against circumstances related with the horrendous mishap… however, do it slowly. You may choose to return to work, however, go only for a couple of hours from the outset and afterwards develop it gradually.
9. Try not to utilize medications and liquor to adapt. They will just exacerbate it. Attempt to discover different approaches to unwind.

Tips for Supportive Family and Friends

1. Invest energy in the affected individual and ensure that they are safe.

2. Offer help and hear them out, regardless of whether they asked for the help or not.
3. Try not to take it personally if they need to be distant from everyone else in some cases. Try not to judge their reactions to the traumatic experience unless they are at risk for serious harm.
4. Reassure them by stating that you are sorry for what they have been through and that you are trying your best to help them in any way you can.
5. If you were part of the traumatic event, take the time to talk to them about what happened. It is very important to keep in mind that there is no need for blame. The main point is just to give time and space to vent feelings even if it means going through emotional situations.

Ways to Help Children Dealing with Trauma

As with adults, children get over trauma with time. However, children need a lot more love and care given their age inability to process their feelings. Here are some ways in which you can help a child.

Talking about the circumstances surrounding them is important. In particular, explaining why things are happening is important. By trying to help them understand what they are going through, you can avoid feelings of despair, isolation, fear and even guilt.

It's important to reassure children that they are loved and safe.

1. Talk to children about what they are going through. Even if they are young, it is important to be open about their feelings especially fear and insecurity. Children need to be aware of what's happening even if you need to bring it down to their level.
2. Some kids may need a lot more attention and care especially during bedtime.
3. Do not attempt to repress their feelings in any way. Meaningful play is a great way in which children can process their feelings. Attempting to "be strong" may only foster negative feelings inside the child.
4. Whenever possible, take time to do things as a family. By consistently engaging in fun and enjoyable activities, the child will be able to dissipate their negative feelings.
5. It is important to keep the child within an age-appropriate role. Delegating too much responsibility to a child, such as caring for a parent who is dealing with a traumatic experience too may become overwhelming for the child. Also, it is important to avoid becoming too overprotective following the incident. The main goal is to establish a sense of normalcy as soon as possible.
6. Usually, the remedy for children going through such situations is love and understanding. This may get somewhat complicated if the child is lashing out in inappropriate behavior. If this were to be the case, then you may need to seek professional help in order to aid the child in dealing with their feelings.

Effective Treatments for PTSD?

An effective treatment is not intended to "cure" a sufferer by helping them erase the traumatic incident from their mind. In fact, the effectiveness of treatment is measured in the degree that the sufferer is able to process their feelings, understand why things happened and be able to move on. While this doesn't mean forgetting it happened, it does mean that the sufferer is able to accept what happened and move on. On the whole, the sufferer may never get completely over the incident. But, they will be able to lead a healthy and productive life.

Cognitive Behavioral Therapy (CBT)

Cognitive Behavioral Therapy is a perfectly viable alternative for treating PTSD. It can be conducted as a standalone therapy or in tandem with medication.

Cognitive Behavioral Therapy includes:
1. Progressive and incremental exposure to the source of trauma.
2. Education on the condition, its symptoms and how to deal with feelings.
3. Replacing negative thoughts and feelings regarding the situation.
4. How to manage fear, anxiety, and stress through effective techniques.

Chapter 10: CBT Can Help in Mental Health Disorders

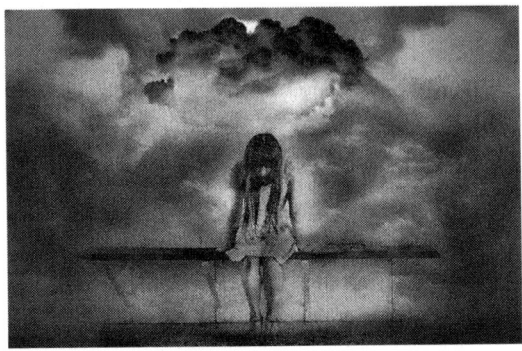

Anxiety

A significant initial phase in overcoming or learning to live with a mental health issue is to become educated about it. This type of education involves learning about what the condition entails and understanding that you, or even a loved one, are not the only ones who might be struggling with this condition. In fact, education in this area helps to develop a support network that can be helpful in overcoming the issue.

If you, or a loved one, are experiencing incessant anxiety attacks would start by learning about what an anxiety attack is. In finding out more about anxiety, one would find that, ultimately, while an anxiety attack is terrifying, it is a brief experience and it will end.

A CBT therapist can assist you in finding the right information you need on the subject while help you deal with your anxiety or any other mental health concern through other reliable sources found in bookstores and on the internet.

Reasonable, Realistic Thinking

When dealing with negative emotions, it is important to spot them as they occur. When you spot them, you can begin to help yourself identify them. As you gain practice and experience identifying these negative emotions, you can then embark upon the process of replacing negative feelings with positive ones. This can help you break the association between an incident and negative feelings.

Negative emotions that are damaging and hurtful can give way to more positive ones that will allow you to process your feelings

- **Negative**: I am such a failure. I always mess things up.
  Positive: I am not perfect, but I know that I will improve with time. I'm human and I will learn from my mistakes through experience.

- **Negative**: I can't get a hold on my anxiety. I don't know why I am unable to control myself.

    Positive: It's alright to feel anxious and edgy. I know that I need to work on improving this but with help, I can get a handle on it. There is nothing I can't do.

Steps to Rational Thinking

1. Consider what you're thinking of letting yourself know. The greater part of us are not used to focusing on the manner in which we think, despite the fact that we are always influenced by our thoughts. By setting your attention on your thought patterns, you will be able to have a clear idea of the thoughts that commonly enter your mind.
2. As you become more aware of your thoughts, your ability to identify negative thoughts will become much easier. For instance, if you feel miserable pondering your grandma who's been doing combating malignant growth, this idea shouldn't be tested in light of the fact that it's totally normal to feel dismal when contemplating a friend or family member enduring. In any case, you'll be able to pick up on negative thoughts any time the creep up on you. That way, you'll be able to avoid any negative reactions when you find yourself in need of interacting with others around you.
3. Pay attention to any changes in your emotion, regardless of how little of a change it might appear to be. It pays to be vigilant of your feelings so that you can keep a close eye on the onset of such feelings. When it does occur, ask yourself why you feel the way you do and what you can do to help you feel better about it.
4. Once you become able to identify your feelings, it will be a lot easier for you to detect triggers and become alert to the onset of such thoughts and feelings as they occur. It certainly helps to determine if your feelings are reasonable or completely irrational. Often, negative and anxious thoughts are the product of unsubstantiated fears. To combat this, the best way to go about it is to challenge your fears. For instance, are your fears really as bad as you think? After all, the likelihood of the worst-scenario is generally very slim.
5. Finally, in the wake of testing a negative idea and assessing it all the more impartially, attempt to concoct an elective idea that is increasingly adjusted and practical. Doing this can help bring down your trouble. Notwithstanding concocting reasonable articulations, attempt to think of some fast and simple to recall adapting explanations. That's why realizing that the most logical explanation is usually the likeliest one. This will help you avoid becoming alarmed for no reason.
6. One effective strategy is journaling. By keeping a record of your thoughts and feelings, you can keep track of the instances in which you feel this way and how often such feelings set in. Ultimately, this will help you see progress or determine if there has been a regression of any kind.

Relaxation Strategies

Finding effective relaxation strategies are always useful when dealing with anxiety and stress. As such, CBT espouses the use of techniques that can help you get a handle on your feelings in addition to managing the onset of sudden episodes. You'll be able to manage your feelings more effectively as you gain a better understanding of your particular circumstances.

Two methodologies regularly utilized in CBT include deep breathing, that is, controlled bursts of inhalation and exhalation. When you do this, you take a deep breath and hold it for a short period of time such as 5 seconds. Then, you release the air in a controlled manner. Additional procedures to achieve relaxation involve tuning in to quiet music, contemplation, yoga and a back rub.

It's imperative to acknowledge, in any case, that the objective of relaxation isn't to stay away from or wipe out nervousness (since stress is not dangerous) but to make it somewhat simpler to cope with these feelings.

Step-by-Step Instructions to Prevent a Mental Health Relapse

1. Exercise is important for your mental and physical health and when you stop exercising, you may find that you're having the same issues as before. However, if you keep with it, you will have a better mentality, a better outlook on your life, as well as having a better emotional life. All of which can help you avoid a relapse.
2. Continue rehearsing what you have learned. In doing so, you'll be able to avoid regressing back into your previous state. Please remember that consistency is the name of the game. By being consistent, you can approach your negative feelings effectively and address them immediately when you detect their presence
3. It is also essential to understand when you are feeling the onset of such feelings, for instance, when you are under a great deal of stress or pressure. Additionally, it makes a rundown of caution signs (e.g., progressively on edge thoughts, visit contentions with friends and family) that reveal to you your uneasiness may increment. When you recognize what your admonition signs or "warnings" are, you would then be able to make an activity arrangement to adapt to them. This may include, for instance, rehearsing some CBT abilities like quiet breathing or testing your negative reasoning.
4. Keep in mind that, similar to just like anyone else you might meet, you are a work in progress. That is why you need to embrace the possibilities that the future affords. If you cling to your old thoughts and beliefs, it might actually make it harder for you to make significant advancements in the way you can deal with overcoming your feelings.
5. If you have had a slip by, attempt to make sense of what circumstances drove you to it. This can enable you to make an arrangement to adapt to difficult circumstances later on. Remember that it's not unexpected to once in a while have slips and that you can gain so much from them.

6. How you consider your slip by your actions is important as well. Focus on your hard work and avoid feeling those negative feelings. If you are feeling those negative feelings bubbling up remind yourself that you're worth it and that you're not a failure or a disappointment. You're an amazing person and you deserve to remember this. You should also remember that everything you have learned through this program (like how to stop your feelings of anxiety) is hard to be unlearned. You've done the work; you just need to keep going.
7. Keep in mind that failures are typical and can be survived. Setbacks are common and should not be the basis for beating yourself up over them. The main thing is to try and stay as positive as you can.
8. Lastly, reward yourself whenever you feel that things are going well. There is no need for any lavish rewards, but any kind of positive reinforcement can be useful in order to help you stay within the right frame of mind.

Confronting Fears: Exposure

It's entirely expected to need to keep away from the things you fear since this decreases your uneasiness for the time being. For instance, if you find yourself getting overly anxious about closed spaces, such as the case of claustrophobia, you can challenge yourself by taking a short elevator ride, such as going from one floor to another. This measured confrontation allows you to have very limited exposure, but exposure, nonetheless. That is one of the core tenets of CBT, being able to face your fears in a measured approach.

The initial step includes creating a plan by which you can expose yourself to your fears in a measured and controlled manner. That way, you won't run the risk of overwhelming yourself. For example, if you are afraid of bugs, you can begin by watching videos about insects, seeing an insect in a zoo behind glass, and being in the room with someone holding an insect. When you have a list, organize it from the least frightening to the most frightening.

Beginning with the circumstance that causes you the least tension, more than once participate in the type of situation that you fear. This could be something like simply looking at images of spiders and work your way up until you are finally able to bring yourself to being in the presence of a spider. This is why CBT is about progressively working yourself up to ultimately facing your fear. Eventually, this will represent an experience in which you have officially overcome the fears that have been haunting you.

Depression

Battling depression is intense. Fortunately, there are numerous ways you can battle depression and win. What works one day may not work the following, so you need the same number of instruments in the tool kit to adjust and deal with whatever depression has caused you.

Here are a few ideas for battling depression:

1. Set Small Goals

- Depression can cause the most straightforward tasks to appear to be overwhelming, so you will need to try and separate things into smaller and more specific tasks. For instance, rather than questioning how you will get all of your work done this week, begin to examine this stressor more effectively by making a list of each task you need to accomplish and plan for how to best ensure you accomplish it.
- Each time you complete a task, give yourself credit. Basically, getting up when battling depression is an achievement and if that is everything you can do in a day, that is alright. Push yourself, but don't beat yourself up if you can't keep up with your typical pace.

2. Give Yourself Credit

- We realize that it is so difficult to battle depression, so we feel compelled to pressure this as much as possible – be grateful for any means and progress you make, regardless of whether it takes longer than you thought.
- Healing from depression requires some serious energy. The new knowledge and skills you acquire, though, will be with you and available to serve you at any time moving forward.

3. Concentrate on The Basics

- *Sleep, diet, physical exercise* –make an honest effort to take care of these as they can have a serious effect on your capacity to effectively overcome depression.
- Make a point to think 'physical movement' and not 'work out.' Taking a short walk, running errands, or anything that gets you up and moving counts. Getting outside and into the sun can likewise help. Here are five straightforward tips on maintaining your progress.

4. Stay Away from Or Limit Alcohol and Other Substance Use

- A portion of the tips above is tied in with adapting to depression by entertaining ourselves. Drinking and other substance use may feel like an approach to distract, separate, or numb yourself from the torments of depression, yet it is anything but a sound method to do it and will consistently transform into a more serious issue.

5. Continue Doing Things

- This may appear to be hard from the start since you most likely won't have a similar measure of energy or motivation you ordinarily do, yet part of battling depression is basically giving your mind another thing to consider (and asleep from negative thoughts).

6. Talk to a Therapist

- Talking to a therapist about depression is similar to going to a doctor to talk about your cold symptoms. If you want to get the most helpful information for battling depression, you should talk with a therapist.
- Keep in mind, therapy isn't just a place to complain and cry; it's associated with realizing what's fundamental to your depression, growing new skills for dealing with the stuff that life throws at us, and progressing in the direction of improving and making the most of your life. With regards to depression, there is not a viable alternative for looking for expert help – if you're feeling discouraged, connect with a therapist when you can. It's that clear. Study talk therapy and how to discover a therapist.
- Try to concentrate your thought anyplace else – take a walk, try something new, or meet a friend for coffee. The primary concern here is that you need to abstain from lying about and wallowing in hopelessness throughout the day. When you get moving, you'll naturally discover you have more energy than you thought you would.

7. Connect with Friends and Family

- A ton of folks hides feeling depressed from the very individuals that could help the most.
- Discussing what's causing you stress or weighing you down can help decrease the impact of these thoughts. Allow those who are near to you to help.

8. Testing Negative Thinking

- Being able to understand and identify when depression is weighing you down is the initial step toward healing. When you are feeling depressed, a wide range of negative thoughts can cloud our minds, so it's essential to have the option to simply hold these thoughts and let them go.

9. Keep Some Humor in Your Life

- Discovering ways to make yourself laugh provides your mind with a break from all the negative thoughts depression brings.
- Regardless of whether this includes talking a friend or watching a funny show or film, it is important to keep some humor in your life.

10. Shift Your Attention

- If your state of mind is overloading you to the point where it feels incomprehensible, try focusing on something different. Abandon what you were focusing on that caused you so much stress immediately and for a short space of time. This can be particularly useful when attempting to manage and defeat self-destructive thoughts. Mindfulness activities can be useful in shifting thoughts away from negative thoughts.

Sleep Disorders

The misery of a sleeping disorder affects around 30% of the population. When sleep troubles begin, it turns into a mental and physical fight. Research and clinical trials demonstrate that a sleeping disorder is associated with decreased personal satisfaction, just as depression is. Therefore, depression can directly prompt sleep issues. Sleep deprivation can likewise prompt feelings of nervousness, disappointment, misery, depletion, and an inability to focus. The more we search for sleep, the less we discover it. Rather than obsessing over trying to sleep, spend that time researching new things you can do to help yourself sleep.

Concentrate on the Body

If you experience consistent difficulty quieting your mind, it very well may be increasingly compelling to concentrate on the body first. You can utilize relaxation strategies, breathing activities, and physical therapy methods. One example of these strategies is to concentrate on your breath and body instead of on negative thoughts and disappointment. To do this, you inhale gradually in through your nose and out through your mouth. This straightforward exercise will naturally relax your breathing and help your body unwind. At that point, after a couple of breaths, begin to breathe naturally again and put a hand on your stomach so you can feel it rising and falling. This is otherwise known as "riding the wave" of your relaxation. Regardless of whether you actually fall asleep or not, your body is very calm.

To work with the brain, CBT can be successful in challenging negative reasoning and any contributing beliefs. A difficult explanation could be, "Despite the fact that I am struggling to sleep, I can work to quiet my brain and body as well as can be expected." Or, "I am struggling with sleep problems and it won't exist forever. I can get through this." You need to accept your emotions, express the realities, and promise yourself that you are doing the best that you can. Keep a log of your sleep and anything that improves it.

Quiet Your Mind

You can take activities to improve the nature of your evening sleep. At the times of your restlessness and pain, you can work to quiet your brain and body using cognizant relaxation, cognitive therapy, and argumentative behavior therapy procedures. I prescribe that you initially counsel your therapist or doctor to guarantee that you have no mental issues, medicinal inconveniences, or drug connections that could be causing your difficulties with sleep.

With regards to sleep hygiene, considers demonstrating that a sleep schedule that incorporates a timeframe to loosen up can be viable. A typical practice is to mood killer all gadgets after 9:00 pm and afterward get dressed and cleaned up for the evening. When prepared for bed, do a relaxation exercise and go through 30 minutes perusing a book before finally shutting your eyes. If you are as yet battling to sleep, attempt to diminish the measure of time you thrash around by getting up and heading off to a calm, agreeable spot in another room or territory of the room to pursue or accomplish more relaxation activities.

Sleep Apnea

Obstructive sleep apnea is a serious yet common sleep issue. Your airway consistently ends up blocked while you

Sleep Apnea is considered to be a very serious sleeping disorder. In consists of insufficient oxygen intake when you are sleeping, and so you wake up gasping for air as you were not breathing. At the point when this happens, you may make gagging noises, or you might wheeze significantly. This is the result of oxygen deprivation in your brain. You will find that this occurs on more than one occasion per night. Additionally, for some sufferers, it can happen many times each night in extreme cases.

CPAP Therapy

Continuous Positive Airway Pressure Therapy (CPAP therapy) utilizes a device which provides a calming does of air as administered by a mask, or small prongs, which fit into your nose.

Options. If you are reluctant to wear a mask during sleep, there are some alternatives.

You can choose to do the following:

- *Attempt positional therapy.* A few people basically experience the ill effects of this condition when they sleep in a supine position. As such, this therapy aims to keep the individual sleeping on their side. This helps minimize the effects of the condition.
- *Surgical procedures.* Surgery may be an alternative is a device such as a CPAP does not work or is not recommended.
- *Wear a dental or oral device.* Make sure the device fits you properly.
- *Experience the weight of the board program.* This alternative involves losing weight. Often, being overweight may be a factor that contributes to the onset of sleep apnea.

Description of Sleeping Disorders

Sleeping disorders are those conditions that keep a person from getting a full night's sleep, that is because it prevents them from falling asleep or it consistently wakes the individual. There are two types of sleeping disorders, those known as "transient" that is temporary, and "interminable" that is, chronic conditions that persist for extended periods of time.

REM Sleep Behavior Disorder

REM sleep is highlighted by the phase of sleep in which you usually dream. You come up short on the muscle loss of motion a great many people understanding while sleeping. At the point when the condition makes threat you or anybody around you, it's paid attention to especially.

You could have an REM sleep behavior issue if you yell, talk, hit, punch, shout, and more while snoozing or even move your appendages in your sleep.

When a person shows issues with REM sleep, the general course of treatment is medication. This is vital in order to avoid serious illness down the road.

Chronic Insomnia

A constant inability to achieve a state of sleep is characterized as Chronic Insomnia. Experiencing issues with sleep for a period exceeding a month can be considered as chronic. This can leave you feeling exhausted the next day as you are not able to rest appropriately. By experiencing a consistent irregular sleeping disorder, you experience a dozing design where you have a couple of evenings of good sleep rotating with numerous evenings of a sleeping disorder.

Transient or Short-Term Insomnia

This kind of sleep deprivation regularly happens in consequence of an upsetting life occasion — for instance, losing a friend or family member or experiencing trouble at work. Also, prolonged periods of stress can set off episodes of insomnia though they may be limited to periods that do not exceed a couple of nights. Ultimately, the individual falls asleep due to exhaustion.

Normal Treatment Types for Insomnia

Medication can be prescribed to help address this issue. For instance, if there is an underlying case of depression or anxiety, then treating this aspect may be enough to help you relax enough to get decent sleep. Sleep meds can be utilized also yet are ordinarily recommended to be utilized on a present moment or as-required premise.

Non-therapeutic strategies, for example, cognitive behavior therapy, hypnotherapy, sleep confinement, and relaxation methods, can likewise be utilized to treat sleep deprivation. Lifestyle changes, for example, evading caffeine and liquor, are additionally exhorted.

Restless Legs Syndrome

Restless Legs Syndrome (RLS) can be understood as an involuntary leg movement that occurs while you are sleeping. This can lead to feelings of unpleasantness and discomfort leading you to spend precious energy or building up tension in your thighs, hamstrings, and calves. This may also send other unpleasant sensations to other parts of your body.

Basic Treatment Types for Restless Legs Syndrome

- Medications and CBT can be prescribed as a treatment for RLS.

Narcolepsy

Narcolepsy makes you all of a sudden fall asleep whenever and regardless of your current circumstances. In general, the sufferer cannot control dozing off in random situations, for example, you could start to doze off while eating. Individuals with narcolepsy can't direct their sleep-wake cycle.

General Course of Treatment for Narcolepsy

- The most common course of treatment for narcolepsy is a strict sleeping schedule and medication.

Substance Use Disorders

When thinking about how to manage someone who is addicted and how to manage addiction, it's essential to think about the idea of addiction. Addictions don't occur in storehouses. They occur in networks loaded up with cherishing individuals. At the point when addictions strike, those relatives and friends need to find a way to get the individual they cherish into treatment programs that can help.

Families have a huge influence in the recuperation of a someone who is addicted. Each and every one of these individuals needed to battle back against that addiction, and chances are, about these individuals had relatives and friends pulling for their possible recuperation. If you're the adored one of somebody battling with addiction, you may have numerous inquiries and concerns, for example, how to manage a medication someone who is addicted (managing addiction). Some other potential concerns include:

Managing Dependence and Addiction

1. Find and attend support groups for families of addicts
2. Help families manage the behavior of their loved one who is an addict
3. Help parents of addicts

These relatives and friends likewise need to deal with their very own wellbeing, so they can give the support addicted individuals need to recover. These are tips that can assist families with doing just that:

1. Associate with getting peers.

- It is difficult to live with and additionally support somebody who has an addiction. An addiction in a nearby relative can fill in as a distressing life circumstance that continues for a considerable length of time, and that long-haul brokenness can make it difficult for families to impart obviously. There's a

square of questions between each individual from a family contacted by addiction. The uplifting news is, there is help for groups of addicts.
- Associating with friends may help, especially if families utilize a confided in program. The thought here is to give help to groups of medication addicts. These projects additionally give a protected, nonjudgmental space for relatives to use so as to learn, talk about, and defeat a dependence unfurling in their middle.

2. Instruct and promoter.

- Stress and depression can come from a wide range of sources, yet once in a while, relatives feel the attacks most intensely when they originate from the friends, business partners, and inaccessible relatives they see all the time.
- These attacks originate from all sides. To certain individuals, addictions truly are a type of shortcoming, and these individuals have no issue with pointing out that belief in casual discussions. To other people, addictions are something relatives ought to either fix or overlook.
- Tragically, as well, some language that promotes addiction stigma originates from the therapeutic network. As the Fix calls attention to, groups will, in general, use terms like "clean" and "dirty" when they're discussing dependence, and they may allude to the "war" on drugs.
- It's difficult to remain positive in a situation like this, yet families can be a contributor to the change. They can share a portion of the learning they've gathered from private research, support gatherings, and therapy sessions. They can inform the individuals around them regarding their family's work to defeat an addiction, and they could shift the country's discussion about dependence.
- Pushing in the interest of habit is daring, but on the other hand, it's a crucial and wellbeing insisting activity. As opposed to remaining quiet and raging, families that make some noise are improving, and those discussions could wonderfully affect a family's state of mind.

3. Plan dinners and eat them as a family.

- In the present, turbulent world, it's very simple to eat independently. One partner gets a burger in transit home, while other snacks on the plate of mixed greens at work, and the children get and heat readymade nourishments they can discover in the cooler.
- While timetables can get tight when families are managing addiction-related arrangements, a family feast enables everybody in the family to reconnect toward the finish of a day that may have been distressing, forlorn, and troubling. Every feast expands upon the work done in family therapy, and the custom of eating together can be truly relieving, as well. Indeed, even one feast together every week could have an incredible effect.

4. Schedule private therapy sessions.

- While lifestyle adjustments can be a major help for families in emergency, addictions can cause profound rifts and wounds that nothing, but therapy can heal. That is the reason why it's crucial for individual family members to meet with individual therapists that can assist them with overcoming and comprehending their own issues. For a few, those sessions may include various pressure busting discussions.
- A private therapy session is a sheltered spot for focused on relatives to empty and talk transparently. There's no judgment or fault here. There's only a feeling of receptiveness and thoughtfulness, but on the other hand, there's a lot of work done.
- Private sessions regularly use skill-based methods, in which these parental figures get familiar with how to manage damaging thoughts and beliefs created during long stretches of addictive behavior. They may figure out how to reflect to deal with pressure, or they may deal with decisiveness abilities. They may do gathering work including outrage the board, or they may figure out how to relinquish mutually dependent practices, so they won't feel liable for the poor decisions of others.
- It requires some investment to go to an individual therapy session, and frequently, there's homework to finish between the sessions, as well. However, this private and individual opportunity arrives with various genuine advantages. Relatives who invest their energy in these sessions may get the help they need so as to help other people, and they may discover the quality and resolve that has been absent up until this point.

5. Oversee desires.

- At the point when a dependent individual enters treatment and the family sets out on family care, the feeling of expectation everybody feels can be overpowering. Finally, the addiction issue is being tended to. At last, things will show signs of improvement.
- Lamentably, it can set aside a long effort for the progressions and examples related to dependence on true change. In some cases, that moderate shift prompts frustrations.
- The key is to concentrate on the work some portion of recuperation. It is a procedure, and it accompanies various entanglements. Individuals in early recuperation may commit errors and they may not be their optimal selves; however, families can even now make the most of their time and their fellowship. Regardless of whether things aren't up to a Norman Rockwell level, they can even now be lovely.

6. Go to family therapy sessions.

- Managing an addict is rarely simple. Similarly, as a dependent individual change over the span of an addiction, so does the family. Life partners, kin and guardians of addicts frequently assimilate a considerable lot of the outcomes. They can't speak straightforwardly about the issue that is hurting them, so they end up not discussing a lot of anything by any means. In the interim, these equivalent relatives can accuse themselves in light of the fact that the addiction is still in play, despite the fact that they need the issue to stop.

- These quiet and accuse games can injure a family when help is urgently required. They might not have the devices to help somebody in dynamic recuperation, and they might not have the energy to support themselves. In any case, there are care groups for groups of addicts accessible. If you have inquiries concerning how to manage medication, someone who is addicted, these gatherings can give you the help you need.
- A family therapy program is intended to separate that impression of doubt, blame, and stress. Families that were once characterized by outrage and by habit can be changed into tight, well-oiled units that help each other, no matter what.
- Family therapy sessions can require significant investment, and it very well may be a touch of enticing to skirt a session or two, especially for families with various clashing arrangements and motivation. Nonetheless, this is work that is crucial to the soundness of everybody included, so those gatherings ought to be kept if at all conceivable.

7. Get regular exercise.

- Beginning the day with a quick run or ending the day with a couple of laps in the pool may not be each family's concept of an incredible time, however, these exercise sessions could provide serious benefits. Exercise has the demonstrated capacity to lessen pressure and depression.
- Exercising and working out help to encourage the brain to release "feel-good" neurotransmitters known as oxytocin and dopamine. Brisk exercise sessions can assist families with releasing their stress and worry in restorative manners that don't hurt others and or themselves. Rather than complaining, they can run it off. Rather than pacing nervously, they can do yoga. It's a superb method to keep on track with healing, and it's relatively simple to begin.

8. Learn however much as could reasonably be expected about addiction.

- Consistently, research groups conduct research studies about substance abuse. They're studying how these substances connect with the cells inside the brain, and they're utilizing that information to grow new medications that may one day either treat or counteract addictions.
- That is the kind of information that can help a family's feeling of expectation. With every new piece of information they're learning, they may feel increasingly sure that the addiction can be both treated and defeated.

- Training can likewise assist families with escaping habitual pettiness. As opposed to accepting that the individual's addiction comes from shortcoming, resolution, or determination, they may figure out how addictions come from changes in mind science and electrical motivation adjustments. That information may assist families with letting go of their annoyance, so they can concentrate on mending.
- There is a wide range of online assets that can assist families with learning, and most current book shops are loaded up with books about the science of addiction and the science behind dependence treatment. Families that are lacking in assets may scoff at purchasing PCs, information plans, and books, however, they likewise have alternatives.

9. Stick to a proper sleep/wake plan.

- Probably the most wrecking scenes of medication misuse and addiction occur in the profundities of night. It's during this time individuals with addictions meet sellers, overdose, stagger home from gatherings, or generally get into circumstances that relatives must correct. It's nothing unexpected, at that point, that a few families in the recuperation procedure battle with sleep. Portions of their minds are continually trusting that the following night emergency will emerge.
- Normal sleep misfortune can be a staggering mind-set executioner. Individuals need to stay in bed request to feel their best, and families helping with recuperation should be at the highest point of their games.
- Making a normal sleep plan, in which sleep times and wake times are immovably fixed, can make preparations for profound sleep. At the point when those hours move around, the mind realizes exactly what to do.

10. Keep in contact with individual delight.

- Overseeing desires is a little simpler when families are answerable for their very own joy. That implies each individual from a recouping family needs to set aside some effort to accomplish something that is relaxation and makes them happy. These are exercises that can make the member feel upbeat. They're side interests that are done to save a feeling of viability and worth, and they could support emotional well-being, as well.
- At the point when life is loaded with exercises that appear to be difficult to finish and advance is difficult to see, a side interest that produces something unmistakable can be an incredible solace.

Chapter 11: Identifying Unhelpful Behaviors

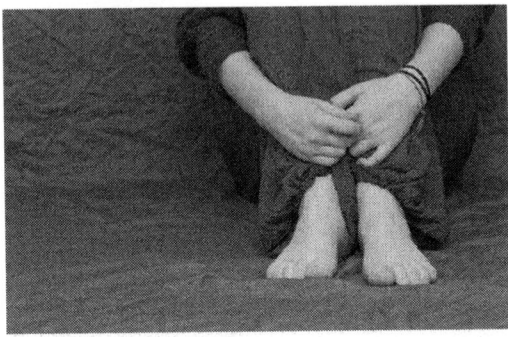

At the point when you have a negative idea or belief or showcase a negative behavior, it frequently makes an example of broken behavior that props your skeptical mindset up in a sort of endless loop or 'circle'. These cycles are called 'keeping up procedures' by therapists.

One of the key concentrations in Cognitive Behavioral Therapy (CBT) is attempting to understand and identify the sorts of thoughts, emotions, and practices you are having that are preventing you from liking yourself and your life.

Attempting to identify these cycles of unhelpful behavior is a key piece of your first couple of sessions of CBT, where you and your cognitive therapist will do a behavioral investigation and together discuss your examples so you would then be able to capture and change them.

How about we take a look at the most widely recognized sorts of 'keeping up procedures' that CBT advising identifies.

1. Avoidance

- It's exceptionally common when you are feeling anxious to need to flee from the circumstance that is making you feel tense. This is the reason why if you endure social anxiety, you will, in general, stay away from social circumstances entirely and will choose instead to isolate themselves and be alone. Or, on the other hand, you might go out but avoid eye contact, remain in a seat on the outskirts of the gatherings, and make frequent escapes to the bathroom. Avoidance will only allow the problem to continue to exist

2. Hairsplitting

- The hairsplitting circle is a typical one if you experience the ill effects of low confidence and certainty. You set yourself practically unthinkable exclusive requirements so as to demonstrate your abilities and worth. "If I'm impeccable, at that point I can't be futile." In any case, by setting such unusually elevated expectations you can never accomplish, you rather strengthen that you are

"pointless" and "not commendable." Your low confidence is kept up and even strengthened.
- Keep in mind, affirmation is critical. If you perceive any of these kinds of thoughts or instances of practices in yourself, you have made a significant initial phase in attempting to break your cycle of useless behavior. Take a stab at observing when and how frequently you think such thoughts or carry on in such a manner and notice in what circumstances the cycles happen. By identifying when you are participating in a circle, you can start to change the procedure of occasions and all the more critically deal with how you think and carry on.

3. Decrease in Activity

- This is the most widely recognized keeping up procedure with regards to depression. Frequently, when you are depressed, you experience negative thoughts and physical symptoms; for example, a decrease in energy. These symptoms tend to prompt withdrawing from activities that typically give you feelings of joy and accomplishment. You might even find yourself only doing the bare minimum each day.
- Tragically, this can make you feel even more depressed, as you are detaching yourself from what generally gives you pleasure. Additionally, withdrawing from activities you typically enjoy often results in losing connections with people who you typically enjoy being around, and people who could ultimately support you through your depression. It can become such a habit to isolate yourself when you are depressed that, often, people end up finding basic tasks like brushing their teeth and showering to be absolutely overwhelming.

4. Checking/Hypervigilance

- This is another basic behavioral cycle if you endure anxiety and depression and furthermore happens with sufferers of Post-Traumatic Stress Disorder. It happens when you are stressed; you could have a genuine disease and regularly filter or are hyper-cautious to manifestations which you accept affirms you have the ailment. This procedure makes you increasingly touchy to getting on consummately ordinary real side effects and translating them as an affirmation of sickness. This at that point expands your tensions and stresses which prompts further filtering and checking, and the endless loop is made.

5. Inevitable outcomes

- If you have contrary beliefs about others' dispositions towards you, you might just at that point inspire responses from those individuals which seem to affirm your unique negative belief. For instance, the desire that others will be forceful and antagonistic towards you may imply that you stroll around with very cautious behavior, which really elicits animosity from others and affirms your belief that others are forceful towards you.

6. Wellbeing Behaviors

- Security practices happen when you need to shield yourself from something you fear. They are frequently identified with tension. If you endure social uneasiness, instances of this sort of behavior incorporate concurring with everything the other individual says, talking unobtrusively, adhering to 'safe' discussions, worrying to control shaking and utilizing liquor and medications to build certainty.
- While it is justifiable to attempt to adapt to unsavory feelings of uneasiness, these practices can really wind up drawing out feelings of tension. This is on the grounds that the genuine issue stays uncertain and is permitted to proceed. For example, in spite of the fact that you figured out how to feel less restless the last time you hosted to go to a gathering since you got intoxicated on liquor, you are as yet going to have uneasiness whenever you have a get-together to go to.

7. Calamitous Misinterpretation

- If you experience the ill effects of tension about your wellbeing or potentially OCD you may be inclined to this useless behavior process, where you misjudge in essence sensations as proof of progressively genuine physical and mental sickness. Uneasiness indications, for example, expanded pulse, discombobulation, palpitations (heart shudders), and brevity of breath are translated as progressively genuine dangers, for example, respiratory failures, strokes or that you are going to "go distraught
- The aftereffect of reasoning such thoughts is that regularly more uneasiness is produced, and the side effects intensify, which seems to negate the up and coming risk to your prosperity.

Chapter 12: Develop A Positive Mindset

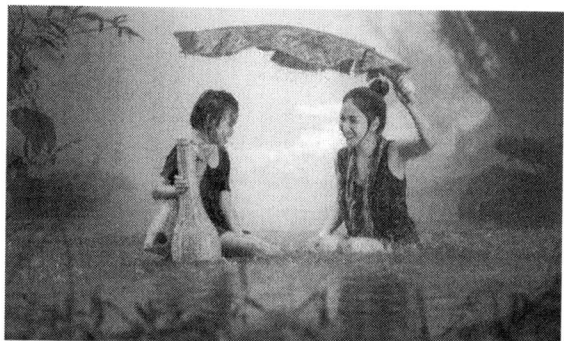

If you have a by and large negative tendency towards life, you will find that your mind will search for and amplify what is negative around you. For example, you may get yourself furious over not winning the lottery, yet you know measurably, the odds of something to that effect happening are practically nothing.

If you take a look at the world around us, individuals seem to be adopting increasingly negative mindsets. Regardless of whether individuals are negative about their nation's leadership, about the negative news they see on TV, about the climate, or even about their sport's team losing. The main concern is that individuals are progressively having a negative disposition towards life, including our vulnerable youth.

The methodology you have towards life matters a great deal. You have undoubtedly known about mantras like 'think positive vibes.' You may consider how precisely you ought to have inspiration in your life; and how to develop the little you have, or even develop it without any preparation. Fear not; we have you secured. Here are a couple of tips on the most proficient method to create and keep a positive attitude everlastingly streaming in your life.

1. Read a Book

- Books are a priceless asset available to you. They educate, energize, challenge, and even lift your spirits. Something you can do if you are feeling particularly stressed or down is dust off your bookshelf and read a book. There are innumerable books out there, accessible either in electronic or printed copies. There are plenty of pros and cons to pursuing either an electronic or printed version, but at the end of the day, a book is a book regardless of its form.

- When searching for a book to pursue, search for ones that will lift your energy, and leave you feeling good. There are moving books that are exclusively made to provide you with steps to acquire a positive mentality. If you are uncertain about such books, you can request help from the book shop you choose to get your books from. You can likewise request advice from your friends and family regarding any books that would give you a positive outlook on life. If you read a book and think that it's helpful, don't be shy! Recommend it to anyone who you think could benefit from it.

2. Have an Emotional Outlet

- Individuals are naturally emotional creatures. The difference is that some people are better at expressing emotions, and some are better at concealing them. In any case, we are, at the core, emotional beings. When you have comprehended your emotions, and furthermore comprehended that some are outside your ability to control, you have to clear a path for you to discharge your negative emotions.

- Let's, for example, say you've had an unpleasant week. Rather than keeping everything inside and pushing it to the back of your mind, you should search for an approach to release it. Individuals have different outlets for their emotions; some of the well-known ones include boxing, swimming, running, etc. At the point when you need to release harmful or negative emotions, search for an activity where you can drive all that emotion to.

- If you let negative emotions bubble up in you, you will just wind up having a negative attitude. Besides, it is unfortunate to hold onto things that could possibly hurt you. Now and again, individuals who cling to negative intuition wind up being discouraged or much more fearful.

3. Smile

- This is ostensibly probably the least difficult advance to keeping a positive personality. A smile can go far into developing energy in your regular day to day existence. When you smile, you not only exercise your facial muscles, you're also increasingly responsive and more approachable.
- A smile will convey to somebody that you're anything but difficult to talk and to identify with, and you may even discover individuals who were straight and inflexible with you begin to be somewhat more open. A smile is a straightforward accessory, but an amazing one regardless.

4. Live in the moment

- Numerous individuals have a belief of either living in the past or living in the future. When you live in the past, you will tire individuals with stories from years ago, wishing it could manifest to the present. Then again, if you live in the future, you will wind up underutilizing your time, pondering how extraordinary things could be, or what will be.

- Probably the most ideal approaches to build up a positive attitude is to live in the present time and place. At the point when you do, you will have the option to expand the open doors that are accessible. Additionally, when you live in the present, you're ready to tailor your connections and develop them.
- Nonetheless, it is essential to understand that both the past and the future have a spot in the present. The past helps you to remember the things you've learned, and the successes you have had. The future, as well, is important. It keeps you on track regarding the different things you might want to achieve.

5. Give circumstances a chance to happen without anyone else

- Each individual needs to have control over a specific degree. A few people need to control everything, while some are generally content with what there is. What you have to comprehend, is that you can't control each circumstance. What you ought to do, is enable the circumstances to normally run their course.
- You can't control the climate, yet you can control how you respond to it. At the point when the sun is excessively sweltering, you should dress suitably, and welcome the climate. At the point when a kindred partner gets an advancement you have been peering toward, don't get all desirous and jealous. Rather, allow them to enjoy all that life has to offer and sit tight for your turn.
- Be that as it may, you should, in any case, hold control somewhat. For example, don't neglect to set an alarm and trust that the universe will wake you up. It is essential for one to find a healthy balance between having control over their lives and letting life take its course.

6. Love and accept yourself

- Probably the best quality anybody can gain in the voyage of positive mentality is that of cherishing oneself. At whatever point individuals discuss love, they more oft than not consider feeling love. While feeling love has its place in setting a positive attitude, there's a whole other world to adore than simply feeling.
- For this situation, the affection we're discussing is an adoration for the easily overlooked details. At the point when you can discover love in the easily overlooked details about your day, you will wind up having a simple day. On the flip side, when you abhor everything that continues during the day, you will have one taxing day.
- Something other than cherishing your condition, you have to adore yourself. At the point when you adore yourself, you will put resources into satisfying yourself. Valid, there are things that will attempt to disturb your day, yet when you cherish yourself, you will disregard a large portion of these things.

7. Stick around positive individuals

- You are the aggregate of your friends. If you stick around contrarily disapproved of individuals, you will undoubtedly wind up being negative yourself. Friends assume a major job in what we do, and how we do it. If you stroll into a bar, you will discover individuals grouped together, having a brew or two. If you research further, you'll discover the vast majority of these bunches share something for all intents and purposes. It is possible that they are coworkers or went to class together. As a general rule, you'll find if there's an individual from the gathering that doesn't fit in, they will be sidelined, or they will grow bored of the gathering and leave for a more engaging one – in their eyes.

- At the point when you stick around positive individuals, there's a plausibility of two things occurring; one, you get baffled by their affable nature and leave the gathering, or two, they impact you into their reasoning. If you need to be a positive mastermind, you should effectively look for after a gathering that is positive and attempt your level best to stay by the gathering.
- It will surely not be simple, and change doesn't occur without any forethought, yet the adventure is well justified, despite all the trouble. Once more, if you see somebody battling with energy, you can draw in them, and attempt to have them join the gathering.

8. Enjoy a reprieve

- Practically all individuals have schedules that characterize their days. For a great many people, they wake up, get down to business, go on with their work, get off work, get some dinner, sleep, and rehash. At the point when you fall into such a daily practice, it tends to exhaust, risky and practically difficult to have a positive mentality.
- To make a positive mentality, you should, occasionally, enjoy a reprieve from your repetitive everyday practice. You can accomplish something unconstrained that will re-invigorate you and help you return on track.
- When taking a break, you don't need to do anything unrestrained, you can simply accomplish something as basic as going out to see the films, tuning in to music, viewing the nightfall, or even simply unwind at home. Whatever makes you want to step out of your daily schedule, pull out all the stops. Insofar as it doesn't overstep any laws.

9. Mind your language

- Truly, your language decides a great deal when you're attempting to develop a living attitude. What you state is either to a great extent impacted by what you feel, or it goes to impact what you feel. Think about this sentence, "Today is complete chaos, I woke up late, I'm late to work and nobody ever values my exertion." The sentence is antagonistic, the individual talking the above has just made the end that the subject day is terrible, hence, they are bound to concentrate on each and everything that won't go their direction.
- Presently, think about this sentence, "Today is a decent day, I woke up late, yet I'm happy to have woken up by any stretch of the imagination. I may have been late to work, yet I'm fortunate I have a vocation to go to, and I wasn't terminated. The individuals around may not value my endeavors, yet despite everything, I'll

work as well as could be expected; on the grounds that I must do as such." This individual has quite recently had a pretty much that day to the individual above; in any case, the subsequent individual has chosen to concentrate on the integrity in the day, instead of the disagreeableness.
- If you strolled into an office and found the two above individuals working, it's extremely simple to differentiate the main individual from the subsequent one. At the point when you have spoken positively about your day, you wind up valuing the little things and finding an explanation or two to push yourself past the day.

10. Reward yourself

- Probably the hardest activity is to remunerate yourself. Commonly, individuals will discover great in other individuals however not in themselves. If you need to be a scholar, you should discover great in yourself first, and reward yourself.
- Remunerating yourself can be deciphered from numerous points of view. In the wake of a monotonous week, you can compensate yourself by taking the end of the week off and relaxation. You could even accomplish something as basic as getting dessert or spending time with friends.

Chapter 13: Develop Self-Discipline

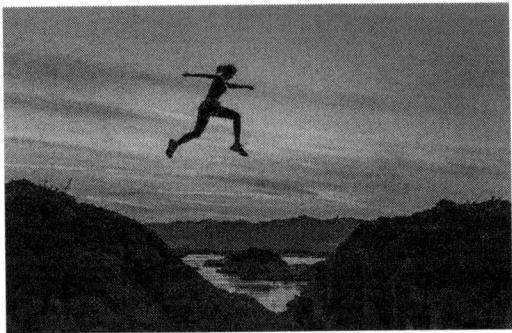

1. Discover a strategy that works for you for conquering tarrying.

- There are a million techniques out there for conquering tarrying. A few people give themselves counterfeit cutoff times. Others break errands into littler lumps and take them individually. Others utilize a reward framework.
- It doesn't make a difference which methodology you use for conquering hesitation, insofar as you have one and it works. What's more, do it normally.

2. Measure your advancement.

- There's an old business proverb that goes, "What you can't quantify, you can't improve. What's more, what you do gauge for the most part improves."
- There's a fact in that. As opposed to setting an obscure or vague objective, if you can put some measurement behind it, you'll have a vastly improved possibility of succeeding.

3. Think about reflection.

- A great many examinations have demonstrated that contemplation diminishes nervousness and expands balance and self-discipline.
- It's difficult to make reflection a regular practice, but at the same time, when you do, it has a massively positive impact on all parts of your life.

4. Reveal your beliefs and examples that lead to you getting to be undisciplined.

- When you fail miserably at self-discipline, how and when does it occur?
- Is it more often than not after work? Is it harder to focus at home, versus at a café? Is it when you don't get enough sleep?
- On the other hand, in what condition would you say you are generally disciplined?

- Know about what works and what doesn't. Afterward, you can place yourself in circumstances where you are increasingly disciplined.
- "If you can work out the example, you can set up circumstances that will enable you to work best," Croft said.

5. Articulate the greater reason behind each endeavor.

- If you have an unmistakable understanding of your objectives and how this endeavor works in conjunction with them, you are significantly more prone to finishing it.
- The greatest wellspring of self-discipline is to have the motivation to carry out the responsibility. To get this going successfully at scale, you need clear objectives you are completely adjusted behind. That will guarantee you generally have an unmistakable reason behind the errands you take on.

6. Remove temptations and distractions.

- For a significant number of us (myself included), our cellphone is our greatest interruption. In this way, when you have to center, put it in silent mode or put it in another room.
- What's more, focus on your workspace. Expel the TV from where you work. Try not to have food there. Keep it clean. The fewer distractions and temptations you have around you, the better outcomes you'll get.

7. Build up great beliefs by beginning little.

- There is an addiction to pull out all the stops and to attempt to revamp your life medium-term. Be that as it may, by beginning little and simple, you have a vastly improved possibility of really fusing another belief into your everyday practice.

Chapter 14: Improve Self-Esteem

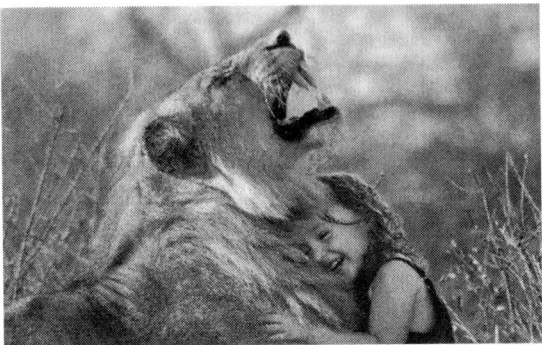

With regards to your self-worth, just a single assessment genuinely matters — your own. What's more, even that one ought to be deliberately assessed; we will, in general, be our very own harshest pundits.

Some individuals choose to explore the world around them and their connections in order to find evidence of their self-constraining beliefs. This attitude is proof that being your own judge can lead to a much harsher imagen than the one others may have.

So, here are some steps which you can follow to help you with your self-worth.

1. Change the story.

- Our personal narrative is important. This narrative is a reflection of the links we have made between our perception and opinion of ourselves. Thus, changing our narrative can lead to a more positive valuation of ourselves and our worth in the world.
- There are instances in which we have programmed negative thoughts into our minds. For example, ideas such as "you're not good enough" can be implanted into the depths of our psyche. Under such circumstances, we may end up accepting such thoughts as the truth. That is why replacing these ideas with positive ones can lead to a successful outcome.
- Familiarity preparing in positive insistences (for instance, recording the same number of positive interactions you have with yourself can drastically reduce the symptoms of depression, among other conditions. Bigger quantities of composed positive explanations are associated with more noteworthy improvement. While they have terrible notoriety on account recently night TV, positive certifications can help.

2. Interactions with others

- *Volunteering to aid those who are in greater need.* "Being of assistance to others helps remove you from your own struggles temporarily. You find yourself getting out of your own head for a while. When you can help another person, it makes you less centered around your very own issues."

- There is a lot of truth to the idea that what we put out into the world is what we will receive from it. You can try this out by making a point of going a full day putting positive ideas into practice whenever you come into contact with someone. Something as simple as being polite can have a significant effect on your interactions.

3. Abstain from falling into the look at and-despair bunny gap.

- Instances of negative self-worth will influence your life and psychological well-being just as different zones in your life, for example, work, connections, and physical wellbeing.

4. Keep in mind that your circumstances do not define you

- Lastly, being able to tell the difference between your personal identity and the circumstances around you are critical to the safe establishment of development. With that security, one is allowed to develop with delight, not fear of disappointment, on the grounds that disappointment doesn't change center worth.
- We are altogether brought into the world with unbounded skills and opportunities for development. Sadly, we are limited by a false belief that we are unable to do anything as a result of our inevitable, unfortunate life experiences. In this way, with diligent work and self-love, negative thoughts and beliefs we hold about ourselves can be unlearned.

5. Be deliberate

- It is important to make a conscious effort to change. We can't make any significant changes in our lives if we don't believe they are necessary. When you are aware that things are not working out, then you will empower yourself to make the changes you need. Otherwise, it may be virtually impossible to get anything done in a significant manner. Please keep in mind that your head can play tricks on you. So, you need to get past them.
- By engaging in an honest exercise of self-analysis, you will find that there are serious aspects in your life which you might have overlooked. When you are honest, you will have the courage to point out, to yourself, what needs to be changed and what needs to be kept.

6. Exercise

- Numerous studies have demonstrated a relationship between exercise and higher self-esteem, along with improved psychological wellness overall. Exercise allows you to center your day around self-care and releases "feel-good" chemicals in the brain to improve your mood. Different types of self-care, for example, appropriate diet and adequate sleep, have likewise been shown to effectively affect one's self-esteem.

7. Forgiving

- Is there would someone say someone is in your life you haven't excused? An ex-accomplice? A relative? Yourself? By clutching feelings of sharpness or hatred, we keep ourselves stuck in a cycle of cynicism. If we haven't forgiven ourselves, disgrace will keep us in this equivalent circle.
- Forgiving self, as well as other people, have been found to develop self-esteem, maybe on the grounds that it associates us with our intrinsically cherishing nature and advances an acknowledgment of individuals, regardless of our imperfections. This is a reference to the Buddhist contemplation on forgiving, which can be rehearsed whenever: "If I have harmed or hurt anybody, intentionally or unwittingly, I ask absolution. If anybody has harmed or hurt me, intentionally or unconsciously, I excuse them. For the manner in which I have harmed myself, purposely or unwittingly, I offer forgiving."

8. Channel your inner hero.

- Everyone is a virtuoso. In any case, if you measure a horse by its capacity to write a book, it's going to carry on with as long as it can remember accepting that it is dumb. We as a whole have our qualities and shortcomings. Somebody might be a splendid performer, yet an unpleasant cook. Neither one of the qualities characterizes their center worth. Perceive your abilities and traits along with the feelings they cause in you. Often, we fall prey to insecurity thereby developing feelings of uncertainty in the manner in which you shake offers a progressively sensible viewpoint of yourself.
- Ask yourself, "Was there a period in your life where you would do well to self-esteem? What were you doing at that phase of your life?" If you have difficulty identifying your one of a kind gifts, request that a friend call attention to out to you. Once in a while, it's simpler for others to see the best in us than it is for us to see it in ourselves.

Chapter 15: Develop Self-Acceptance with Self Talk

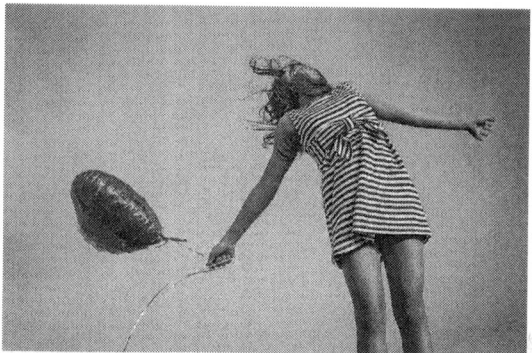

Why is Self-Acceptance So Difficult?

Can you remember a time in your life when you made a mistake and thought things like:

"I'm constantly messing up."

"What's wrong with me?"

This type of reasoning is totally normal, and many experience difficulties with self-acceptance in their lives. However, many treat self-love as a reward for their day. What this means is to think about it like this. You have a horrible day and you need to have some time for yourself. This can look like the following:

- A nap
- A bath
- Your favorite television shows

and other things of this nature. This can be true if you have a good day as well. Everyone needs self-love and self-care and it can help improve your mood and, as a result, your life.

Why Self-Acceptance is Important

Basically, you can't deal with others until you deal with yourself first. At the point when you really, genuinely love yourself, you can navigate the world with more profound empathy for other people, creating a profound feeling of satisfaction and delight from the act of giving.

Self-love is, in this manner, your fuel and foundation. If it's not there, your whole life will be rocky and meaningless. Be that as it may, if you genuinely love yourself, life pushes ahead effortlessly, and everything becomes tolerable.

You'll have more prominent flexibility to withstand any difficult life occasion or individual difficulty. Depression, nervousness, stress, and the pursuit of perfection will disappear and be replaced by the positive thinking that self-love causes. You will always be aware of the fact that difficult times will pass, and you will do so by repeating this mantra in your head:

"I am alright, because I will treat myself kindly regardless of the circumstance."

What Is True Self-Love?

It's not selfishness or vanity. It's not contingent on wanted results. Also, it is anything but an overstated feeling of significance or exemplary narcissism.

Self-Love is Transparent

It's a definitive responsibility to become acquainted with and acknowledge yourself as you are. This will allow you to totally and completely experience life as it transpires. It also enables you to constantly look for approaches to physically, mentally, and profoundly grow from life experiences.

Genuine self-love is giving yourself unconditional positive regard and appreciation. It's reminding yourself that you have the right to have all your own needs met while thinking about yourself as worthy of those needs being met. It's completely knowing, regardless of what you do or don't to do, that you'll still love yourself and be consistent with what your identity is.

How Do You Comprehend Self-Love?

The great poet Oscar Wilde wrote, "To love oneself is the beginning of a life-long romance."

This quote implied that self-love is not a goal that is accomplished and then maintained forever—it is a relationship with yourself that requires consistent practice.

Be that as it may, before we get to everyday self-love strategies and activities, this is what you have to know:

You are the focal point of the universe — everything starts and finishes with you. You will be with yourself forever. Which means you need to work from a position of self-love, instead of self-hating.

You care for yourself the most — No one else is keen on you — your prosperity, security, wellbeing, satisfaction, and presence — more than you. Nobody knows better than you what makes you happy or what hurts you the most. Since no one understands you more than you, it is simply a fact that you also know what decisions are best for you to make. No one can provide you with a better life plan than you.

The love you look for exists inside you — Love from other individuals cannot possibly satisfy you if it develops or mirrors your very own self-love. What's more, cherishing others can actually start from self-love: a reflection or development of the love you have for yourself.

Self-Love Techniques

Self-love is certain, warm, and consistent. It is the finished acceptance of who and what you are. It is simply appreciating and accepting yourself.

It's simply the genuine help, care, and empathy you give yourself that in the end create improved wellbeing, incredible self-esteem, satisfaction, absolute consistency, and prosperity. Self-love is an essential need, a crucial positive worth that prompts internal harmony and joy.

Here are self-love procedures you can use to start expanding your self-love:

1. Clear your mind

Watch and comprehend your present beliefs and values, and the genuine inspirations driving them (ensure you don't borrow or communicate other individuals' beliefs and qualities). If your beliefs and qualities are not serving you or your life goals, question why you are holding onto them.

2. Explore your spirituality

Confidence is simply an act of self-love, regardless of what religion or framework you subscribe to or practice. At the point when you explore your spirituality, it will take you on an adventure of learning things about yourself that can ultimately contribute to your self-confidence. Furthermore, those new thoughts, feelings, interests, and crude emotions will cause you to value yourself for being truly who you are. This will improve your intuition and help to settle on choices that you feel in your gut are right for you.

3. Put a lot of time into self-care

Put as much time as possible into your self-care routine; eat well, work out, get enough sleep, work on your relationships and professional connections, and make sure to make time for entertainment, events, and relaxation. At the point when you feel and deal with your body appropriately, you'll have ideal energy and all of your needs met, which expands upon self-esteem. Self-esteem and self-love are connected at the hip, so taking an interest in things you're great at directly improves your mood and well-being.

4. Be aware of your inner voice

You continually live with an inner voice that is communicating with you almost constantly. It is normal for your inner voice to become your inner critic sometimes. Become mindful and aware of how you treat yourself based on these inner thoughts. Focus on your self-talk and how it affects you. Dispose of the disparaging thoughts and direct your brain and activities to positive practices.

5. Set limits and protect yourself

Identify what is and isn't beneficial to you and use this information to protect yourself. Absolutely never endure mistreatment. Bring the right individuals into your life who mirror your own self-worth and reputation. Live deliberately with purpose and intention.

Chapter 16: Stop Overthinking; Change Negative Thinking

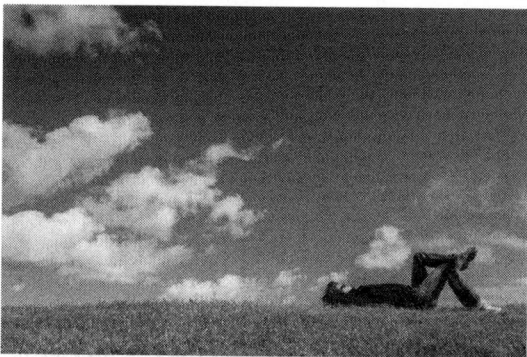

What is Overthinking?

Overthinking is one of those situations in which you make a mountain out of a molehill. For instance, you take a simple encounter with an individual, that perhaps didn't go quite as well as you hoped, and you begin to find fault in places where there isn't. You concoct these ideas about how improper and inadequate you were when simply, the other person was just having a bad day. It's nothing personal. Yet, you make it out to be a huge deal.

This is why you need to deal with the onset of negative emotion in a productive way. Otherwise, you will fall prey to all sorts of ideas that may creep in.

For example, when you're tragic, stressed or restless, your mind will, in general, consider increasingly miserable occasions. You glance through a contorted focal point where you see each circumstance simply more uneasiness or stress. One idea prompts many different thoughts that make you more troubled or increasingly restless. This can lead to an increasingly difficult period of uneasiness in which you may not be able to get a handle on your emotions. This can lead you to make poor choices such as giving up on someone or something.

Overthinkers become deadened with their feelings of fear and questions, in light of the fact that the main picture they have of themselves is ones in which they've fizzled, committed an error or basically come up short. These thoughts linger in the mind until the fester to the point where the individual is rendered insecure with themselves.

Overthinking is different from essential stressing. Worriers stress over things that have NOT occurred. They stress over theoretical circumstances. As such, an overthinker will play a situation over and over in their mind. They dissect every interaction looking for a way to justify its outcomes. Worriers, on the other hand, may become obsessed with something that might not have even happened. The mere thought of something occurring is enough to keep them up at night.

There is good news, though: it doesn't have to be this way

Occupy yourself. Quickly change course and find another activity which can get your mind off this situation. It can be anything! Even getting a drink of water can be enough to reset your brain. Ideally, you can do something which can make you feel happy and makes you feel satisfied. Watch something interesting; laughter is medicine, after all.

Start a gratitude journal. Record your thoughts daily or near-daily (negative or positive), your experiences, wins, and losses, and after that, record things you're appreciative of. Look at your lists. Next time you feel particularly sad or stressed, read over the things that you have determined you are thankful for.

Show your appreciation. Being appreciative is a great way of focusing on the positives in your life. Taking a few minutes each day to show your appreciation is a great way of keeping negative thoughts at bay.

Support Group. A support group is made up of individuals who feel the same way as you do and who are going through the same situation as you are. Alternatively, a support network can be your friends and family in whom you can lean on.

Don't let self-pity get out hand. You can avoid this by setting a time limit. When you have feelings of self-pity, it's alright to acknowledge them and embrace them. But you need to let them go. Otherwise, they may take over and keep you from getting on with your day.

Warmly greet challenges. If you continue trying to change negative thoughts and attempt to push them away, they will follow you like your shadow. Warmly greet your negative thoughts. Let them know, 'Come here and sit with me. I won't leave you', and you will understand how they rapidly vanish. Thoughts are terrified of you. If you get terrified of negative thoughts, then they will control you. Warmly greet challenges, as they often contain important lessons.

Become an observer to your thoughts. You can't stop an idea or predict an idea before it comes. What's more, when it comes, it likewise leaves right away. If you are an observer to the idea, it essentially drifts away and disappears. Be that as it may, if you grip onto it, at that point, it remains with you. Thoughts can come and go and do not have to become a core part of your being.

So, to put it simply: when you fly over the clouds, or when you go past the clouds, you see that the sky is immaculate. When you observe your thoughts as passing ideas, if you do not hold onto them and instead let them travel in and out of your mind, you will be rewarded with clarity of some kind.

Get Busy. When you begin to think negatively and you feel yourself holding onto those negative thoughts, do something. If you just sit, you will continue thinking. Moving the body can distract the brain from these negative thoughts. Your energy can be directed elsewhere.

Improve the course in your body. If your head is loaded up with such a large number of thoughts, sleeps on the floor and continue rolling and you will see the course in the body improves. At the point when dissemination improves then the mind feels much improved.

Chapter 17: Take Care of Yourself and Your Environment

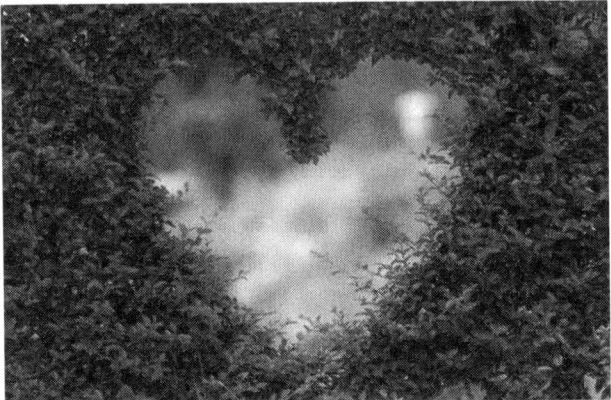

Are you mindful of the effect that you have on nature? If not, increase this type of mindfulness. If you already are, that is great; however, you can keep increasing your mindfulness in other areas of your life, as well. For those that don't have the foggiest idea, thinking about nature doesn't require you to turn into an ecological expert. Simply be eco-aware and eco-friendly!

6 Reasons to Take Care of Your Environment

1) Your incredible extraordinary and extraordinary incredible extraordinary grandkids will value it.

- Except if you have some superpower that I am uninformed of, you won't live until the end of time. All in all, what kind of world would you like to leave for your future family?
- Future ages may confront threats because of issues brought about by us. You should make sacrifices and plan something to keep it from occurring.
- Yet, there must be the look forward, there must be an acknowledgment of the way that to squander, to demolish, our normal assets, to skin and deplete the land as opposed to utilizing it in order to build its convenience, will bring about undermining in the times of our kids the very success which we should by right to hand down to them amplified and created.

2) Earth is our home.

- There are numerous ways you can demonstrate that you care about the condition of the planet we live on every day. Probably the most well-known ways are the three Rs: reduce, reuse, and recycle. Regardless of how little or insignificant your activities may appear, they matter. It just takes one individual to begin a movement that could prompt a significant ecological leap forward.

3) Biodiversity is significant.

- Biodiversity alludes to the assortment of plants, creatures, and other living things in our universe. It tends to be adversely impacted by traditional powers and human exercises.
- We have a large number of the fundamental needs that we have to endure in light of biodiversity. Nourishment, water, shelter, and air. There are regular procedures that have been shaped by different species to provides or influence these needs. If something happens to a specific life form, an undesirable chain response may happen. That may prompt lost biodiversity, which may adversely influence our needs.
- We should treat each piece of biodiversity as invaluable while we figure out how to utilize it and come to understand what it means to humankind.

4) A perfect domain is basic for solid living.

- If you couldn't care less about nature, odds are it will wind up dirtied. It'll be dirtied with contaminants and poisons, which may destructively influence your wellbeing.
- As per the US EPA, open-air contamination is related to heart and asthma assaults, bronchitis, and untimely mortality. What's more, our indoor condition is two to multiple times more harmful than our open-air condition.
- Additionally, water contamination can prompt gastrointestinal ailment, conceptive issues, and neurological issues.
- In spite of the fact that we have treatment frameworks and different systems to battle these issues, no one can really tell what issues may happen. Air continues us and water is an essential need, so we ought to do what we can to forestall contamination.
- At the point when the earth is wiped out and dirtied, human wellbeing is inconceivable. To mend ourselves we should recuperate our planet, and to recuperate our planet we should recuperate ourselves.

5) It's an impression of your character.

- One of my life mantras is, do unto others as you would have them do unto you.
- Nature gives us such a significant number of things for nothing in return. It gives us clean air, clean water, beautiful scenes, stunning perspectives, and the rundown goes on. We take such a great amount from nature, but what do we give it in return? Contamination?
- The least we can do is demonstrate our appreciation by caring for and protecting our planet and all of its nonhuman inhabitants.

- What we are doing to the forests of the world is, sadly, a mirror impression of what we are doing to ourselves and to each other.

6) The general temperature of Earth's environment is increasing.

- Truly, little changes in the normal temperature can prompt successive events of risky climate patterns and destructive storms. Indeed, a dangerous atmospheric deviation and environmental change are real.
- Prepare to have your mind blown. We are, to a great extent, responsible for them in light of the fact that our actions have caused multiple, ever-expanding holes in the ozone layer that expose our planet to increasingly warm temperatures.
- Environmental change may influence human wellness, agriculture, water assets, woods, wildlife, and shorefront regions.
- When we think about our children and our own future, we are motivated to try our best to make positive changes. This can be achieved by finding a positive way to impact the effects of climate change, for instance. So, we need to be in touch with the issues that are represented by this threat.

Chapter 18: Staying Focused on Your Goals

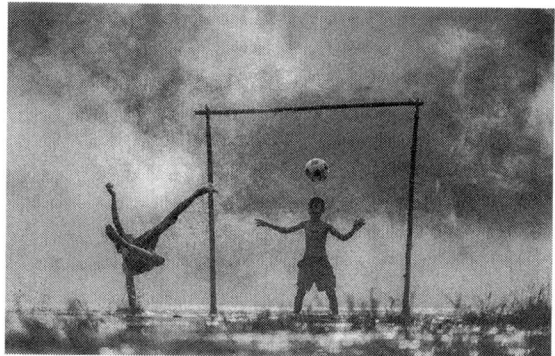

Often, we are compelled to set out to do one thing or another. Yet, we may not always be keen on following through. There is any number of reasons why we may not be able to follow through. This can be the result of negative feelings such as fear and insecurity, or even laziness and procrastination. This is why it is of the utmost importance to identify these issues and correct them.

Here are some great ways in which you can go about finding an alternative to these factors which may be keeping your eyes off your goals.

Make a Dream Board

This technique consists of making a type of collage with pictures and messages (they must be visual) that are related to the way you can achieve your ultimate objectives all the more plainly. Undoubtedly, it will motivate you to make moves towards achieving your goals. It likewise serves to help you to remember your objectives consistently as you see the board daily.

A dream board is meant to provide you with a motivating message that you will help you every time you feel overwhelmed, I look at my dream board and remind myself of why I am doing what I am doing.

Create and List Goals

If you simply set one immense objective, it very well may debilitate, particularly when you don't accomplish it after a brief time. At the point when that occurs, a few people may linger on the objective out and out which is very shocking.

I think that it is supportive to break a major objective into littler objectives. Much the same as when you set out on a long and arduous journey, you make small stops along the way to sleep/recover all through the excursion. Be sure about for what reason you're seeking after the objectives

If you keep abandoning your objectives midway, maybe you were never genuine in them in the first place. When you are genuinely committed to your goals, you will feel compelled to keep going despite you're the little setbacks along the way.

I would pay little mind to the snags until they give way and I'm getting a charge out of my rewards for so much hard work.

I once had a training customer who might set out on numerous new business adventures just to stop inside the initial 2 to 4 months. He didn't understand why. Then, I found out that the issue had been due to the fact that he had gotten bored. All things considered, he was at that point procuring great cash with his present place of employment and that gave him little motivation to move out of his customary range of familiarity. From that point onward, I asked him to put more energy into the business plan acting as if it was the first day of his new venture. Since then, he has been able to translate this philosophy of taking things one day at a time into a successful business venture.

Make Plans

The old adage, "if you fail to plan, you plan to fail" rings truer than ever. If you don't have a firm plan in place, that is a clear idea of how you plan to achieve a goal, the likelihood of actually achieving it will become much lower. So, it's vital that you find a way to make your plans as clear and direct as possible. This will give you a fighting chance.

Learning the Power of "No"

Do you find yourself putting off your goals for the sake of others? It's fine if you like to help out others whenever you can. However, if you continue doing this and do it too often, something is off balance. You can't expect to be successful by putting your own goals and ambitions in the back burner. Personally, I experienced difficulty saying "no" to others. When I realized that putting myself before others wasn't a selfish attitude, I began to realize that there is a balance between being helpful and committed to my own outcomes. So, please try to strive to find such a balance.

Tracking Your Outcomes

It's significant for me to track the outcomes of what I do on the grounds that otherwise, it feels like my activities are not having any kind of effect. Thus, every time I chip away at an objective, I will identify 1 to 2 execution measurements, and track those measurements day by day/week by week.

They illustrate the relationship I have with my ultimate goal since they let me examine whether I'm on track or off track. They let me assess whether I need to change my activities or not. You can never really have a clear picture of where you stand until you are able to clearly see the progress you have made.

One other important benefit of tracking your outcomes: seeing how far you've come will help you find the motivation you need to keep going. This can be the greatest motivation of all.

Focus on 1 to 4 Objectives

If you continually experience difficulty adhering to your objectives, you might be pushing yourself too far. Pick 1 to 4 objectives that are most important to you and stick to them. Try not to trouble yourself with some other objectives until these objectives are accomplished or if your needs shift. For me, my top need objective is to advance my business as much as I can every day. In this way, I guarantee all my daily activities are all geared toward attaining the goals I have set out to accomplish. When I shuffle crosswise over 5 to 6 objectives and gain little ground in them.

Start a Journal for Recording your Goal Interests

Journaling can be a simple and easy way for you to keep track of your progress and your thoughts. It might be a little embarrassing to go back and look at the way you have evolved. But then again, it can be a reminder of how far you have come in such a short period of time.

Conclusion

Thank you for making it through to the end of *Cognitive Behavioral Therapy for Anxiety*. This book was produced with a great deal of thought and care in mind. We hope it has been useful and informative. There is a great deal of information which you can now put into practice in your daily life.

So, what is the next step?

Please take the time to make the most of each opportunity that every new day affords you. When you are able to harness the power of every new day, you will find it easier to get up and make the most of it. After all, there is nothing that is holding you back. Aside from real and credible obstacles, which you can overcome, the biggest limitations are usually in your mind.

This is why making the most of the information, techniques, and strategies that we have discussed in this book can certainly make the most of your opportunities to become the best that you can possibly become.

Overthinking

Stop! Change Your Thoughts, Declutter Your Mind and Rewire Your Brain. Mindfulness Technique to Relieve Anxiety, Stop Worrying and Think Positively. Problem Solving Tips for a Happier life

By Albert Dales

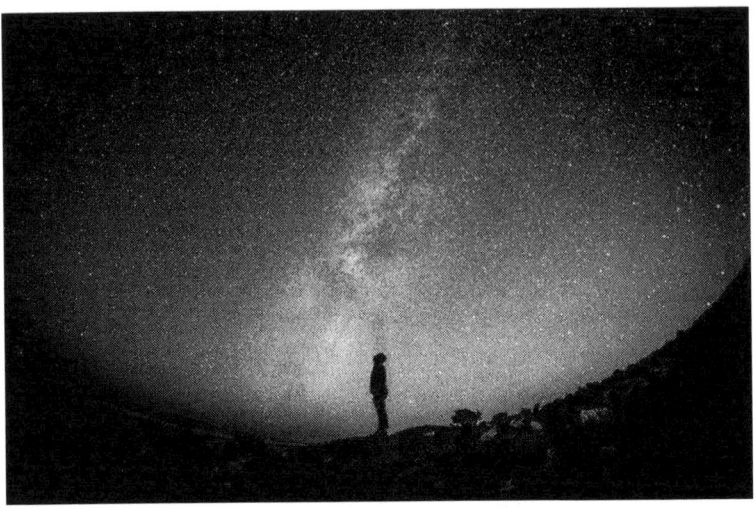

© Copyright 2019 by Albert Dales - All rights reserved.

The content contained within this book may not be reproduced, duplicated or transmitted without direct written permission from the author or the publisher.

Under no circumstances will any blame or legal responsibility be held against the publisher, or author, for any damages, reparation, or monetary loss due to the information contained within this book. Either directly or indirectly.

Legal Notice:

This book is copyright protected. This book is only for personal use. You cannot amend, distribute, sell, use, quote or paraphrase any part, or the content within this book, without the consent of the author or publisher.

Disclaimer Notice:

Please note the information contained within this document is for educational and entertainment purposes only. All effort has been executed to present accurate, up to date, and reliable, complete information. No warranties of any kind are declared or implied. Readers acknowledge that the author is not engaging in the rendering of legal, financial, medical or professional advice. The content within this book has been derived from various sources. Please consult a licensed professional before attempting any techniques outlined in this book.

By reading this document, the reader agrees that under no circumstances is the author responsible for any losses, direct or indirect, which are incurred as a result of the use of the information contained within this document, including, but not limited to, — errors, omissions, or inaccuracies.

Table of Contents

Introduction 151
Chapter 1: What Is Overthinking? 152
Chapter 2: What Are the Symptoms of Overthinking? 154
Chapter 3: Signs You Are an Overthinker 156
Chapter 4: Types of Overthinking 158
Chapter 5: Causes of Overthinking 160
Chapter 6: Relationship Between Overthinking, Anxiety, Stress and Negative Thinking.. 162
Chapter 7: Dealing with Negativity... 164
Chapter 8: Nature of Negative Thoughts 166
Chapter 9: Anxiety, Change Negative Thoughts 168
Chapter 10: Embrace Positive Thinking 170
Chapter 11: Benefits of Positive Thinking... 172
Chapter 12: How to Increase Positive Thinking 174
Chapter 13: Declutter Your Mind 176
Chapter 14: What Is Mental Clutter?... 178
Chapter 15: Causes of Mental Clutter 179
Chapter 16: Practical Tips on How to Declutter Your Mind.................180
Chapter 17: Declutter your Environment 182
Chapter 18: Space Clearing 183
Chapter 19: Minimalism 185
Chapter 20: Less is more 186
Chapter 21: How to Stop Overthinking... 187
Chapter 22: Stop Over-analyzing Things 189
Chapter 23: Stop Information Overload 191
Chapter 24: Stop Being a Perfectionist 192
Chapter 25: Stop Procrastination -- Analysis Paralysis -- Causes and Solutions 193
Chapter 26: Set Deadlines.. 195
Chapter 27: Create a To-Do list 196
Chapter 28: Evaluate Your Time Usage.. 197
Chapter 29: Limit Your Media Consumption 199
Chapter 30: Plan Your Meals Wisely.. 201
Chapter 31: Simplify your Life and Live in the Present 203
Chapter 32: Slow Down and Rewire your Brain to Be Yourself...........204
Chapter 33: Create Good Habits 205
Chapter 34: Do What you Love 208
Chapter 35: Embrace Positive Influences with Positive Thinking 209
Chapter 36: Remove Negative Influences Cut Off Destroying Thoughts 210
Chapter 37: Getting Rid of Toxic People..211
Chapter 38: How to Stop Overthinking with Mindfulness Meditation . 215
Chapter 39: What Is Mindfulness Meditation? 216
Chapter 40: How to Meditate Your Worries Away 220
Chapter 41: Mindfulness in Everyday Life.. 223
Chapter 42: A Simple Mindfulness Meditation Practice to Relieve Stress and Anxiety.. 227
Chapter 43: Mindfulness Exercises for A Good Sleep 229
Chapter 44: Active Problem Solving, Think Smarter 232
Chapter 45: Critical Thinking to Improve Problem-Solving and Decision-Making Tips 236
Chapter 46: Focus on the Problem You Are Solving.............................238
Chapter 47: Find Simple Solutions 239
Chapter 48: Make Fact-based decisions...240
Chapter 49: Stop Overthinking for an Easier and Happier Life 242
Conclusion 243

Introduction

Congratulations on purchasing *Overthinking: Stop! Change Your Thoughts, Declutter Your Mind and Rewire Your Brain. Mindfulness Technique to Relieve Anxiety, Stop Worrying and Think Positively. Problem Solving Tips for a Happier life* and thank you for doing so.

The following chapters will discuss the best ways you can get around the problems associated with overthinking and procrastinating in order to manage your time and energies a bit more wisely.

Overthinking is one of those things in life which may be causing you unpleasantness every time it creeps into your mind. In fact, it might even be limiting your abilities to make the most of your time and effort. Needless to say, overthinking is one of those things which may be holding you back.

Most people spend a lot of their time overthinking and failing to realize that they can utilize their time in a more effective way. There are many reasons for overthinking, but what people do not realize is that it is as dangerous as any fatal disease.

That is why this book has been written with every intent to help you focus on the important things in life; the things which you truly treasure such as spending time with your loved ones and dedicating time to your favorite activities.

Great care has been taken to produce a book which has been useful and informative. Please take the time to focus on each of the chapters as they are filled with nuggets that will surely give you insights you can apply to your everyday life.

There are plenty of books on this subject on the market, thanks again for choosing this one! Every effort was made to ensure it is full of as much useful information as possible, please enjoy!

Chapter 1: What Is Overthinking?

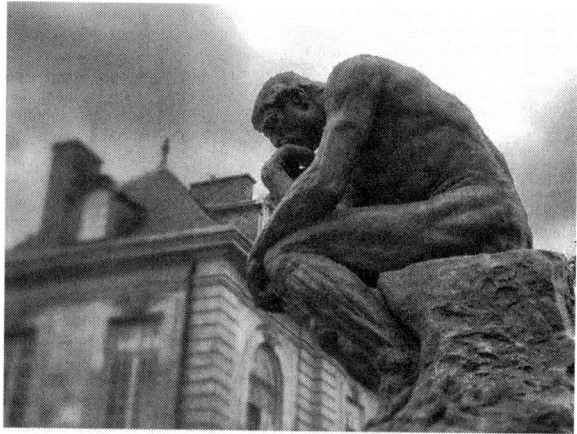

Overthinking is one of the most common reactions that we tend to have as individuals. Often, we mull over things that have happened, or we believe are going to happen. Of course, it is a valuable skill to have, to reflect and think about the things that have occurred in our lives.

However, it is one thing to reflect with the purpose of learning and growing from the past, and it is another completely different thing to constantly go over and over painful situations that we can't do much about.

Then, there is the dreaded future. When you overthink the future, you are often invaded by thoughts of what could be, or what might not be. You might find yourself constantly concerned about events that, upon rational examination, are unlikely to happen. Yet, your mind is overly active, worried about grave consequences.

In the present, overthinking might take the form of waiting too long to make a decision. You might find yourself being hesitant about what to do, or what to say. Then, before you know it, your opportunity has passed, and you are left with nothing but regret about having missed an opportunity due to your inability to act.

For example, you have been offered the job of your dreams, but it requires you to move to a new city. Naturally, you are inclined to do your homework and conduct research on the new city and company. However, you become paralyzed by thoughts about not having enough information on the new job. You are overly concerned about making the wrong move. Then, you think about past situations in which you may a wrong choice. Soon, you are so hesitant to act that you simply cannot work yourself up to saying "yes" or "no". In the end, your inability to act has led the company to pass on you and give the job to someone else.

As a result, thinking things too much, dwelling on the past for too long, or concerning yourself with the future in excess may lead you to miss the wonderful opportunities that life has for you TODAY.

Chapter 2: What Are the Symptoms of Overthinking?

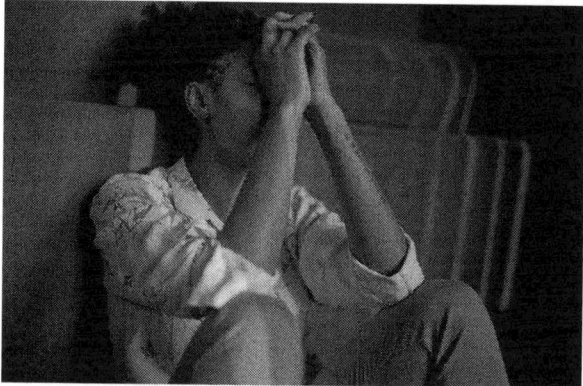

From time to time, we all become consumed by a problem or situation which we can't stop thinking about. When that happens, there is no choice but to try and manage our feelings as best we can.

Here are some clear signs that demonstrate you may be going through an overthinking episode:

1. A basic quality of overthinkers is that they see the world in high contrast. This means that everything that happens is a tragedy. They are always thinking about the worst-case scenario even when it isn't even close to being that bad.
2. They crave for affection, yet they don't always get it. Often, overthinking is just a ploy to get attention. While this isn't always the case, it might be worth asking yourself if it is just the comfort that you seek.
3. They pay attention to others' assessments as well. Considering the opinions of others is crucial in understanding your feelings and what you can do about those issues which worry you.
4. Overthinking is often characterized by a pessimistic attitude. While it's perfectly normal to worry about things now and then, pathological overthinkers tend to be glass-half-empty folks.
5. These individuals may turn into a burden to their closest friends and family. This is especially true if overthinkers are unable to function properly in their usual, day to day activities.
6. An overthinker attempts to locate importance in all things. Indeed, everything is urgent, everything is a life and death struggle, and everything is headed toward a tragic end.

7. You are overthinking if something is at the forefront of your thoughts and you persistently go over it. If you find yourself that you can't let something go, chances are you are simply overthinking things.

8. Experience the ill effects of sleep deprivation. It is common for overthinkers to lose sleep on a regular basis. While it's normal when you have something important to worry about, the chronic overthinker will experience sleep deprivation issues as a result of their pathological worrying.

9. Overthinkers recollect each and every word and detail from a discussion. If you find yourself keeping a play by play account of your conversations, then there is a very good chance you fall under the category of overthinkers.

10. Overthinkers have trouble relating to others. These folks will find it hard to build lasting relationships especially if they are bent in seeing the worst of every situation.

So, if you happen to find yourself overly concerned about things, worrying excessively, or simply losing sleep on a consistent basis, perhaps it's time to look inward and find out what is really at the root of your overthinking tendencies.

Chapter 3: Signs You Are an Overthinker

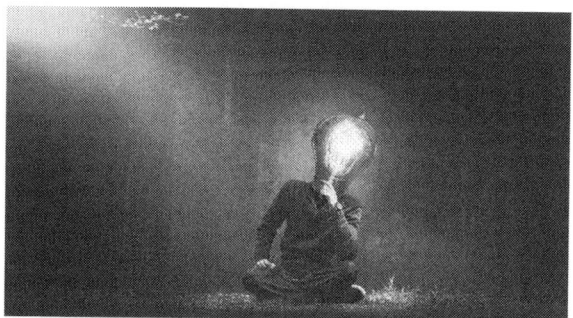

1. **Chronic fatigue.** The brain is at its maximum capacity when overthinking takes hold of your attention. Since the brain is a power-hungry organ system, it consumes a great deal of your usual energy. Hence, you may find yourself constantly tired bordering on exhaustion. This is why you often need more sleep than most folks.

2. **Overanalyzing everything.** The chronic overthinkers make something out of everything. Even when someone makes a very innocent comment, the overthinker will find something and blow it out of proportion. Often, it is just a ploy to get the attention they crave.

3. **Dread of disappointment.** The knit-picking tendencies of the overthinker lead them to constant disappointment. Since it is virtually impossible for them to take anything at face value, they will try to find the catch in everything. This leads to constant disappointment.

4. **Failure to be in the now.** The overthinker is generally concerned about the past and focused on the future. This leads them to forget about living in the present, that is, enjoying life's most precious moments, and the people around them.

5. **Continually re-thinking themselves.** In other words, the overthinker is constantly second-guessing themselves, making unreasonable criticisms about themselves and the things they have done or failed to.

6. **Constant headaches.** Given the fact that the brain is at full blast, the overthinker is generally prone to headaches. It is only when these folks are able to calm down that they find peace and solace in the world around them.

7. **Chronic sleeping disorders.** Since overthinkers are prone to insomnia, they tend to be sleep deprived until their bodies shut down. At that point, they may oversleep as the body attempts to recoup precious rest.

8. **Stiff muscles and joints**. A chronic overthinker is in a constant state of stress. This may lead to maintain a consistent state of stiffness in joints and muscles. Hence, aches and pains throughout the body are very common.

9. **Living in dread**. There is the overwhelming sensation of impending doom no matter how cut and dry things may be. After all, there is always the possibility that something could go wrong regardless of how far-fetched it may be.

If you can relate to these characteristics, then it would be a great idea to find a person in whom you can trust, who can listen to you, so that you can ventilate at least some of your feelings as often as you can.

Chapter 4: Types of Overthinking

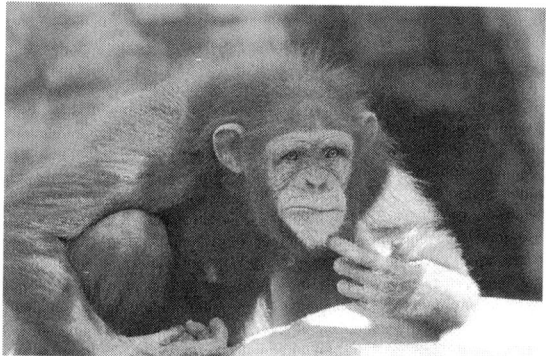

Overthinking is a point of view that is excessively mind boggling bringing about sat around idly, chance because of inaction and low-quality choices.

Thinking about an excessive number of variables in a choice without separating and gauging significance.

Blaming the basic leadership process so as to abstain from something you would prefer not to do.

Disregarding something you definitely know.

Sitting around idly and assets pondering a choice that shouldn't be made at this point.

Seeing issues where they don't exist.
Slowing down on a choice because of missing data.

You wind up making each circumstance in your life about 100x more difficult than it must be.

You can't release anything since you're persuaded that if you simply keep running over the subtleties a couple of more occasions, you'll at long last reveal some new comprehension of the circumstance or it will some way or another change the result.

You've most likely never been secure with a thing in your life. You've drawn nearer everything from picking a school and an accomplice to your outfit toward the beginning of the day and brand of bread at the market with equivalent degrees of tension.

You're always saying thanks to the companions who stick around to hear you think about similar subtleties of a circumstance or relationship over and over, and however you never truly land at a different end, only the demonstration of overthinking is sufficient for you.

Rest is the most difficult part of your life since laying quietly in obscurity is the main time you aren't diverted enough to not have the option to sink into dashing considerations.

If somebody ever parts ways with you/decays to go out with you, you persuade yourself this is a direct result of a hundred irrelevant stumbles you made.

You wind up tormenting yourself over each other worn-out side remark somebody makes in light of the fact that clearly there is some significance to be revealed, it's unmistakably simply an issue of considering it until you discover it.

Chapter 5: Causes of Overthinking

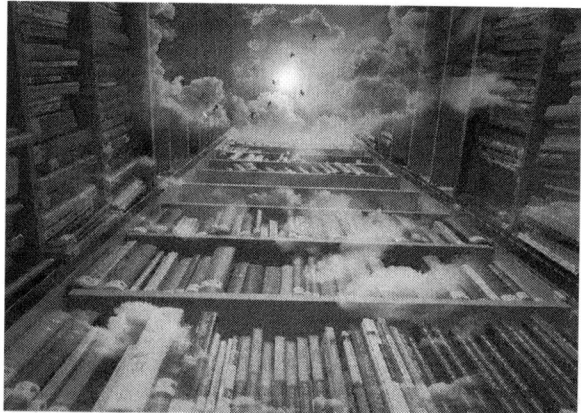

Overthinking is a purely psychological response to stress. That is basically it. When a person is stressed out in a situation, they tend to think about, ponder, and analyze it.

Now, a healthy approach would be to find a solution for it, deal with it and move on. However, the human psyche isn't quite as cut and dry. That means that depending on a person's innate traits, they will dwell on issues longer than others.

As such, a person who is far more analytical will find the need to deconstruct events in their mind so that they are able to understand what happened and why it happened. In this regard, the need to find the root cause of the issues which occur in life lead the individual to become engrossed with certain event. Over time, this constant attention to certain events leads to a full-blown obsession.

Here are three of the most common underlying causes of overthinking:

1. Generally speaking, overthinking stems from feelings of insecurity. For instance, if an individual has abandonment issues, they may tend to feel as though everyone is bound to leave them at some point. By the same token, someone who has been profoundly hurt in the past may become so wary of others that they feel the need to distance themselves from others in order to keep themselves safe. As a result, they are always looking over their shoulder, trying to figure out who is lurking by.

2. Other times, a chronic overthinker is simply seeking attention from those closest to them. This is due to the fact that they feel neglected or disregarded. Hence, the overthinker may begin to fabricate ways in which they can take advantage of a situation solely for their personal benefit.

3. Then, there is the very real possibility that a person is simply faced with a situation which they don't know how to deal with. Thus, this leads them to ruminate over an issue which they can't let go due to their lack of understanding. When this happens, it is of the utmost importance to seek help before a small issue gets out of hand.

While there may be countless reasons why a person will become obsessed with events in their lives, it is important to have a support network that can provide emotional support whenever the individual is confronted with a situation that causes them a high degree of stress and anxiety.

Chapter 6: Relationship Between Overthinking, Anxiety, Stress and Negative Thinking

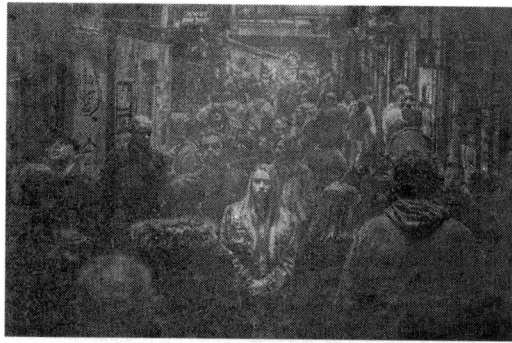

As we have discussed earlier, overthinking a specific issue that has got all of your attention is actually quite natural. For example, you are planning to move to a new home. In this case, it is perfectly natural to be overly concerned about such an important event. However, a healthy individual will let go of the issue once it has been completed.

The overthinker may choose to knit pick the event of moving to the point where they go over minutiae in order to seek problem areas to dwell. This is why overthinking has a clear correlation with stress, anxiety, and pessimism. In fact, overthinking tends to create a negative feedback loop; a negative issue leads to stress which leads to anxiety which leads to overthinking which leads to more stress which then leads to more anxiety which leads to more overthinking.

Do you see where this is going?

As such, we are going to pinpoint some of the specific attitudes which tend to fuel that negative feedback loop:

1. **Overgeneralizing**: This is taking one model and saying it's valid for everything. Search for words, for example, "never" and "consistently." Example: "I'll never feel typical. I stress over everything constantly." Reality: You may stress over numerous things. However, everything? Is it conceivable you are misrepresenting? In spite of the fact that you may stress over numerous things, you additionally may find that you feel solid and quiet about different things.

2. **Cataclysmic reasoning**: This is accepting that the most noticeably awful will occur. This sort of silly reasoning frequently incorporates "imagine a scenario where" questions. Model: "I've been having migraines of late. I'm so stressed. Consider the possibility that it's a cerebrum tumor?" Reality: If you have bunches of migraines, you should see a specialist. In any case, the chances are

that it's something increasingly normal and far less genuine. You may need glasses. You could have a sinus disease. Perhaps you're getting pressure cerebral pains from pressure.

3. **Concentrating on the negative**: This is once in a while called separating. You channel out the great and spotlight just on the terrible. Model: "I get so apprehensive talking out in the open. I simply realize that individuals are considering how awful I am at speaking." Reality: Probably nobody is more centered around your presentation than you. It might search for some proof that beneficial things occurred after one of your introductions. Did individuals hail a while later? Did anybody disclose to you that you worked admirably?

4. **Win big or bust reasoning**: This is additionally called dark or-white reasoning. Model: "If I don't find an ideal line of work survey, at that point I'll lose my employment." Reality: Most execution audits incorporate some helpful analysis—something you can chip away at to improve. If you get five positive remarks and one useful recommendation, that is a decent survey. It doesn't imply that you're at risk of losing your employment.

5. **What "should" be**: People now and again have set thoughts regarding how they "should" act. If you hear yourself saying that you or other individuals "should," "should," or "need to" accomplish something, at that point you may set yourself up to feel awful. Model: "I must be in charge constantly or I can't adapt to things." Reality: There's nothing amiss with needing to have some authority over the things that you can control. Yet, you may cause yourself nervousness by agonizing over things that you can't control.

Chapter 7: Dealing with Negativity

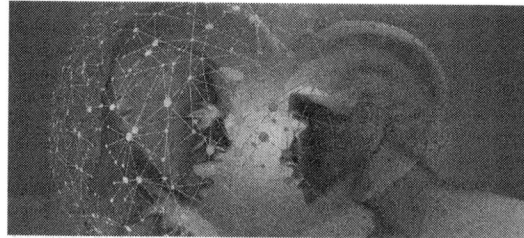

One of the most important things which any overthinker can do is accept that they are just that, overthinkers. When the overthinker sees the world for what it is, they begin a transition from focusing on the negatives of life to focusing on the brighter side of life.

The following is a list of actions that an overthinker can take in order to facilitate the transition from a pessimist outlook to a more positive one.

1. Be Peaceful and Smile

Smiling is one of the easiest and most effective ways to get you in a positive state of mind. Of course, you shouldn't do it unless it actually feels natural to do so. Nevertheless, smiling can help you trigger positive emotions inside you. This can then lead to a more optimistic outward projection. The end result may very well be that others catch your vibe making it far easier for you to get along with the circumstances around you.

2. Try not to Take it Personally

Learning not to take things personally is a great way to ensure emotional health. The fact of the matter is that the overthinker tends to take everything personally. What this means is that the overthinker will be concerned with trying to catch all the angles because everyone is out to get them. So, if your colleague doesn't respond, it's not because they hate you; it could be that they are simply upset over something else that happened to them. End of story.

3. Remain Patient to Create Space

Patience is a virtue. Overthinkers tend to be very short of it. This is especially true if there are situations beyond your control. Often, this tends to be the bane of the overthinker. For example, they have sent a job application and are sitting by the phone waiting for a reply.

Yet that reply may take a while...

Hence, impatience takes hold of the individual leading them to concoct all kinds of scenarios. These fabrications may very well drive the individual mad until the situation is finally resolved. That is why one of the most important qualities which an overthinker can work on is patience. As patience is fostered, the overthinker will be able to begin getting a firm grip on their thoughts and emotions.

Managing Your own Negativity

Learning to handle negative energy is an essential skill for all folks. So, here are some effective ways which can help you balance out your negative energies.

1. Use humor

While we don't mean taking things lightly, it is essential to try to find the humor in life whenever appropriate. Humor can often diffuse some of the tensest situations you can find yourself in.

2. Keep in mind, you are not your emotions

You are not governed by your emotions; you have full control over them. As such, don't be afraid to take the bull by the horns. You are totally in control of what you feel. Don't run away from your feelings; embrace them and try to learn from them.

3. Acknowledge that these emotions are temporary

Feelings come and go. Even if something is incredibly painful, the old adage, "time heals all wounds" is perfectly apropos. So, give yourself time to heal and let go of the negativity in your life.

Continue with Openness and Intention

Openness is more about giving yourself permission to feel what you feel. Don't run away from your feeling. That is only pushing the can down the road. When you feel ready, confront your feelings and learn from them. This will lead you to gain vital insights into your own self.

Chapter 8: Nature of Negative Thoughts

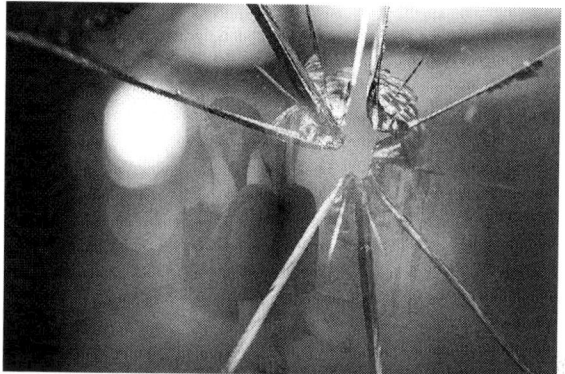

By changing your musings, you can change your emotions. While occasions are frequently outside of your control, you can figure out how to control your contemplations along these lines making increasingly positive passionate encounters.

We should take a gander at the attributes of negative programmed considerations to all the more likely comprehend their temperament.

1. Catastrophic commonly and foresees or expect a terrible result.

You consequently accept the direst outcome imaginable which makes upsetting feelings. Those disastrous considerations are frequently a significant wellspring of nervousness.

2. Its own.

You customize and appoint fault to yourself for things that aren't generally your deficiency. Adverse programmed thinking drives you to customize and acknowledge fault for things that are not so much heavily influenced by you.

3. Involve explanations like "should", "must" or "should."

Explanations that are confined with these words, especially when coordinated toward yourself, can prompt sentiments of self-fault, dissatisfaction, blame, outrage, and disappointment. These words ordinarily are unbending and don't permit space for modification for circumstances that change.

4. It's inescapable and tenacious.

One negative idea normally prompts another negative idea except if it's interfered. You can either nourish it so it keeps on flourishing or starve it by not proceeding to give the cycle what it needs to endure.

5. They generally make you feel awful about yourself.

These contemplations never leave you like yourself. You stress over not being sufficient now and never feeling adequate ever again. This makes sentiments of misery and vulnerability.

6. They are found out.

You structure ongoing examples of programmed musings that are difficult to perceive and in this way change. You can't change something you're not mindful of.

7. They will in general act naturally subverting.

At the point when a negative idea sneaks in, you start to feel frightful or stressed which affects your behavior. One of two things can occur. You don't make the move you have to take to accomplish a decent result in light of the fact that your dread has immobilized you. Or on the other hand, your activities are contrarily affected by the musings you have so the outcomes are undermined which further fortifies your negative programmed considerations. The idea of the cycle is horrendous.

8. Believable regardless of how outlandish they show up.

Programmed considerations have a convincing quality to them and you will in general structure your enthusiastic experience dependent on these contemplations.

9. They are one-sided.

You will in general markdown the positives and just feature the negatives. Because something you wanted didn't work out, doesn't imply that nothing will ever work out.

Hearing your programmed considerations is the initial phase in dealing with your most extraordinary feelings. Attempt to identify the idea you had preceding the beginning of your feelings. What were you thinking just previously and during the terrible inclination? Tune in to your inward discourse and hear what you're letting yourself know. You may think that it is supportive to begin an idea diary to record your musings. This will assist you with bettering comprehend the job your considerations play in your passionate encounters. After some time, you'll start to doubt your programmed musings and begin to address how substantial and genuine these considerations are. To diminish the recurrence of excruciating feelings, you have to tune in to what you think and ask yourself how legitimate these musings are. Keep in mind, what you think about last makes what you feel.

Chapter 9: Anxiety, Change Negative Thoughts

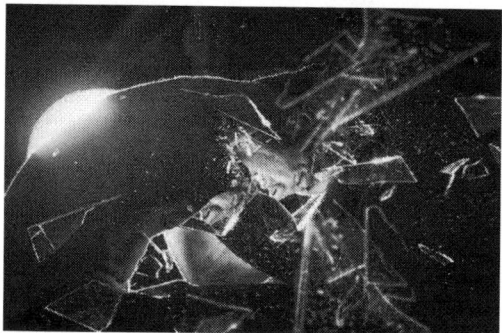

Anxiety is generally brought on by negative thoughts and vice-versa. When you dwell on the negatives, anxiety tends to shoot through the roof. Hence, the following strategies will help you get a handle on your negative thoughts thereby curbing your anxiety.

Thought Journals

Thought diaries chip away at a similar reason. They offer you the chance to get outside of your musings and get a progressively target viewpoint on them. First, you identify the substance of your negative musings, and after that, you record them in your diary. This makes you mindful of your considerations, gets you outside of them and enables you to survey them and choose whether or not they are valid.

Contemplation

Contemplation implies analyzing past, and current, events in order to distill valuable lessons from them. If you simply dwell on how miserable a situation made you feel, then you will only be fueling negative feelings inside of you. So, the next time something negative happens, don't be afraid to sit down and deconstruct why it happened. Then, take the most valuable lessons and put them to good use.

Intellectual Behavioral Therapy and Cognitive Restructuring

Psychological rebuilding is a procedure where you identify your negative idea examples and afterward question them. As such, subjective rebuilding is a procedure where you research your negative musings and build up that they are not valid.

There are five phases to intellectual rebuilding:

    1. **Question** - This is exactly what it seems like. Evaluate your negative considerations if you think they are not valid. Challenge them. If you will, in general, think you are a disappointment, review to mind times when you

were not a disappointment. If you will, in general, imagine that you are constantly a disappointment in social circumstances, review to mind events in which you and someone else felt near each other. By and by, this is tied in with figuring out how to quit accepting your negative musings.

2. **Identify and Record** - The main activity is to identify your negative musings and record them in a diary. Also, record the circumstance where you had every episode of negative contemplations and how the musings made you feel. This will begin the way toward isolating yourself from your negative considerations.

3. **Practical Goals** - Negative considerations are frequently the handmaiden of having ridiculous pictures of and objectives for yourself. It is possible that you should be extraordinary in all that you do. Or then again you may request that yourself be somebody you aren't. This sort of mental self-view is an arrangement for negative contemplations. You will regularly be a disappointment in your own eyes, and this will offer ascent to negative musings. Create sensible objectives for your work life and your public activity. This will diminish your negative mental self-portraits and negative musings.

4. **Positive Thoughts** - When negative considerations come up, supplant them with positive contemplations. "I enjoyed myself at that last gathering I went to". "Last week's gathering, everyone thought my marketable strategy was brilliant, and we utilized the arrangement with a couple of slight modifications."

5. **Examine** - Analyze the considerations in your idea diary. Search for examples in the subjects of your musings. Do your contemplations make negative pictures of yourself? What are the negative pictures they make? Try to perceive what sorts of circumstances trigger your negative considerations. The vast majority of all, investigate the musings to check whether they are truly valid.

Chapter 10: Embrace Positive Thinking

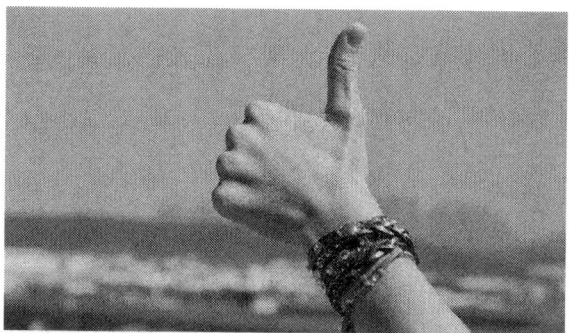

What makes somebody think emphatically? Maybe a couple of us are that upbeat vagabond, whistling and kicking through harvest time leaves cool as a cucumber in light of the fact that our lives are regularly punctuated with extraordinary trouble and despondency. Be that as it may, how would we get back up again in the wake of having the breeze thumped out of us? Positive reasoning is something that really takes work. The best individuals are the ones that can likewise recognize the truth about life; a beautiful brilliant gift, not without affliction.

The indiscriminately hopeful individual doesn't see this and when they experience an issue, which they unavoidably will, it floors them. They didn't see it coming, how right? For they are indiscriminately idealistic!

You need a touch of cynicism to enable you to explore the world. Else, we wouldn't see the threat that is surrounding us, and we wouldn't have the option to investigate a scene in any incredible profundity if we constantly held a kind of Disney perspective on the world. What's more, we as a whole realize that is not how the world is. Yet, when things are going admirably, we should figure out how to outfit that and appreciate those minutes, since like the terrible minutes the great ones are brief as well. So, building up the capacity to see them when they are available is significant for your prosperity and emotional well-being.

You absolutely would prefer not to be the interminable doubter, that individual can never observe any great in anything and they are continually trusting that something wrecking will occur so it can reaffirm their perspective that life is 'a story told by a bonehead, brimming with sound and wrath, signifying nothing'.

Also, they are not extremely charming to be near, indeed, an innately contrary individual is debilitating to be with. Furthermore, it must debilitate to be in their headspace. Never open to the likelihood that decency and bliss are surrounding us. Be that as it may, you must be available to see it; your eyes can't perceive what the psyche doesn't accept.

Opening yourself up to positive considerations really expands the odds of positive alluring results happening in your life and consequently change how you see the world.

Can any anyone explain why a constructive individual pulls in other folks? For what reason would we like to be in their organization? What is it they have that is irresistible? What's more, how can it be that about every single fruitful individual has a positive perspective on the world and have a principal faith in themselves? What's more, by what means can we as a whole build up an uplifting mentality?

Think about the accompanying tips:

1. How would you like to think? What is impeding those musings discovering unmistakable quality in your life? It is regularly as basic as saying; 'I will be certain today. I will be available to the plausibility of something extraordinary occurring for me.' Negative musings can nearly end up like a companion to us, we can be hesitant to release them since they are so recognizable. Regularly we get trapped in a negative example of musings. It tends to be difficult to see an exit from deduction skeptically.

    In any case, when we take a gander at how we think and why we figure a specific way we can begin to improve our point of view with the goal that it permits us the capacity to see the miracle of our lives and how to grasp the great occasions.

2. Think about how you think. Tune in to your considerations, ask yourself a significant inquiry, is the manner in which I'm thinking valuable or liable to realize a positive result or not.

3. Remember contemplations originate from you; you are responsible for them. It can regularly feel like we are a detainee to the huge number of arbitrary contemplations coursing through our brains. Be that as it may, we choose which ones are significant and important for us. Become better at altering your contemplations; focus on the ones that will improve your life, not those ones that keep you down.

Chapter 11: Benefits of Positive Thinking

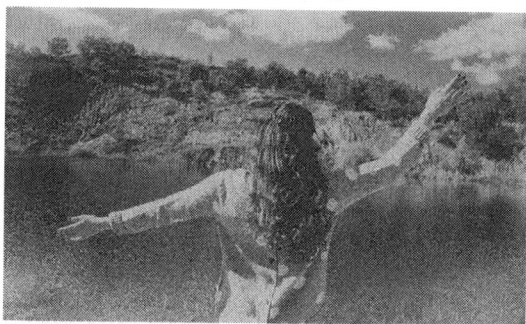

Why have an uplifting standpoint in life, since you can? Since there's a great deal in it for you. That is the reason. Keep in mind, positive reasoning is believing that is naturally advantageous. This is the thing that makes it 'positive' in any case.

You've just observed the 10,000-foot view perspective on the three essential advantages: positive reasoning causes you accomplish something you need, encourages you feel better (or if nothing else better), and it's helpful and quickly improves your life somehow or another.

Be that as it may, you can burrow down further to identify progressively specific advantages that are likewise worth increasing in value. In view of this, here are a few advantages of reasoning all the more emphatically:

More achievement: having more vitality, progressively confidence, and increasingly self-assurance prompts more achievement

Better rest and wellbeing: increasingly quiet, positive feelings imply less unpleasant, negative feelings that can negatively affect your body; the outcome is you appreciate the medical advantages of positive reasoning, including better nature of rest

A progressively beneficial life: the more you increase the value of your life with positive reasoning, the more advantageous life is for you

More noteworthy certainty: the more you trust you can accomplish things (a typical type of positive reasoning), the more self-assurance you have

More satisfaction and happiness: the more positive worth that you find in life, the more joyful you become, and the more you appreciate life

Feeling more grounded: as your certainty and confidence increments because of positive reasoning, you likewise feel more grounded and all the more dominant

More vitality: positive reasoning frequently persuades and stimulates you to accomplish things

More genuine feelings of serenity: the better you feel by and large with positive reasoning, the more significant serenity you have

Higher confidence: the more worth you find in yourself with positive reasoning, the higher your feeling of self-esteem

Increasingly agreeable cooperation with others: the more you appreciate life and worth yourself, the more you will in general appreciate social connections

More noteworthy clearness of brain: since you have a decision, it bodes well to think in legitimate, adequate positive ways that advantage you as opposed to in negative manners that hurt you; this is an advantage of positive reasoning great worth considering

Does thinking positive have any kind of effect?

Completely. You simply figured out how you can profit by positive intuition from numerous points of view, so sure reasoning truly works for improving your life.

The most significant inquiry, at the present time, is this: would you like to think positive contemplations and turned into an increasingly positive scholar?

This is on the grounds that the most significant factor for turning into an increasingly positive mastermind is to just need to think all the more emphatically, and to be definitive about making a move to think progressively positive considerations, paying little mind to whether any other individual needs you to think all the more decidedly or not.

With this lucidity of the brain, you are as of now well on your approach to growing increasingly positive perspectives about things.

Along these lines, if you have just realized what positive reasoning is, your following stage is to study how to think all the more emphatically and how to remain positive regardless of the conditions.

Chapter 12: How to Increase Positive Thinking

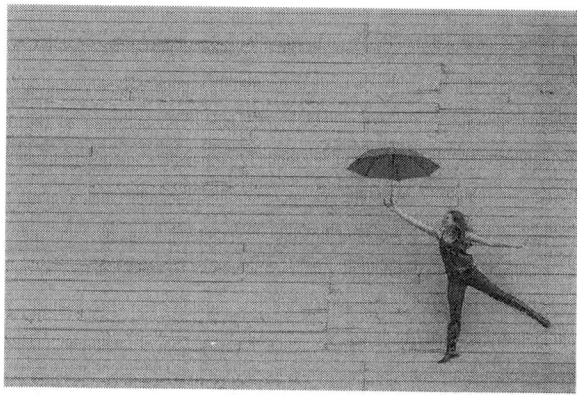

1. Start littler than you might suspect – The "floss just 1 tooth" – approach

Make your propensity so little that you can't state no. If you do this, to begin with, you can concentrate more on structure a propensity, as opposed to on results or how huge your propensity is.

Another regular propensity that too few individuals really do is flossing day by day. So, my recommendation is simply to floss one tooth the principal night.

Obviously, that appears to be so ludicrous a great many people giggle. Be that as it may, I'm absolutely genuine: if you begin exceedingly little, you won't state no. You'll feel insane if you don't do it. Thus, you'll really do it! That is the point. As a matter of fact, doing the propensity is substantially more significant than the amount you do.

At this moment I'm simply observing one extraordinary minute I saw, toward the finish of every day. Once in a while it just takes a couple of words to share this, occasionally it's two sentences. I've fused it into my day by day routine with regards to sharing what I completed the Buffer group, so it's anything but difficult to recall and simple to do.

Beginning little has helped me to join the training into consistently so it's turning into a propensity, without stressing over what a major assignment it is.

2. Set up your condition

Leo Babauta consistently has extraordinary exhortation on structure propensities, and this is one of my top picks. Naturally, we attempt to assemble new propensities (or even break old ones), with huge effects on our current conditions. Condition for this situation incorporates the individuals we invest energy with and the messages we hear or let ourselves know, just as our physical condition.

The stunt here is to guarantee your condition is as helpful for you proceeding with your new propensity as could be expected under the circumstances.

3. Attempt to Meditate – 3 minutes is sufficient

Ruminating is valuable for the body and brain. It does not just improve care and positive reasoning while you're doing it, however, it has been appeared to diminish sickness and improve care and sentiments of direction in life as long as a quarter of a year subsequent to being rehearsed every day for a brief period.

Beginning little works for contemplating, too. Think about only 3 minutes, to begin with, which is anything but difficult to do and supportive in building up a solid propensity. Subsequent to setting up the propensity for half a month, you can gradually build the length of your contemplation sessions to a sum that gives you the most advantage.

4. Observe 1 positive minute consistently

Seeing the positive things that occur in your regular day to day existence has been demonstrated to be an effective strategy for expanding your positive reasoning. This doesn't simply happen when you're doing the activity: the impacts can, in reality, last any longer.

One movement that is frequently said to improve energy is to record (or offer with somebody) three things you're thankful for toward the finish of every day.

Chapter 13: Declutter Your Mind

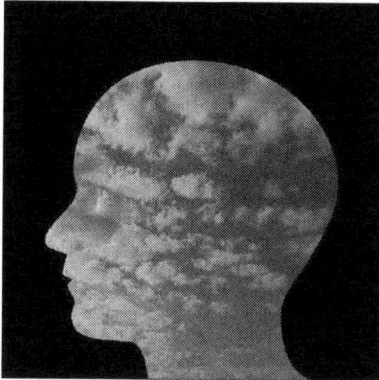

Thinking about how to declutter your brain? Having a bustling personality can make you feel pushed, restless and overpowered. Fortunately, we've assembled a rundown of approaches to declutter your brain.

1. Put pen to paper

At the point when you're attempting to keep mental tabs on everything that is going on, your contemplations are probably going to get confused. Keeping in touch with them down will assist you with prioritizing what's most significant, which will make you feel less focused. You can check significant dates and updates on a schedule or in a scratch pad, and scribble down your musings on anything that is stressing you in an individual journal. It doesn't make a difference whether you utilize an application or simply get a pen and paper. In a stretch, even the back of your hand will do (however it's not our first decision).

2. Keep at it

Work a portion of the tips recorded above into your regular day to day existence to enable you to offload mental mess. Ensure you get a touch of 'personal time' each day with the goal that you can slow down appropriately. Much the same as tidying up your room keeps it from transforming into an all-out dump, reflecting, composing, ruminating and conversing with others consistently will help anticipate the development of messiness in your brain.

3. Be careful

We've all heard that reflection is a decent method to clear your brain and unwind. What you might not have heard is that there are a huge number of approaches to be careful. This implies you can search for a way that suits you. Some regular things to attempt are yoga, exercise and profound relaxing. Some not really normal approaches to rehearse care are washing up, snuggling up or chilling by the seashore. Do whatever works for you.

4. Identify the issue

It's difficult to fix something if you don't know what's up. Know about admonition signs that your psyche is getting to be stuffed. Some normal things to watch out for are issue resting, poor fixation and not able to unwind.

When you've perceived that your psyche needs a spring clean, the following stage is to discover what's adding to the messiness. Invest significant time to think about how you're feeling. This will assist you with identifying what's worrying you, and why. After some time, you'll improve at detecting the notice indications of a jumbled personality and have the option to halt things from the beginning pleasant and early.

5. Converse with somebody

Conversing with a confided in companion or relative, regardless of whether on the web or eye to eye, can be an extraordinary method to clear your psyche, discharge a few feelings and get whatever's irritating you out into the open. It additionally gets a new take on an issue that is got you puzzled and is worrying you. If you're truly battling, recollect that you don't need to handle your issues without anyone else. There are loads of different experts accessible to chat with about whatever's stressing you.

Chapter 14: What Is Mental Clutter?

Mental clutter is the stuff that occupies room in our mind, yet keeps on living without rent as we feed, dress, and generally deal with life. The stuff sends us on aimlessly throughout life, and in the long run, leads us down a street that goes no place quick. If we let it, mental clutter will move in and take lasting habitation in our psyche. With a little work, we can figure out how to rinse our psyche and push ahead.

Generally speaking, the mind's optimal state is one in which it is able to focus on the task at hand. For instance, if you are reading a book, then you are able to read that book without your mind making it impossible for you to concentrate on the book.

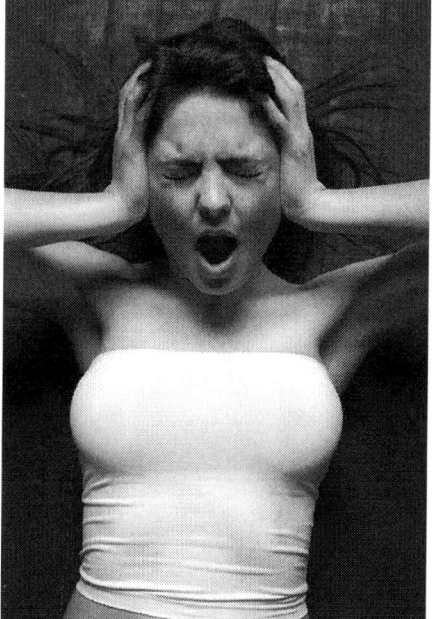

This is the crucial point in which you can determine if your mind is actually cluttered: you cannot focus, much less concentrate, on anything. What this means is that when you attempt to do something, your mind is always taking you back to that which is occupying the most of your mental real estate. In fact, mental clutter can get to be so bad, that it can limit your ability to carry on with a normal life. While this may seem extreme, the fact of the matter is that it can certainly get to be that complicated.

Dealing with mental clutter is like dealing with a cluttered garaged. At some point, you are going to have to throw some stuff out and keep the stuff that is actually useful. In other words, there will come a time when there are things that you need to let go of. In other words, there are things which you are going to have to let go in order to free up precious real estate for the things that actually matter. As you become more adept at this, you will begin to recognize which things you need to hold on to, and which things you need to deep-six.

Chapter 15: Causes of Mental Clutter

In order to help you sort out the clutter, it is important to recognize which things are worth keeping and which are not. In short, anything that causes you anguish, pain, stress or plain unpleasantness needs to get the heave-ho. Those things which fill you with happiness, joy, and satisfaction need to be treasured for what they are.

As such, there are 3 kinds of mental clutter that are especially harming, and which you need to drop like a hot potato:

Negative self-talk

Our convictions about ourselves, others, and the world can significantly influence what we state about ourselves, others and our conditions. These conviction frameworks start from numerous encounters we gather over our lifetime. Twisted conviction frameworks can likewise develop because of horrible encounters or interminable dismissal.

Stress

Stress is fear's first cousin. Stress is constantly situated toward what's to come. Indeed, in some capacity, we accept that through our stressing we can really keep certain occasions from occurring and control our future. I am not proposing inactivity or inaction as the fix. We do be able to settle on decisions—yet we can just settle on those decisions with the best data and direction we have at the time. Stress pushes our deduction into absolutes and keeps us from seeing unmistakably. At the point when we start thinking in highly contrasting, there is next to no space for inventiveness or critical thinking.

Blame and ruminating over past slip-ups/decisions

The blame game is bad enough when you play it with others. It is even worse when you play it with yourself. If you constantly blame yourself over everything that happens, there will come a time when it will gnaw away at you so much, there won't be much left. So, take responsibility when it is warranted and learn to accept that there are things that are simply beyond your control.

By learning to identify these prime culprits of overthinking, you will be able to stop them in their tracks as they approach your life. By getting rid of them, you will be able to give yourself a fighting chance at decluttering your mind.

Chapter 16: Practical Tips on How to Declutter Your Mind

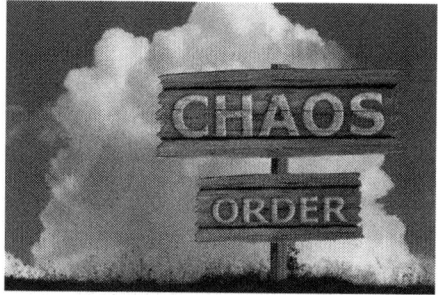

So, now that we have figured out what mental clutter is, the question begs:

How could we escape this cycle?

It begins with a cognizant decision to change. Behavior change begins with our reasoning. Dealing with your considerations is a continuous, everyday procedure.

Keep in mind you past and develop from it.

Help yourself to remember how you adapted or left a specific circumstance before. You can expect that on occasion you will slip once again into old examples. This is ordinary—those examples have been developing for a considerable length of time. Stress and blame specifically are difficult feelings. At the point when you get yourself in an old example, ask yourself, "How's my self-talk?" If you wind up drenched in tension, separate your stresses into 2 classifications: those you can control and those you can't.

Track your considerations.

Watch the words that leave your mouth (I'm certain that perusing with life partners will have a potential volunteer to help). How frequently do you end up saying words like, "can't," "generally," "must," or "never?" These are absolutes that keep us stuck.

Guide yourself to Stop!

Whenever stress rings a bell, or you verbalize it for all to hear, guide yourself to Stop! Supplant negative considerations with positive ones. One case of a positive idea is a token of what you do have rather than what you need. This isn't just about cash yet, in addition, your aptitudes, gifts, capacities, companions, family, and supporters.

In essence, making a concerted effort to clear your mind of clutter is a tremendous first step which you can take toward getting a handle on overthinking. As you begin to sort out through the fluff, you will be able to make better sense of your life and, most importantly, about the people around you. Bear in mind that if there are people feeding that clutter, then it might be time to move away from them.

Chapter 17: Declutter your Environment

Thus far, we have focused on clutter on a psychological and emotional level. However, we are yet to talk about decluttering at a practical level. What this means is that no matter how much you strive to clear up your mind, you will always be haunted by your surroundings. As a result, you need to also declutter your environment.

Decluttering your environment means getting rid of things that no longer serve you. For example, it might mean getting rid of old newspapers and knickknacks which no longer serve a purpose. It may also mean giving away old clothes that don't fit or getting rid of painful mementos.

It also means moving away from people who are affecting you both physically and emotionally. In some of the most extreme cases, some folks need to move to a new home, city or get a new job. Indeed, your environment plays a huge role in how you feel and fueling your overthinking patterns.

A good way to go about this is to become methodical in cleaning up your personal space on a regular basis. This personal space includes your space at work and at home. If you resolve to clean up every once in a while, you will find that you are also clearing up space in your mind. By seeing the clutter gone from your physical surroundings, you will be able to gain a sense of peace and openness.

By the same token, clearing up space from people who may be cluttering your life will also give you that sense of openness and liberation. As a matter of fact, having "too many" friends can be a source of stress and anxiety due to the perceived social commitments that you must comply with. Consequently, you may be adding an unnecessary source of stress in your life.

By whittling down your list of friends, you will find that sharing with those friends whom you truly value and cherish will actually help you to heal that which ails you.

Chapter 18: Space Clearing

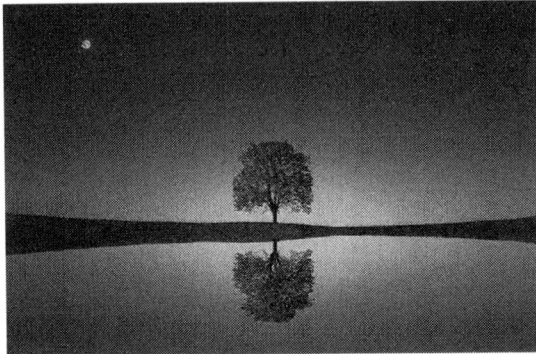

Space clearing means clearing the space on a vitality level. It is old craftsmanship drilled day by day in numerous old societies and there are various ways and materials utilized for space clearing.

The purpose of the requirement for space clearing is straightforward: similarly, as on a physical level you see the residue and earth gathering in your home because of everyday exercises, the equivalent occurs on a vitality level. You may not see the "residue and earth" of human feelings, however, they do gather in any space, so it is ideal to get them out routinely.

By and large, it is prescribed to do an exhaustive space clearing session at any rate once per year in your home, or after serious occasions with negative vitality, for example, a separation, for instance. It is likewise imperative to space clear a house that you simply moved in, particularly if it is a dispossession house.

A light type of space clearing can be utilized each time you clean your home on a physical level, just as when your clutter clearing sessions.

Locate your top pick, most pleasant method for space clearing and use it frequently. For instance, I realize that numerous individuals are hesitant to smirch their place, yet they happily utilize basic oils for a similar reason. For those hesitant to utilize the real wise smear sticks, you will be glad to realize that you would now be able to purchase a smirch stick in fluid from, in a manner of speaking. Which means, there are air splashes imbued with the vitality of sage smirch sticks, and clearly utilizing an air shower is a breeze!

Another way I totally love is to utilize the "blessed wood" from a tree that develops in South America. It has the most beautiful, purifying and uplifting aroma, feeling the vitality of Palo Santo is an unadulterated joy. Alongside savvy and lavender, presently I generally use Palo Santo sticks, as well.

By and by, I want to utilize a mix of space clearing types day by day. I do get a kick out of the chance to smear, yet rather than a major smirch stick group, I think that it is progressively charming to utilize separate little stalks of sage. Sage feels profoundly purifying and establishing to me.

After the savvy, I utilize a stalk or two of lavender similarly, and the smell is simply superb, calming and tranquil.

Simultaneously I have a little tealight light consuming and generally have my fundamental oils diffuser going, as well. This may sound muddled as you read it, however, I guarantee you it is exceptionally simple, brisk and agreeable.

Examination in different ways and find what works for you. For the day by day or week after week use, you need a simple space clearing arrangement that inevitably turns out to be right around a propensity.

Chapter 19: Minimalism

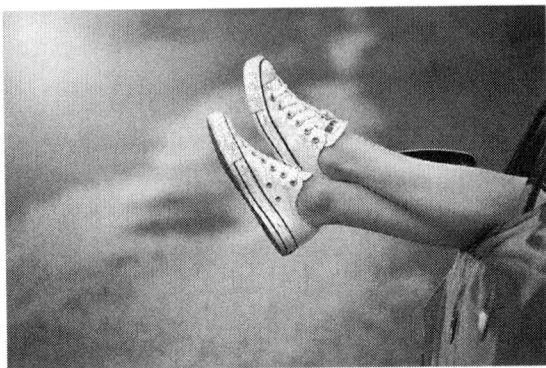

Minimalism is as much a lifestyle choice as it is a mindset. Minimalism means to go through life with things, and people, which really matter most to you; the things which you really need to live. What this means is that you need to have your priorities perfectly clear in your mind.

Furthermore, minimalism should not be confused with frugality or downsizing. For instance, it doesn't mean giving up your car simply because it's wasteful to drive a car. The fact is that if you can't afford to own a car, then, by all means, get rid of it and find the right solution for your budget. But this also means that you don't need to break the bank and buy the most expensive car on the market... even if you can afford it. If you are perfectly capable of getting by with a regular car, then that's where you need to be. While it might be tempting to go drive around in an exotic sports car, the truth is that you can do without it.

Hence, minimalism is about setting your priorities straight and spending your time, money, and efforts and those things which are conducive to achieving your goals and aims. As such, simplifying your life also removes distractions and sources that lead to overthinking.

Think about it along these lines: the less stuff that you have to think about, the less sources of worry you will have. Plain and simple. Of course, there are things which are essential in all of our lives. You need to identify what they are. By the same token, you need to identify those things which are not.

Another great way of framing minimalism is this: minimalism is the result of decluttering your life. When you get rid of all the fluff, you are left with the essentials that you need to live the lifestyle that you want... without unnecessary clutter taking up precious real estate in your mind.

Chapter 20: Less is more

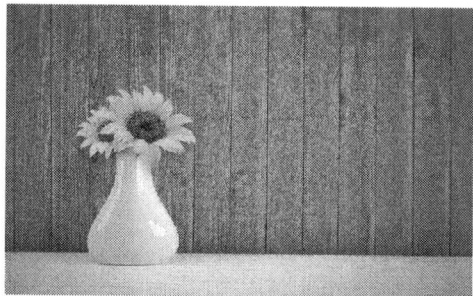

This is a tried and true adage. Indeed, "less is more", especially when you are talking about curbing the possibility of overthinking. When you declutter and adopt a minimalist lifestyle, you become more efficient.

In a traditional sense, efficiency is doing more with less. This is particularly true in manufacturing. In fact, manufacturing is built on trying to reduce the consumption of materials and eliminating any kind of waste or residue.

If we translate this into real life, you will find that you can, in fact, do so much more with less. You are able to accomplish so much when you declutter and minimalize your life.

Let's consider this example.

You dedicate a certain amount of your waking hours to the various activities which compete for your attention. However, if your attention is pulled into 25 million directions, you will find yourself lacking the ability to focus on a single issue. This will lead you to take far longer to get something done than it should actually take you.

In this case, less is more when you are able to get more done in less time.

How is that possible?

It is perfectly possible when you declutter your mental real estate and allow your mind to focus. This might mean locking yourself up in your office and forgetting about the world around you for a couple of hours. Yet, if you are able to do this, you will be able to get more done in two hours than you would have been able to do in two days.

So, don't be afraid to declutter and whittle down on all those unimportant things which are competing for your attention. Also, when you become more efficient, this opens up time and space for yourself, your family and your personal pursuits. However, this begins with your ability to declutter and make the most of your most productive times. It might mean going to bed a bit later or getting up a bit earlier, but you will be far better off for it.

Chapter 21: How to Stop Overthinking

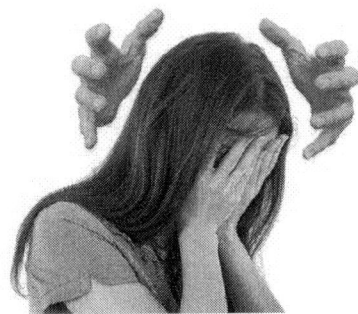

Overthinking a choice isn't just inefficient and thwarts you from gaining any ground, it can likewise cause some genuine wellbeing results, including expanded nervousness and melancholy, low quality of rest, and undesirable adapting abilities, for example, voraciously consuming food.

What's the one thing on your plate that you've been putting off settling on a choice on? Regardless of whether it's a basic choice, for example, picking which conduit cleaning organization to procure or an increasingly intricate one, for example, whether to acknowledge a new position offer, sitting on a choice can make you have an inclination that you're incapacitated. You let yourself know, "no more, simply pick one and proceed onward." But the subsequent you settle on a decision, considerations of "am I making the best decision?" begin to flood in.

Attempt these procedures to maintain a strategic distance from the negative outcomes of overthinking:

Timetable your reasoning time

One of the issues overthinkers frequently face is pondering their issues throughout the day, or at troublesome occasions, for example, during a significant gathering. To stay away from this, planning a specific time where you give yourself the opportunity to consider the issue you have to settle on a choice about. If considerations about the issue creep into your cerebrum before your booked reasoning time, letting yourself know "No, I'm going to consider that after supper, not during this gathering" can assist you with pushing those musings away, realizing you'll return to it later.

Put a cutoff time on your considerations

To evade over-ruminating about a choice, give yourself a time period to consider it. By letting yourself know, "I'm going to settle on this choice by 10 p.m. today and whatever I choose will be fine" signifies you are giving yourself consent to consider it, yet not enabling it to take over different pieces of your day.

Solicit yourself what a sensible sum from time is to think about this issue. If it's a little issue, for example, what paint shading to paint your office, maybe a cutoff time of 15 minutes is adequate; while a bigger choice, for example, regardless of whether to acknowledge a new position offer in another city may warrant two or three days of an idea.

Take a break

You know the articulation "dozing on an issue," well, that is on the grounds that occasionally we're better at taking care of an issue when we're not considering it. Once in a while, we settle on better choices when we let those thoughts permeate in our cerebrum. Giving the latent pieces of your mind a chance to work through the issue can give the appropriate response a chance to come to you when you're not anticipating it.

At the point when you get yourself overthinking about an issue, attempt to change the divert in your mind by proceeding onward to another subject or changing your physical space by taking a walk or moving your workstation to a gathering space to chip away at something different.

Know the difference between critical thinking and stressing

While for the vast majority of us, overthinking originates from a dread of the results of making a move An or B, the individuals who are constant overthinkers regularly accept that they can take care of an issue by proceeding to pound away, considering it. In any case, stressing isn't equivalent to effectively taking care of an issue. While harping on an issue, thinking "this is awful, I can't deal with this" or repeating things that occurred in the past are a useless utilization of your time, pondering what steps you can take to improve the circumstance or effectively thinking about an answer for the issue are useful toward pushing ahead. Getting to be mindful of when your reasoning is unhelpful and when it's effectively critical thinking can assist you with ensuring your time spent reasoning isn't simply adding to your pressure.

Chapter 22: Stop Over-analyzing Things

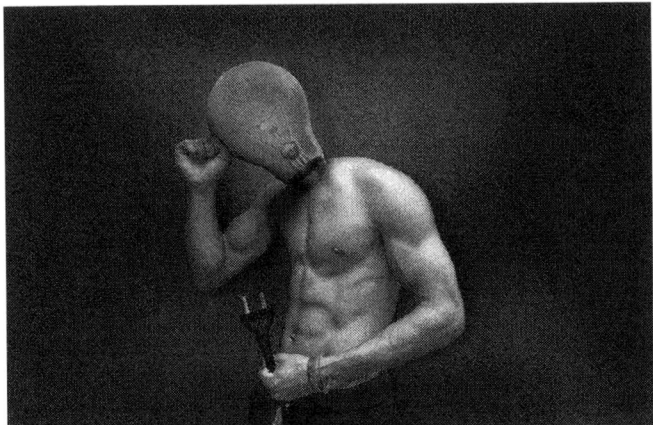

This is easier said than done.

It should be said that there is a fine line between due process and over-analyzing. So, how can you tell the difference? How can you tell the difference between doing your due diligence when something happens and when you are obsessing over it?

The answer is actually quite simple: when you find that thinking about an event begins to interfere with your usual activities, then you are overthinking. This particular event is taking over your attention. If this type of attitude renders you inoperative, you've gone too far.

Here is an example:

You had an argument with your boss. A discussion over a seemingly innocent issue got out of hand. You and your boss got upset and had a heated discussion about the situation.

Thus, you begin to fear the consequences of this situation. You begin to fabricate ideas of being fired or being seriously reprimanded. Perhaps your boss hasn't been too concerned about it, but you are now losing sleep over the prospects of what could happen.

Overthinking begins to take hold when you are unable to think clearly about anything else. If you don't take the necessary steps to remedy the situation, the thoughts occupying your attention will begin to fester inside of your psyche.

The solution might be as simple as walking into your boss's office and talking about the situation. Unless your boss is an unreasonable tyrant, they will be open to discussing the situation. It might mean having to apologize; perhaps your boss may feel compelled to apologize as well. At the end of the day, if you work things out, you can iron out any hard feelings.

As you can see, being proactive is one of the most important steps which you can take to nip overthinking in the bud. As you begin to think about things in terms of possibilities rather than problems, you will begin to discover the many ways in which you can curb overthinking and give yourself a fighting chance against overthinking.

Chapter 23: Stop Information Overload

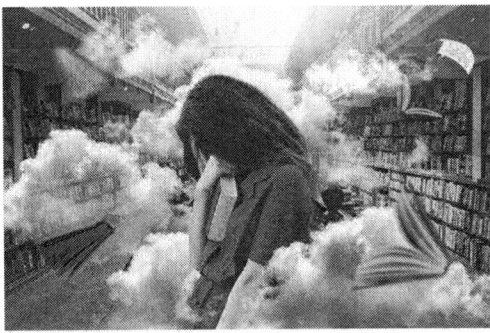

Information overload can happen in a heartbeat. One minute, you're going about your usual business. Then, all of a sudden, things happen, you get a call, emails pour in and you are overloaded with information. Stress shoot through the roof and anxiety kicks into high gear as you need to deal with multiple issues at the same time.

If this sounds familiar, then you're not alone. In fact, it is quite common to see information overload at every turn. It can be daunting to think that you have no alternative but to deal with what's coming at you.

Well, there is an alternative. Always ask yourself, "what's the most important thing I could be doing right now?"

When you train yourself to always think along these lines, you will be able to make yourself productive and stay clearheaded despite the flurry of information and occurrences around you. By being clear on the most important thing for you at any given time, you will be able to sort through the flurry around you.

When you're not clear and what your top priorities are, it is easy to get tangled up with things that are not a top priority. The fact of the matter is that most of the time, many of the things which you are on your plate are not ultra-urgent. With that in mind, avoiding information overload is far easier than you think.

So, always keep your top priorities in mind. That way, when the action gets fast and furious, you need to stay focused on the most important task at hand. By resisting the temptation to multitask, you will be able to do more with less. As you become more and more efficient, you will see your productivity soar and your self-confidence spike. Please bear in mind that you don't need to do everything right away. Most of the time, you can negotiate deadlines and get help when you need it.

Chapter 24: Stop Being a Perfectionist

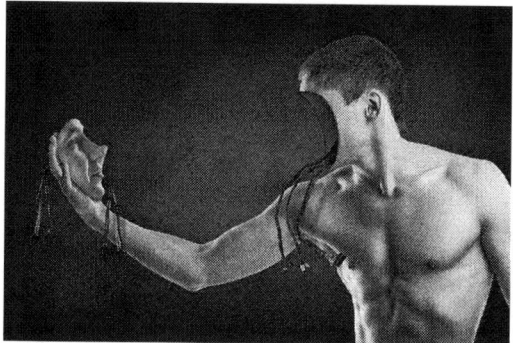

We all want to be the best. We all want to have the best. We all want to be the greatest. And while it's great to be ambitious and search for excellence, it can lead to putting undue pressure on yourself.

There is a very fine line between being a positive perfectionist and a negative one. When you are a positive perfectionist, you strive for excellence while admitting that mistakes are a part of the learning process that involved achieving greatness. On the other hand, being a negative perfectionist will lead you to become unreasonable and intolerant to mistakes.

So, what does that imply?

It implies that there needs to be a balance between tolerating mistakes and becoming a toxic individual. When you tolerate mistakes within a reasonable level, especially from yourself, you are able to grow and learn. When you reach a toxic level, you put so much pressure on yourself, and others, to be perfect, that it just eats away at you.

A great example of this can be seen in parents who place unrealistic expectations on themselves and their children. These types of parents expect perfect grades, perfect behavior and perfect appearance from their children. Over time, this can become a toxic environment for a child. It may lead them to develop self-esteem issues while leaving the parent emotionally exhausted from all the pressure they put on themselves and their families.

The dark side of perfectionists leads them to criticize everything they do and second guess themselves at everything turn. Needless to say, that is hardly an environment which is conducive to personal growth and development. In short, we need to cut ourselves a little bit of slack, acknowledge when we haven't done out best and come back the next day determined to be better. When you are able to put past failures behind you and learn from them, you will be able to truly grow as a person.

So, take the pressure off yourself; you're already doing a great job.

Chapter 25: Stop Procrastination -- Analysis Paralysis -- Causes and Solutions

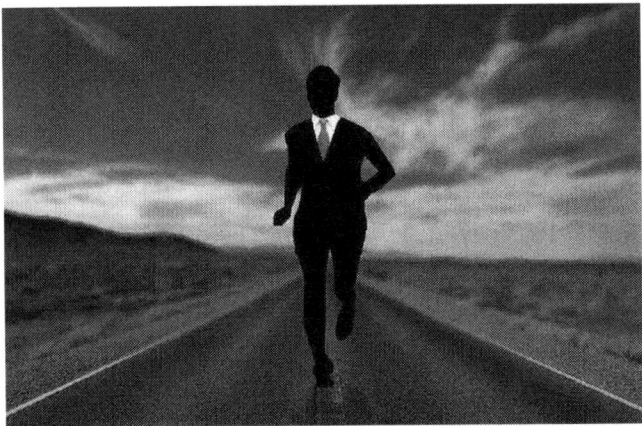

Procrastination, in short, means putting things off. What's wrong with that? Well, putting things off generally builds up pressure until one thing, or another blows up.

Think about this way: you see a crack in a wall in your home. Do you get it fixed or leave it that way? You could do nothing about it. However, it will eventually break and cause far greater damage than you had anticipated.

So, here are some great ways in which you can deal with procrastination and the paralysis that comes from over-analyzing things.

1. Try not to Believe Everything your Mind Tells You

It is perfectly true that your mind can play tricks on you. So, don't be afraid to listen to your gut every once in a while. You will find that listening to your gut feelings can validate a lot of your first impressions.

2. Change the Channel

Often, taking a timeout from the hustle and bustle of your daily routine is enough to help you regroup and gain the focus you need to solve the issues at hand. Don't be afraid to take a step back and breathe.

3. Know The Difference Between Thinking and Overthinking

When your thoughts are geared toward finding a solution, being proactive and dealing with situations, you are thinking. When your thoughts are about worry, concern, and fear, you are overthinking.

4. Try not to Make Mountains Out of Molehills

Everything that happens in life isn't the end of the world. While it is always a good idea to be prepared for the worst-case scenario, the fact of the matter is that you will rarely have to deal with the worst possible outcome. When you take a look back at life, you will realize that things could have always been worse.

5. Timetable Some 'Stress Time' Into Your Day

No, we don't mean you should make time for stress; what we mean is that it is okay to get stressed out. When that happens, take time to decompress and detox from the stressful situations in your day.

6. Become Consciously Aware

Living in the present is one of the most valuable attitudes you can take. Don't worry about the past because it's gone. Don't worry about the future because it hasn't arrived yet. Concern yourself with the present, the rest will fall into place.

7. Settle on Time-Limited Decisions

Set a timer for your decisions. If something requires your immediate attention, then do it. Then, you can determine when something needs to be done based on its priority and urgency. That will help you set effective timetables for your decisions.

8. Set the Mind Back in Its Place

At the end of your day, do take the time to unwind and relax. Sometimes, it only takes about 15 minutes to regroup, relax and get prepped for the next day. Don't neglect downtime as it is important for the recovery of your energy and focus.

Chapter 26: Set Deadlines

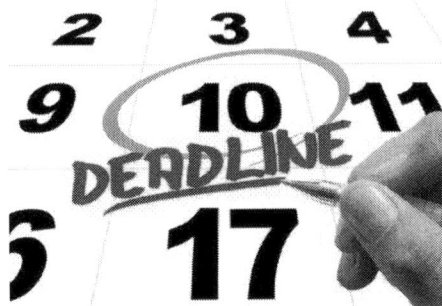

Deadlines are not meant to constrict your life. They are meant to set boundaries by which you need to work with. Imagine if we didn't have deadlines in life; nothing would ever get done.

Think about that.

If you didn't have to pay your bills on a certain day, would you ever pay them at all?

As such, deadlines help us to organize ourselves in such a way that we are able to make the most of our time in a productive manner. By setting deadlines to important decisions and actions that need to be done, you will find that it will create the structure that you need in order to keep your goals moving forward.

By the same token, healthy scheduling means that you are able to set realistic timelines for your personal goals while managing work and school in a way that you can comfortably handle the load. If you find that you simply cannot cope with everything on your plate, then it might be time to rethink your approach and let go of things that are not conducive to your overall goals and aims.

Think about it this way:

You need to make a decision regarding your car. It is getting older and may need to be replaced soon. So, you set a deadline: "I will get rid of it the next time it breaks down" or "I will get a new car at the end of the year". As you can see, these deadlines don't necessarily involve time and date. What they do involve in a marker in which you have prompted yourself to act. So, when your car does break down, you know it's time to act. This gets rid of overthinking and hesitation. You know when you need to act.

Perhaps the biggest benefit of deadlines is that you can hold yourself accountable. So, if you don't meet your deadlines, then there must be a reason for it. You can then analyze why things didn't go down the way you intended them to as opposed to beating up yourself over it. That way, the next time you set a deadline, you know it is within reason.

Chapter 27: Create a To-Do list

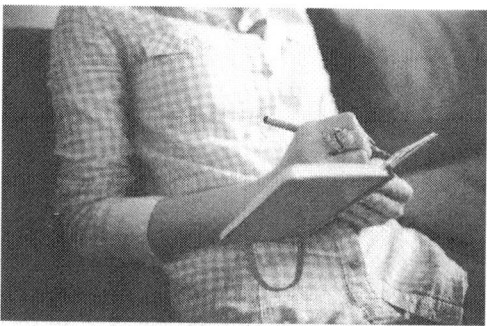

You might be thinking that To-Do lists are old-fashioned and old school. The fact of the matter is that they are relevant tools so long as you use them for what they are intended: to help you prioritize your activities.

Have you ever heard the expression, "that will go atop the To-Do list"?

The reason for that expression is due to the fact that the top of the list involves the actions which have the highest priority. If something gets shoved down to the bottom of the pile, then it means it is not as important as others.

When you go about creating a To-Do list, you are essentially ranking your activities from the highest to the lowest priority. This entails making an educated assumption as to what needs to be done, and when it needs to be done, and what can wait.

Another important value to the To-Do list is that it helps to create personal accountability. When you see that the To-Do list just keeps piling up with unfinished items, then you need to ask yourself if the items on that list really need to be there. If they do, then you need to analyze why they haven't been done.

Often, clearing a To-Do list might mean consciously making an effort to set time aside and drilling down. Many times, this is the solution to an unfinished list. If something doesn't make sense, or you know it doesn't belong on the list, then it might be a good idea to deep-six it.

Furthermore, keeping a written list such as in a notebook can help your brain fixate the things that need to be done on that list. As you actually write things down, you will be able to help your mind focus on what needs to be done. That takes the guesswork away, reduces stress and nips overthinking in the bud. You know what you need to do; so, it is only a matter of getting down to business.

Chapter 28: Evaluate Your Time Usage

This can be tricky especially if you are prone to distraction. When you get easily distracted, you can be sidetracked from activities which really matter. By the time you come to realize, precious time has ticked away on something which wasn't urgent or important.

In order for you to track your time usage, it is a good idea to make a conscious effort to take note of the time you spend on various activities. Here is a quick list of activities which you can rather easily track the time you spend on them:

- Commuting
- Watching TV
- Playing games
- Social media
- Socializing
- Sleeping
- Running errands

All of these activities, while important to a certain degree, can be tracked rather easily. In particular, commuting and sleeping are two activities that need a specific amount of time allotted to them. If you neglect sleep, you will pay the price over time. If you spend too much time commuting, then you might have to reevaluate your options.

The fact of the matter is that time allocation is a zero-sum game. This means that you have to take away from one activity to give to another. This is why prioritization is so important. When you realize what's truly important, such as sleep, you won't neglect giving it the time it deserves.

As you make a concerted effort to track the time you spend on your various activities, you may be startled to realize how much time you actually devote to activities that don't have much bearing on your goals. For example, you need to evaluate the impact that playing video games have on getting you a promotion at work. Nevertheless, if you play video games as a means of unwinding, then doing so in a productive manner will be helpful. Doing so in an unproductive manner will simply take attention away from what truly matters in the long run.

Chapter 29: Limit Your Media Consumption

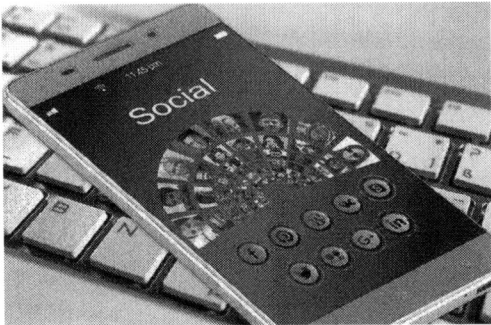

Rehearsing care is a famous New Year's goals this year. Care as a hunting term scored a 98 a week ago on Google. The score speaks to the pursuit of intrigue comparative with the most noteworthy point on the graph, so care is certainly a present pattern. Similarly, contemplation scored 100 a week ago. Both pursuit terms scored close to 50 only five years prior.

I started reflecting a year ago and have thought that it was useful in various manners. It hasn't quite recently decreased pressure; I've additionally turned out to be increasingly engaged and beneficial at work. Contemplation is dubious, particularly for apprentices. More often than not, I utilize guided contemplation applications or digital broadcasts to enable me to center.

Quiet is an application I use, and every day it delivers a themed guided contemplation. So far this year, the majority of the topics have included basic New Year's goals, for example, substance misuse, indulging and negative musings.

The present topic was the careful utilization of media. Every contemplation closes with a statement, and the present was from self-improvement creator Mark Manson.

"Boundless access to learning brings boundless chance. Be that as it may, just to the individuals who figure out how to deal with the new money: their consideration," he composed.

Endless news sources and online networking channels, accessible every minute of every day on advanced cells, all go after our consideration. A considerable lot of these data sources are composed to mix an enthusiastic reaction to energize snaps or remarks since commitment is media cash.

A great many people realize that, yet they regardless enable themselves to get cleared away in the ebb and flow of feelings created by news waterways. If you read about deplorable events, rapes, and offending political spikes before you even get up, you'll likely convey those negative feelings with all of your days long, and they will drain the delight out of your day. Do this for a long time, and you'll before long find you're carrying on with a life bereft of bliss and satisfaction.

Restricting media utilization isn't simple. As somebody with a news-casting degree who has made her living in media and substance for a large portion of her life, it's very a battle for me. If you battle with careful media utilization as I do, here are three hints I've discovered supportive.

Join Facebook gatherings

In the course of recent months, I've joined Facebook bunches for exceptional needs guardians in my general vicinity, female entrepreneurs, online business suppliers, and otherworldly development. Posts from these gatherings currently overwhelm my news channel, diminishing the number of posts that don't create any positive or accommodating data, similar to companions or relatives contending about governmental issues. It's likewise decreased the time I spend on Facebook, in light of the fact that these gatherings are loaded up with individuals who are living rich, satisfied lives and they share ways I can do it, as well. Rather than getting sucked into careless recordings or negative political discussion, I'm propelled to put down my telephone and live right now.

Start the day accomplishing something imaginative

This tip originated from my Facebook profound development site. Research has demonstrated that if you start your day accomplishing something profitable and innovative, for example, working out, journaling or contemplating, you'll convey that outlook with you for the duration of the day. In like manner, if you start your day accomplishing something receptive, for example, understanding news or reacting to web-based social networking posts, you'll convey that mentality throughout the day. The previous is unquestionably more positive and satisfying than the last mentioned.

Breaking point your news time

One of the nifty devices I'm utilizing this year is a shape clock, which is actually what it seems like. It's a plastic 3D square with times on each side and a clock component inside. Turn the measure of time face up, and the clock will tally down and blare when time is up. I utilize the clock to enable me to concentrate on work errands, but at the same time, it's useful when devouring media. I just give myself 15-20 minutes of news time every day. At the point when time is up, I proceed onward. News locales like CU Insight can be extremely useful when restricting news time since you can rapidly filter an assortment of news sources.

Your consideration is important to cash. When you ace that idea, it will be simpler to all the more carefully expend media and select data that will enable you to live a more joyful and increasingly beneficial life.

Chapter 30: Plan Your Meals Wisely

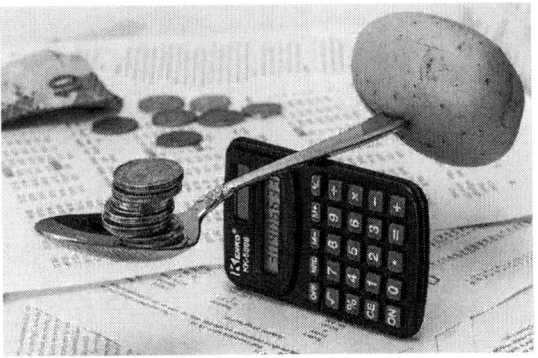

One of the primary ideas of planning is figuring out how to oversee cash admirably. In any case, planning for nourishment can end up difficult as a result of haphazardly eating out or sporadic shopping for food. Truth be told, the spending plan for nourishment is likely the most difficult piece of making a reasonable family spending plan due to the consistently changing business sector and fluctuating costs.

Pursue these tips to make planning for nourishment somewhat simpler:

Plan Ahead – Planning ahead can help spare issues when planning for nourishment costs. Arranging every one of the dinners out constantly means posting your necessary fixings, computing the expense, and constraining eating out. Not exclusively does preparing help with the planning, however, it helps with the shopping for food also in light of the fact that the desires are spread out obviously every week. Supper arranging doesn't need to be difficult, and it can even be adaptable.

Make a List – For any individual who is beginning a nourishment spending plan, causing a rundown of staple goods to can be an ideal method to hold that financial limit under tight restraints. Start by experiencing the storeroom and cooler. Record the vital food supplies under one heading; at that point include everything else into a subsequent heading. By isolating needs and needs with regards to shopping for food, budgeters can wipe out extra superfluous spending. Close to everything, record an expected expense or real cost if known. If the expense is obscure, speculate. If one of the "needs" on the rundown doesn't cost as much as getting ready for, at that point, it is discretionary to buy from the "need" list.

Make it Flexible – Make sure the whole spending plan is somewhat adaptable. If spending isn't as much in another piece of the spending that month, take a day to overdo it a piece and have a pleasant supper out. If the day has been long, utilize a minimal expenditure to get some dessert or cake. If there is another eating routine in the arrangement, fix the nourishment spending plan to incorporate the costs of another nourishment thing. Whatever is done, make a point to be adaptable with the essential shopping for food and nourishment spending plan. It can spare a decent piece of worry later on.

Inexpensive food and café tips – Eating out isn't modest. Furthermore, if you do it as often as possible, the dollars truly add up. A worth supper at a well-known burger chain may just be 5 dollars, however, that is a great deal of cash spent on a moderately healthfully void passage. If you make every one of the three of your day by day squares inexpensive food, you'll be doing harm not exclusively to your cardiovascular wellbeing and your waistline yet to your wallet also.

Chapter 31: Simplify your Life and Live in the Present

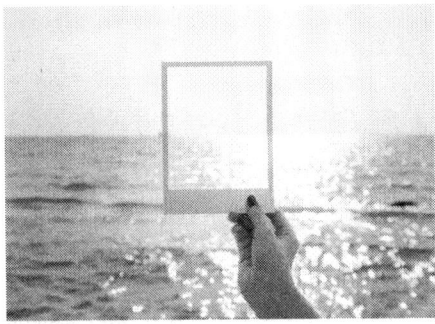

Living in the present in one of the hardest things to do in life. It is not quite so easy to go through not thinking about the past or the future. In fact, we spend most of our lives remembering the past and planning for the future. In the meantime, we tend to forget about what's actually going on at the present time.

When you practice living in the present, you take away overthinking's fuel. Mainly, you are not dwelling on the past and you are not overly concerned about the future. Of course, it makes sense to prepare for the future. But then again, if you are prepared, then there's not much you need to worry about. You have everything you need to be ready. That way, when the future comes, you know what to do.

This is why the present is all about focus. This ties back to prioritization, your To-Do list, focus, concentration and being aware of your situation at present. When you are able to make all of these assessments, you realize that the present is the only thing that matters.

Why?

Because the present is the only thing you actually control. Moreover, when you declutter your lifestyle, it is so much easier to focus on the present simply because you have much less to worry about. If you have a number of balls in the air at the same time, it'll be hard for you to keep track of everything that's going on around you at any given time.

That leads to stress and anxiety… and it leads to overthinking things.

When you resolve to live in the present, you are not leaving the past behind nor are you neglecting the future; in fact, you are empowering yourself to use our most prize possession as efficiently as possible: time.
Time is the only commodity which we cannot get back once it is spent.

Chapter 32: Slow Down and Rewire your Brain to Be Yourself

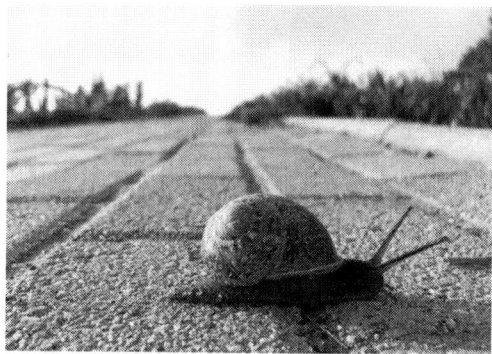

Modern science has shown that the brain is a work in progress. What that means is that it is never fully developed. Of course, from childhood to adulthood, the brain matures enough to allow humans to carry out important biological functions.

This implies that the brain is hardly set in stone once you reach adulthood. In fact, whatever conditions you grew up in can be modified over time. While this takes a concerted effort to do so, it is by no means impossible. You have the power to consciously train your brain to do whatever you need it to do.

In the process of development and maturation, the brain develops its wiring, meaning, that it develops the neurological network that is responsible for activities such as language, critical thinking, motricity, and core biological functions.

For example, the brain is trained to function on eight hours of sleep a night. Yet, you can rewire your brain to function on less. Now, this doesn't mean that it will be functioning at optimum capacity, but it will get the job done. By the same token, you can rewire the brain once more to go back to functioning on more sleep.

So, if you find yourself consciously aware of the negative habits which you have acquitted over time, then the time has come for you to make a conscious effort to retrain your brain to do what you need it to do. This might mean develop new habits or curb older ones.

It does matter. What does matter is that you are able to make sense of the most important functions that you need to do when you need to do it. So, if you resolve to get up earlier and make the most of your day, then you can certainly train your brain to go to bed earlier and get up earlier. While that may not be the easiest thing in the world, it is certainly possible if you really set your mind to it.

This is possible of any habit and any skill you wish to develop in yourself.

Chapter 33: Create Good Habits

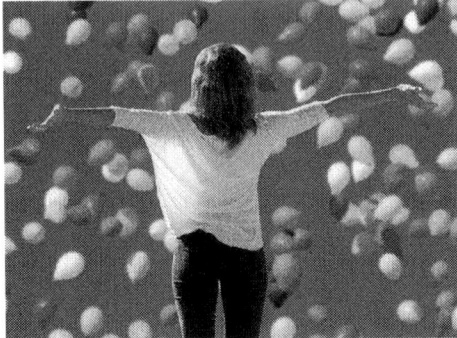

It very well may be difficult to manufacture great propensities.

These thoughts are not by any means the only method to manufacture great propensities — there are a lot of others out there — however, these straightforward advances can enable you to gain ground with a large portion of the objectives you have for your wellbeing, your work, and your life.

That is particularly valid if you need to stay with them as long as possible. Fortunately, there are a couple of basic systems that you can use to construct great propensities and break awful ones.

Also, in light of that, here are 3 things that you can do right presently to manufacture great propensities.

1. Build up an arrangement for when you fizzle.

Dan John, a prominent quality and molding mentor, regularly tells his competitors, "You're bad enough to be disillusioned." The equivalent is genuine when you construct another propensity. What were you anticipating? To prevail as a matter of course from the earliest starting point. To be impeccable in any event, when individuals who have been doing this for a considerable length of time commit errors all the time?

You need to figure out how to not pass judgment on yourself or feel regretful when you commit an error, and rather center around building up an arrangement to refocus as fast as could reasonably be expected.

Here are three systems that may help...

I discover the "never miss twice" mentality to be especially helpful. Perhaps I'll miss one exercise

Set calendars instead of cutoff time.

Disregard execution and spotlight on structure another character.

Make this your new saying: "Never miss twice."

I'm not going to miss two out of a column. Perhaps I'll eat a whole pizza, however, I'll line it up with a solid dinner. Perhaps I'll neglect to think today, yet tomorrow first thing I'll be overflowing with Zen.

Making mistakes on your propensities doesn't make you a disappointment. It makes you typical. What isolates top entertainers from every other person is that they refocus rapidly. Ensure you have an arrangement for when you fall flat.

2. Start with a propensity that is so natural you can't state no.

The most significant piece of structure another propensity is remaining predictable. It doesn't make a difference how well you perform on any individual day. Continued exertion is the thing that has a genuine effect.

Therefore, when you start another propensity it ought to be anything but difficult to the point that you can't disapprove of it. Truth be told, when beginning another behavior is ought to be anything but difficult to such an extent that it's practically ludicrous.

Need to fabricate an activity propensity? You will probably practice for 1 moment today.

Need to begin a composition propensity? You will likely compose three sentences today.

Need to make a good dieting propensity? You will likely eat one solid supper this week.

It doesn't make a difference if you start little on the grounds that there will be a lot of time to get the power later. You don't have to join a CrossFit rec center, compose a book, or change your whole diet at the earliest reference point.

It's anything but difficult to contrast yourself with what others are doing or to want to improve your exhibition and accomplish more. Try not to give those sentiments a chance to pull you off-kilter. Demonstrate to yourself that you can adhere to something little for 30 days. At that point, when you are having some fantastic luck and staying predictable, you can stress over expanding the difficulty.

Initially, execution is superfluous. Accomplishing something amazing more than once won't make any difference if you never stay with it for them since a long time ago run. Make your new propensity so natural that you can't state no.

3. Set aside some effort to see precisely what is keeping you down.

I as of late talked with a lady named Jane. She needed to practice reliably, yet had consistently imagined that she was, in her words, "the kind of individual who didn't prefer to exercise."

Jane chose to bring an end to the propensity down and understood that it wasn't really practicing that troubled her. Rather, she didn't care for the issue of preparing for the rec center, driving someplace for 20 minutes, and after that working out. She likewise didn't appreciate setting off to an open spot and working out before other individuals. Those were the genuine hindrances that anticipated her activity propensity.

When she understood this, Jane contemplated how she could make practicing simpler. She purchased a yoga video and began practicing at home two evenings for each week. She was additionally an educator and her school offered an activity class for the staff after school. She began setting off to that class since it implied that she didn't need to drive elsewhere or put in a great deal of planning time just to exercise.

Jane has been adhering to her exercise routine throughout recent months. She says, "You probably won't have the option to fix all that you don't care for, however making sense of how to function around a couple of those obstacles may give the push you have to get past the halfway point and stick with your objectives."

The individuals who stick with great propensities see precisely what is keeping them down.

You may imagine that you're the "kind of individual who doesn't care for working out" or the "sort of individual who is sloppy" or the "sort of individual who surrenders to desires and eats desserts." But by and large, you're not bound to flop in those territories. Rather than owning a sweeping expression about your propensities, separate them into smaller pieces and consider which zones are keeping you from getting to be predictable.

When you know the specific pieces of the procedure that keep you down, you can start to build up an answer to tackle that issue.

Chapter 34: Do What you Love

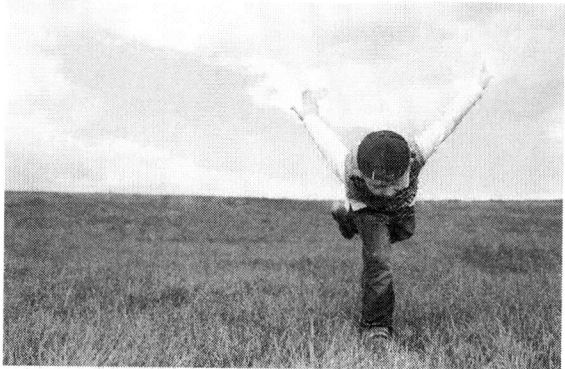

How many times have you heard this one?

Sure, it might sound cliché, but it's actually true. There is something about doing what you love which makes life so much better.

Now, you might have heard this phrase related to work. After all, who wouldn't love to make a living doing what they love the most. Some people do, and some fail in the process.

Of course, doing what you love doesn't necessarily mean making a career out of it. It just means that you are making the most of your time partaking in activities that fulfill you; which gives you a sense of satisfaction and happiness.

For example, some folks find joy in the church. Attending their church service invigorates them and gives them a new lease on life. Others feel that way about sports, hobbies, travel and so on.

When you make a point of doing what you love, you are opening the door to a wonderful life in which you have control over what you wish to do with your time and your efforts. Naturally, we all need to make a living, pay bills and take care of our household. Still, these responsibilities don't preclude our ability to enjoy our lives.

So, make a point of taking the time to do the things that you love. Even if it is just one thing, at least you can make the time you need to enjoy life. Please bear in mind that life is fleeting. The next thing you know, it may be gone forever. The last thing that anyone wants is to live with regret, with a sense of longing for the time that was spent on other things.

After all, how many people have you heard regret not spending more time at the office while on their deathbed?

Chapter 35: Embrace Positive Influences with Positive Thinking

The universe is made up of energy. That energy is both positive and negative. What's more, both types of energy attract each other in such a way that positively charged energies attract other positively charged energy. The same can be said about negative energy.

In a practical sense, this means that when you charge your life with positive energy, the likelihood of you attracting more positive energy increases significantly. Conversely, if you charge up your negative energies, then that is what you shall attract.

Now, if your deal is to hang with negatively changed individuals, then by all means. But if you are looking to make a positive change in your life, then it is positive energy which you seek. This begins with making an effort to positively change your mindset.

To positively change your mindset, you can begin by flipping the narrative around. Let's assume that you have money problems and are in need of more cash. The obvious way to look at this issue would be, "I don't have any money. I need more money".

When you utter the words, "I don't have money", you are making a declaration to the universe that you lack. What this means is that you are embracing a scarcity mindset.

On the contrary, if you reframe the issue as "I have bills to pay. How can I make more money?" you are automatically making an affirmation to the universe that you are looking for opportunities.

Ask and you shall receive.

It's fairly straightforward.

So, make a point of cutting out "negatives" from your vocabulary. Make a point to make positive affirmations in spite of the situation. Stop saying, "I am sick" and embrace "I will be healed".

As Descartes said, "I think therefore I am".

Chapter 36: Remove Negative Influences Cut Off Destroying Thoughts

Negative energy is everywhere. You can find it at every turn. Negative energy can take the form of unhappy people, violent content on television, or even environmental damage. You can see this on a consistent basis. No matter where you go, you will encounter charges of negative energy.

And while there isn't much you can do to stop negative energy from swirling around in the world, there is plenty which you can do to stop it from taking over your mind. In fact, when you find yourself immersed in a negative environment, it is very easy to get caught up in the negativity of the situation.

For instance, you are working in a very negative environment. Your boss and co-workers aren't getting along which leads to an overall unpleasant atmosphere. At this point, you have one of two choices, you either let that get to you, or you don't. Of course, it's not quite that simple.

One of the most effective ways to avoid being brought down by this type of atmosphere is to simply stop it from getting to you. You can learn to recognize the onset of negative thoughts and emotions. When you do, you can nip them in the bud. You can make use of mantras such as, "negative energies can't touch me" or "negative thoughts are like a ship passing in the night".

In other words, don't let negative thoughts pull up a chair and have a seat. If you allow them to do that, you are opening the door to trouble. The main thing to keep in mind is that you are the master of your thoughts and your emotions. The only way something can get to you is if you let it.

However, it is true that a highly negative environment will undoubtedly charge you with negative energy. In that case, it is always a great idea to have ways in which you can unload those energies. That is why pleasant activities are needed at the end of the day. That way, you can simply let go of the energies which are negatively affecting you.

Chapter 37: Getting Rid of Toxic People

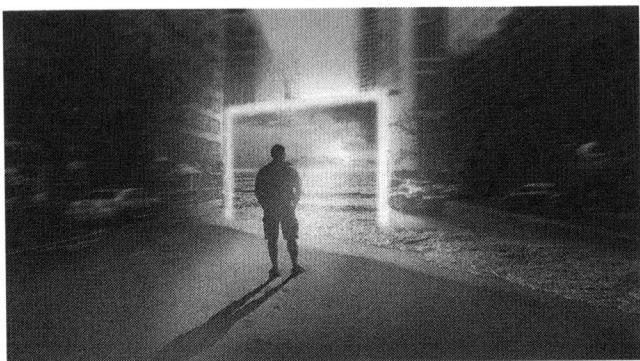

Severally, we talk and spotlight on the significance of evacuating and getting rid of poisonous nourishment, films, and beverages, yet we overlook the significance of expelling dangerous individuals with lethal frames of mind from our lives. Much the same as every single other thing that is harmful in nature, poisonous individuals can harm and taint our lives with mental, enthusiastic and physical infections. Evacuating dangerous individuals can be difficult, particularly when we have a current association with them. Notwithstanding, here are a few hints that will enable you to evacuate any sort of lethal individual from your life:

1. Change your organization

One approach to treat the impact of awful things that have occurred in your life is to start to take in beneficial things. To dispose of poisonous individuals, encircle yourself with capable and beautiful individuals. The lethal individual will have no real option except to pull out.

There was a companion of mine who had a negative and lethal view concerning everything, so as to dispose of him, I warmed up to some folks with a ton of positive vibes. Sooner or later, I saw he barely came around me when I was with them. In the end, he left me.

Besides, through positive relations, you can enhance your shortcomings. You will likewise think that it is simpler to proceed onward from the hurt that negative and dangerous connections could have caused.

2. Be firm

Most harmful individuals resemble parasites, they don't do well without their host. This implies simply instructing them to leave your life probably won't be sufficient in light of the fact that they will consistently attempt to return. It is now that you should rehash your position without jumping. Your activities ought to likewise mirror your words (when you state "leave", you should avoid them yourself).

3. Gain as a matter of fact

After you have disposed of lethal connections, you need to gain from them. Hence, before beginning any genuine fellowship on a relationship, you should check such people for comparative characteristics. This will enable you to dispose of dangerous individuals for all time.

4. Structure plainly characterized limits

In managing poisonous individuals, it is significant that you defined limits concerning what they can do with you and what they can't. These limits must be upheld on the grounds that poisonous individuals consistently attempt to figure out how to sneak once again into your life. For instance, if you intend to restrict connections to simply welcome, guarantee that when they endeavor to raise a point for a discussion, you cut them off.

Obviously, this could be difficult, yet whatever merits doing at all merits progressing nicely. A few persuasive statements for understudies, laborers, educators, among others, express the significance of defining and keeping to limits, regardless of the expense.

5. Try not to be decent to them

At the point when we are attempting to expel an ailment from our body or attempting to get rid of dangerous nourishment or drink, we are not decent to it. The equivalent goes for poisonous individuals. Try not to grin to them, don't be delicate with them, rather, be exacting and solicit them to get out of your life.

This doesn't imply that you ought to turn into an awful or remorseless individual. Simply guarantee that your earnestness and stance leave no uncertainty of your aim in their brains.

6. Try not to attempt to transform them

Commonly, we fall into the snare of reasoning that it is our duty to change dangerous individuals or that they will in the end change. To dispose of them, you should be prepared to acknowledge that they won't change and that it isn't your obligation to endeavor to change their disposition. Interestingly, they generally appear to be happy to take exhortation and to change, yet they don't.

At the point when you quit searching for their salvation, it ends up simpler to desert them. I thought that it was difficult to leave a harmful relationship. This was on the grounds that consistently I woke up persuaded that the other individual was going to change. She didn't. I abandoned attempting to spare her so as to proceed onward.

7. Genuinely let them go (excuse)

Don't simply concentrate on physically disposing of a lethal individual, likewise, dispose of them inwardly. If a lethal individual hurt you, excuse the individual in your heart as you let the individual go. Along these lines, the individual doesn't stay to torment and harm you inwardly, even after they have left physically.

Keep in mind that generous them isn't overlooking that they are poisonous individuals, it is simply to enable your heart to proceed onward from them also. The absence of absolution is the reason numerous individuals are still overloaded from lethal connections that they are out of.

8. Identify the lethal nature

The absolute first activity in the voyage of disposing of dangerous individuals is to have the option to identify such individuals and how they are poisonous. Research has demonstrated a few attributes that will assist you in identifying a dangerous individual. You can view individuals as lethal when:

- They generally request that you substantiate yourself to them.
- They never apologize.
- They are manipulative.
- They are not steady.
- They never assume up liability.
- They are judgmental.

If you are in any type of relationship, where the individual shows any of such attributes (reliably), you are with a lethal individual. Realizing this is the initial step to being free.

9. Maintain a strategic distance from snares of emergencies

Harmful individuals consistently attempt to get again into your life or to remain thereby continually keeping you occupied with one emergency that happens in their life. To dispose of poisonous individuals, you should be prepared to turn away from their purported emergency and to proceed onward with your own life. Overlooking harmful individuals is a powerful method to get them to gather their packs and leave your life.

10. Know and claim your shortcomings and disappointments

Dangerous individuals are aces in the craft of misusing your disappointment for their own narrow-minded intrigue. Nonetheless, when you come to comprehend and acknowledge your shortcomings (with an offer to improve and turn out to be better), their hold over you falls flat. This makes the undertaking of showing them out of your life progressively effective.

Owning your shortcomings likewise incorporates putting stock in yourself and luxuriating in your quality and triumphs. This likewise causes you to see why your life is of an excessive amount of significant worth to permit dangerous individuals in it.

Lethal things are harmful things that can murder us if we don't dispose of them as fast and as proficiently as could be expected under the circumstances. Guarantee that you don't wait or proceed with that lethal companion or in that poisonous relationship anymore. It will enable you to live more. The tips recorded above will help you in escaping harmful connections.

Chapter 38: How to Stop Overthinking with Mindfulness Meditation

Folks who are unfamiliar with meditation believe it is some practice that monks do atop a mountain in the middle of nowhere. The fact of the matter is that you can practice meditation at any time, and in any place you choose.

One of the best to practice mindfulness meditation is when you are feeling overwhelmed by emotions, work, people, problems and so on. When you do this, you will be able to harness your emotions so that you can bring them back down to manageable levels. That way, when overthinking begins to creep in, you can stop it in its tracks.

Here is how mindfulness meditation works:

Let's say the action at work is getting hot and heavy. Naturally, you are consumed by the action and are beginning to have negative thoughts creep up behind you. So, what can you do?

Live in the here and the now.
Think about what the most important thing is at that moment. Think about why you feel why you do. And most importantly let go of the negativity that emerges from being in that situation.

Next, take a deep breath… you can literally count to 10. Each time you breathe in, close your eyes and visualize oxygen entering your lungs and charging your body with positive energy. Slowly exhale while you visualize a small black puff of smoke carry negativity away. This energy will dissolve in the air and disappear.

This practice does not need to take more than a couple of minutes. But that couple of minutes can be instrumental in helping you focus and keep negative thoughts at bay. Before you know it, you will have curbed negative feelings down to their least expression.

This can definitely help you stay focused while you get stuff done. Afterward, you can make the time for some self-care and unwind from the day you've had to deal with.

Chapter 39: What Is Mindfulness Meditation?

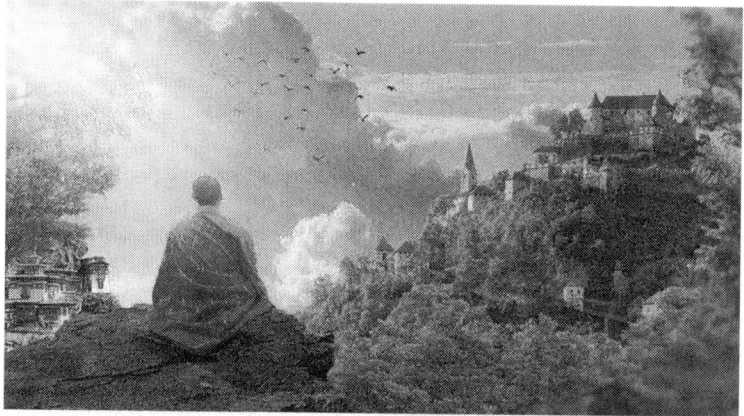

Have you at any point felt pushed, restless, or overpowered by life?

We live in a bustling world. With messages and messages flying all around as you are venturing over your kids' toys and attempting to get the canine sustained while the nourishment on the table is getting cold, you most likely get a handle on worried consistently.

Done effectively, mindfulness will enable you to diminish your pressure and nervousness, limit the measure of time that you spend feeling overpowered, and help you value every little minute as it occurs. In a universe of confusion, mindfulness may very well be the stunt you have to figure out how to have the option to adapt to the frenzy.

Luckily, there is a straightforward propensity you can use to normally quiet yourself down and acknowledge life more. It's called mindfulness. Mindfulness is the act of deliberately concentrating the majority of your consideration on the present minute and tolerating it without judgment. This is an incredible spot to begin if you are searching for the key component in joy.

If these sound like results you'd love to involvement, at that point I prescribe perusing this extreme manual for being careful about the duration of the day. First up, we'll spread the advantages of mindfulness—specifically, how it can decidedly affect both your mental and physical prosperity.

Advantages of Mindfulness

1. Mindfulness diminishes uneasiness

Research has discovered that mindfulness is particularly useful in diminishing nervousness. Rehearsing mindfulness consistently revamps your cerebrum so you can refocus your consideration. As opposed to following a negative and stressing thought down a way of every single imaginable result, you can figure out how to see the truth about your contemplations and simply let them go.

2. Mindfulness improves memory, focus, and execution

Focusing and focusing on the job that needs to be done might be one of the most significant psychological capacities individuals have. Mindfulness is one of the not very many strategies that function as a remedy for mind-meandering and the negative impacts that losing focus may have on you. Truth be told, inquire about understudies has demonstrated that there is an association among mindfulness and focusing both all through the study hall.

Extra examinations have demonstrated that ruminating over a standard premise causes the cerebrum's cerebral cortex (which is answerable for memory, fixation, and figuring out how) to thicken.

3. Mindfulness gives relief from discomfort

Around 100 million Americans experience the ill effects of ceaseless torment each day, yet 40% to 70% of these individuals are not accepting legitimate medicinal treatment. Numerous investigations have demonstrated that mindfulness contemplation can decrease torment without utilizing endogenous narcotic frameworks that are generally accepted to diminish torment during subjective based systems like mindfulness.

Oneself created narcotic framework has as a rule been suspected of as the focal piece of the mind for mitigating torment without the utilization of medications. This framework self-produces three narcotics, including beta-endorphin, the met-and Leu-enkephalins, and the dynorphins. These work together to lessen torment by rehearsing mindfulness.

4. Mindfulness assists with passionate reactivity

Of the considerable number of reasons that individuals more often than not have for learning contemplation, being less sincerely receptive is normally high on the rundown. Being careful or "Zen" compares to moving with the punches in life and being non-receptive to things that may come to your direction.

What's more, there's unquestionably something to this. Mindfulness contemplation has permitted study members to remove their feelings from upsetting pictures and spotlight more on an intellectual errand, as contrasted and a control gathering.

5. Mindfulness decreases rumination and overthinking

One of the most well-known manifestations that join tension is rumination or overthinking. After you start to stress over something, your mind will clutch that firmly and make it difficult to give up. It is anything but difficult to get into an idea circle where you keep on replaying every single awful result possible. We as a whole realize this isn't valuable since stressing over something doesn't keep it from occurring.

One investigation really demonstrated that individuals who were new to mindfulness and started to rehearse it during a retreat had the option to give fewer indications of rumination and uneasiness than the control gathering.

6. Mindfulness makes more joyful connections

Scientists are as yet uncertain this works, yet rising cerebrum studies have demonstrated that individuals who take part in mindfulness all the time show both auxiliary and useful changes in the mind locales that are connected to improved sympathy, empathy, and generosity.

Another advantage of mindfulness is in its impacts on the amygdala, which is the cerebrum's enthusiastic preparing focus. Mindfulness is connected to decreases in both the volume of the amygdala and its association with the prefrontal cortex. This recommends mindfulness may bolster feeling guidelines and lessening reactivity, which are two significant devices for making and looking after connections.

7. Mindfulness improves rest

The unwinding reaction that your body needs to mindfulness reflection is a remarkable inverse of the pressure reaction. This unwinding reaction attempts to ease many pressures related to medical problems, for example, agony, wretchedness, and hypertension. Rest issues are regularly attached to these illnesses.

One investigation of more established grown-ups affirms that mindfulness contemplation can help in getting a decent night's rest. As indicated by this examination, mindfulness reflection can expand the unwinding reaction through its capacity of expanding attentional components that confer command over the autonomic sensory system.

8. Mindfulness eases some pressure

Since individuals are looked with an expanding measure of weight nowadays because of the mind-boggling nature of our general public, they are regularly tormented with a ton of stress. This adds to a wide assortment of other medical issues. Mindfulness can diminish worry by going about as a precaution measure, and help individuals overcome difficult occasions.

9. Mindfulness advances mental wellbeing

Specialists have discovered that IBMT (integrative body-mind preparing) starts positive auxiliary changes in the cerebrum that could help secure against mental infection. The act of this strategy helps support productivity in a piece of the cerebrum that enables individuals to direct behavior.

10. Mindfulness advances intellectual adaptability

One examination proposes that not exclusively will mindfulness help individuals become less receptive; it may likewise give individuals progressively intellectual adaptability. Individuals who practice mindfulness seem, by all accounts, to be ready to likewise rehearse self-perception, which consequently withdraws the pathways made in the cerebrum from earlier learning and permits data that is going on right now to be comprehended in another manner.

Reflection additionally enacts the piece of the mind that is related to versatile reactions to push, which compares to a quicker recuperation to a benchmark line of reasoning in the wake of being contrarily affected.

Chapter 40: How to Meditate Your Worries Away

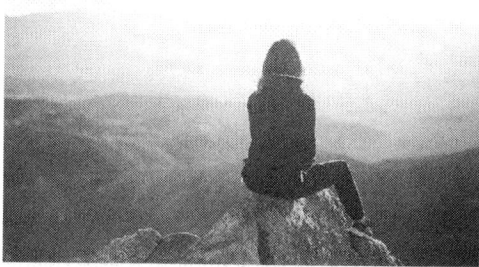

We are instructed to move away from dread—to pick comfort and quick fulfillment over the hard way. But then, we who ruminate are continually picking the hard way. Confidence is a position of a riddle, where we discover the boldness to have faith in what we can't see and the solidarity to relinquish our dread of vulnerability.

Each time I go into contemplation, it is a demonstration of trust, of squeezing into dread and drawing nearer to reality. It is the act of contemplating that has enabled me to look for that reality, to pick the harder way, and to discover sympathy for myself all the while.

As the years progressed, I've gone over a couple of sorts of contemplation that have helped me in the most dread ridden times of my life.

Qigong Meditation

In Traditional Chinese Medicine, it is accepted that dread is put away in the kidneys. In Western medication, it is realized that frightful considerations are minimal more than compound and electrical sign, activated through a mind-boggling system of correspondence in the body's cells. With enough reiteration, those neural pathways are framed and established, causing a similar reaction each time a danger is recognized.

Sit with your shoulders and your feet level against the floor. Spot your hands over your kidneys (at your back under your lower ribs). Picture them and the little adrenal organs over them in your psyche.

At the point when the psyche is looked with a danger, regardless of whether genuine or saw, it revisits those pathways to do similar activities. Furthermore, that is the place qigong contemplation steps in. By rehashing positive musings, you can make and fortify neural pathways, and clear up the kidneys, to assist you with more noteworthy authority over your feelings.

After a couple of breath cycles, lean forward a little as you breathe in, catch your hands beneath your knees, open your eyes, and envision breathing out dread, making a "choo" sound.

Closer your eyes, grin, and breathe in your stomach out envisioning dull blue light and harmony encompassing your kidneys and adrenal organs. Breathe out by driving your stomach back in.

Lean In

The act of reflection is intended to be down to earth in helping us travel during our time with a touchstone of harmony and mindfulness. Similarly, as with any feeling, contemplation can help balance out us notwithstanding trepidation to enable us to comprehend it all the more unmistakably.

As the day progressed, you can enable yourself to meet dread in an increasingly positive manner with the intensity of reflection.

Check-in with your feelings consistently. At whatever point you feel dreadful, let the inclination remain.

Rather than running, adopt a full breath and strategy your contemplations of fear and stress with neighborliness and interest. Be thoughtful to yourself in dread, as you would for a confided in companion.

If you have the opportunity and space, plunk down and inhale into your dread for ten breath cycles.

Dread AS POWER

Dread is stating that this is the ideal time to have the option to do what you're attempting to do. Your body is really setting you up to have a positive result. When you can truly comprehend that dread is a feeling like some other feeling, you can figure out how to oversee it. And afterward, you can accomplish things that the vast majority consider to be exceptional.

To beat my dread of statures, I have grasped the fear, taking a lead shake climbing class where I need to move to the highest point of the divider and free fall mostly down the divider before being securely gotten with a rope.

Through training, receptiveness, and cheering companions and teachers, I have figured out how to inhale through the dread and let go again and again. The dread remains, however my response to it has changed.

Practice it yourself — what is your dread? What little, safe advances would you be able to take to work on disapproving of your breath in that dread? As you practice, what changes do you see after some time?

Chapter 41: Mindfulness in Everyday Life

As we have pointed out earlier, mindfulness is not some practice limited to monks who have taken a vow of silence. This is the type of practice which virtually anyone can do, at any time, and anywhere.

So, here are some additional strategies to implement mindfulness in your everyday life:

1. Sit with your experience

At the point when you center around being careful, you can sit with your experience.

Rehearsing mindfulness through concentrating on your body, psyche, and soul will enable you to turn out to be all the more dominant. The more you do this, the more you shut out the sense of self and the better you will feel in all pieces of yourself.

With shut eyes and a casual body, center around your relaxing. Tune in for sounds that are close by or even far away. Output your body to get a feeling of what is loose and what is holding strain. If you have a tingle, see the tingle however don't attempt to transform it. Simply travel through it.

This is a great practice for simply being careful without attempting to take care of business.

Once in a while, life is awkward like a tingle. Sitting with the experience will enable you to see that things go back and forth.

Nervousness can sneak up in your paunch or you may encounter a snugness in your throat while you reflect.

The brain is telling the body that there are such a large number of activities. At the point when you do encounter strain in the body, you can contact that zone with your hands and inside the state, "This as well." You're recognizing your full understanding without attempting to transform it. This is mindfulness.

Let's assume you're sitting outside in a recreation center; all is well until you see two individuals unmistakably enamored. Abruptly, dejection kicks in and no one is around to facilitate the inclination. This bit of dejection has consistently been in your heart.
It's not constantly enacted however can emerge at any minute. You become feeble and it feels like your heart is sinking. Different occasions you've felt alone are activated and put away vitality from the past strikes a chord.

How would you take care of the issue without calling somebody or utilizing an old device to calm down your contemplations and sentiments?

Basically, see that you took notes. You are the subject and you are what takes note. Those sentiments of the void are objects. Out is to see who is feeling the torment and depression. Give the emotions a chance to go through without fleeing or staying away from them.

Mindfulness doesn't mean getting to be associated with the show of the psyche. It's tied in with seeing the manner in which the psyche and body are reacting with full acknowledgment.

The touchy individual in you who has had numerous encounters will feel apprehensive, destitute, and desirous every once in a while. This is the mind and the conscience affecting everything. You are the person who is careful, you are the inhabiting being who knows.

To take advantage of the piece of you that sits looking out for this human experience, you simply need to remain completely focused.

All of what I'm stating may appear to be exceptionally perplexing for some who have never polished mindfulness. It just requires some investment of not responding and rather watching your experience to comprehend the procedure I'm discussing.

Reflection is an incredible practice for minutes that bring awkward feelings.

2. Attempt this activity

Make proper acquaintance with the one in your brain. Just inside make proper acquaintance. Who makes proper acquaintance and who hears hi? It's you who's talking and it's you who's tuning in.

The most ideal approach to turn out to be free from the steady prattle that is bolstering your horrendous thoughts is to step back. Take a gander at it dispassionately. Musings are only an object of the psyche, something that should drift by and not be clutched or dismissed.

As you're careful and watch the voice, you'll start to see that the greater part of what it says has next to no significance. It complains about the past and utilizes old encounters to attempt to control present and future encounters. This causes a wide range of issues in your life.

If you need to turn out to be free from your own brain, you must be careful enough to truly observe what's happening up there. At the point when you discover that a lot of your activities originating from some nonsensical voice that wants comfort, you can start to settle on different choices.

All in all, mindfulness can mend numerous things yet how would we accomplish it? One of the pathways to calm the psyche and go within ourselves is through contemplation.

3. Everyday contemplation

Contemplation isn't difficult but then its effortlessness threatens many.

This is on the grounds that your self-image wouldn't like to be calmed. It reveals to you that you're excessively occupied, that reflection is inconsequential, and that it's excessively unusual and otherworldly for you.

What's truly going on is that the self-image is terrified of ending up calm. Backing off and going in methods there's the capability of standing up to awkward sentiments. You gave your sense of self the activity of keeping away from distress or saw peril.

At the point when we ponder, there is incredible danger of running into past torment.

Mindfulness through your contemplation enables you to at long last manage old injuries so you don't need to live with them any longer. That implies that they never again have power over you.

To develop mindfulness, you'll need to invest significant energy consistently, yet this shouldn't be a task. The mind will prattle and reveal to you it's exhausted. Simply continue watching the objects of musings and emotions traveling through you.

The more you practice, the more you'll anticipate having that uninterrupted alone time. Consider it daily in the spa or getting a back rub. When you get into it, that focused inclination makes you feel as loose as 40 minutes in a sauna.

While you'll start to experience benefits practically immediately, the more you practice mindfulness, the more noteworthy the advantages will be.

In both the Buddhist ways of thinking and present-day psychotherapy, mindfulness is accomplished through reflection.

There is a wide range of approaches to reflect as well, so don't sit in lotus posture and consume those incense sticks at this time. Reflection is the umbrella for mending and inside your contemplations, you can accomplish numerous things for the body, psyche, and soul.

Mindfulness contemplation isn't tied in with changing or modifying yourself in any capacity. It's tied in with getting to be mindful of what your identity is. As you sit peacefully, things will come up. As you search inside yourself, recollections may come up as if they are a motion picture on a screen.

If you remain in the seat of cognizance without getting sucked in, you can become familiar with a great deal. You'll know if you get sucked in on the grounds that you won't let pictures go. You'll get genuinely included and pressure will begin to develop.

Buddha said that the wellspring of your enduring is attempting to flee from your immediate experience. Remaining in a lovely minute from your past is equivalent to pieces of torment. Clutching things keeps you before and it's essentially not beneficial for your mind.

Chapter 42: A Simple Mindfulness Meditation Practice to Relieve Stress and Anxiety

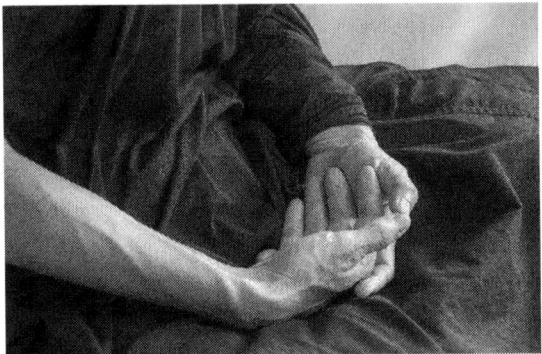

The most fundamental approach to do careful breathing is essential to concentrate on your breath, then breathe in and breathe out. You can do this while standing, yet preferably you'll be sitting or in any event, lying in an agreeable position. Your eyes might be open or shut, however, you may think that it is simpler to keep up your concentration if you close your eyes. It can save an assigned time for this activity; however, it can likewise rehearse it when you're feeling especially pushed or restless. Specialists accept a customary routine with regards to careful breathing can make it simpler to do it in difficult circumstances.

Once in a while, particularly when attempting to quiet yourself in a distressing minute, it may begin by taking an overstated breath: a profound breath in through your noses (3 seconds), hold your breath (2 seconds), and a long breath out through your mouth (4 seconds). Something else, essentially watch every breath without attempting to alter it; it might concentrate on the ascent and fall of your chest or the sensation through your noses. As you do as such, you may find that your mind meanders, diverted by contemplations or substantial sensations. That is OK. Simply see this is occurring and delicately take your consideration back to your breath.

To give considerably more structure, and help you lead this training for other people, underneath are ventured for a short-guided reflection. You can tune in to the sound of this guided reflection, created by UCLA's Mindful Awareness Research Center (MARC), in the player underneath; if it doesn't play, you can discover it here or download it from MARC's site.

Tune into your breath. Feel the regular progression of breath—in, out. You don't have to do anything to your breath. Not long, not short, simply characteristic. Notice where you feel your breath in your body. It may be in your belly. It might be in your chest or throat or in your noses. Check whether you can feel the vibes of breath, each breath in turn. At the point when one breath closes, the following breath starts.

Locate a casual, agreeable position. You could be situated on a seat or on the floor on a pad. Keep your back upstanding, yet not very tight. Hands resting any place they're agreeable. Tongue on the top of your mouth or any place it's agreeable.

Notice and loosen up your body. Attempt to see the state of your body, its weight. Allow yourself to unwind and wind up inquisitive about your body situated here—the sensations it encounters, the touch, the association with the floor or the seat. Loosen up any zones of snugness or strain. Simply relax.

Presently as you do this, you may see that your psyche may begin to meander. You may begin contemplating different things. If this occurs, it's anything but an issue. It's exceptionally characteristic. Simply see that your brain has meandered. You can say "thinking" or "meandering" in your mind delicately. And after that tenderly divert your consideration right back to the relaxing.

Remain here for five to seven minutes. Notice your breath, peacefully. Every once in a while, you'll lose all sense of direction in idea, at that point come back to your breath.

Following a couple of minutes, indeed see your body, your entire body, situated here. Give yourself a chance to unwind much more profoundly and after that offer yourself some gratefulness for doing this training today.

Chapter 43: Mindfulness Exercises for A Good Sleep

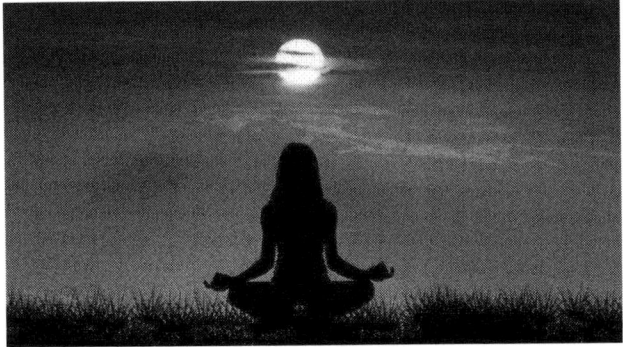

Mindfulness reflection offers a novel and compelling way to deal with feeling guidelines and stress decrease that can drastically improve rest designs.

Normal, customary nervousness and stress can prompt rest issues in youngsters. Youngsters may experience difficulty nodding off or staying unconscious and may wind up on edge about their issue resting. Research demonstrates that mindfulness-based activities significantly increment rest time, lessen a sleeping disorder and lower pre-rest excitement levels. One investigation found that understudies who took an interest in Tai-Chi expanded their mindfulness as well as improved their rest quality. Another investigation of ninth-grade girls encountering poor rest found that mindfulness preparing improved rest beginning, rest productivity, and complete rest time. The understudies hit the sack before and woke before also.

Mindfulness contemplation was initially created as a preparation technique for expanding mindfulness. By expanding mindfulness right now, people can shift their regard for what is, as opposed to stress over what may be. Mindfulness and acknowledgment help introduce the "giving up" that enables rest to normally happen.

Here are a few hints for managing your kids through mindfulness contemplation exercises to help slip them into the joyful place that is known for Nod.

For offspring everything being equal, put aside a couple of minutes before sleep time, in a perfect world simultaneously every night, to take part in a genuine talk. Give the youngster a chance to trust their issues and fears. Offer consolation and compassion, and an embrace or cuddle if fitting. At that point start a mindfulness work out. Guardians and kids can take part in these activities together the initial couple of times, and afterward, later the youngster might be happy with starting activities all alone.

Turning Off Meditation

This can pursue a resting contemplation. Notice the sentiment of the body on the bed. Feel the warm body sinking into the bedding. Notice where the body feels overwhelming and where it feels light. Notice the little toe of the left foot and envision it will rest for the evening. Give it consent to turn off for the evening. Do likewise for each toe on the left foot, at that point the impact point, wad of the foot, lower leg, calf, knee, and thigh. Presently, breathe out and see how the whole left leg is loose, substantial, and warm. Rehash this turning off exercise with the correct leg. Proceed up through the pelvis, gut, chest, and down the arms, into the hands and fingers. Drift off to rest.

Situated Mindful Breathing

Sit on an agreeable seat, reflection pad, or the edge of the bed. Drop the jaw somewhat, let the eyes close. Pursue the breath as it streams gradually in and out. Feel air traveling through the nose and mouth. Notice the stomach and chest rising and afterward falling. Focus on the quiet interruption before every inward breath. If the mind meanders, simply return consideration tenderly to the breath. Profound, delicate, slow breathing can loosen up the body and moderate the heart.

Adoring Kindness Meditation

After careful breathing, an offspring of all ages can get cherishing generosity by thinking about an individual near them who adores them profoundly. Regardless of whether a parent, relative, companion or even somebody who has passed on, they can picture that individual alongside them, grinning and sending adoration and warmth. They ought to wait over the affection that is exuding from that individual's general existence. Feeling that affection, they should now infer a second individual who appreciates them and envisions that individual remaining by them on the opposite side, simply radiating out adoration and security. At long last, they can infer everybody who cherishes and thinks about them—their preferred instructor, their closest companion, their pet—and envision them all assembled, sending wants for joy and wellbeing. They can feel in their heart and chest region all the glow, wellbeing, joy and delight of being cherished.

In the second piece of a cherishing thoughtfulness reflection, a youngster can send that adoration back to every individual, beginning with the first they envisioned. They can feel their very own heart growing, loaded up with happiness and love that streams out to other people.

Resting Mindful Breathing

Untruth serenely in bed and take in profoundly and completely. Feel the lungs load up with air. Notice the chest and midsection rising. Presently breathe out and let the emotions and stresses of the day stream out with the breath and vanish like wisps on the breeze. If stresses emerge once more, acknowledge them without judgment and breathe out them delicately with the breath, seeing them skim away and disappear. Presently envision breathing out to the edge of the sky or skyline and after that breathing from that point once again into the body. This activity can shift the body to a quiet and-interface state.

Chapter 44: Active Problem Solving, Think Smarter

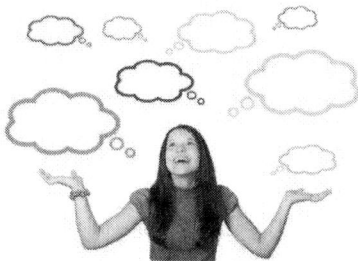

When faced with an issue, a large number of us like to stall or stay away from the issue out and out. Dodging issues is a momentary arrangement. Critical thinking keeps you pushing ahead. It's basic for completing work. Along these lines, the quicker you can tackle any issue, the quicker you can complete the work or audit the answer to guarantee it's right (and return home on schedule).

So, here are some useful tips that can get your creative juices flowing.

1. Investigation

Obviously, look into alone isn't sufficient. Consider inquiring about the field where you've planted the seed of information, yet it's the worked over that nursery, the watering and sustaining that uncovers natural product. That worked is an investigation. It's a method to take what you know and use it to comprehend why something isn't continuing as it should. The examination comes in numerous structures, regardless of whether it's money-saving advantage investigation, hole examination or whatever other structure that encourages you to comprehend your present state.

Systematic aptitudes enable you to see a circumstance and draw based on what is frequently turbulent wreckage, the center issue that is causing the issue. This critical thinking ability gives you a pathway through the issue, so you can create powerful answers for determination.

These scientific aptitudes are not simply useful for triage; however, it helps, yet they can likewise help to precede the issue when you're in the exploration arrange. The issue with research is realizing what is significant and what is not. Expository aptitudes give you the devices to organize viably, as time is consistent with the quintessence with any serious issue.

2. Exercise

There are practices you can do to pick up critical thinking aptitudes and help with your capacity to all the more likely react to issues and fathom them rapidly. For instance, there are rationale thinking tests that help sort out your contemplations obviously, dissect them and pick the best game-plan rapidly. These tests will enable you to perceive and maintain a strategic distance from the run of the mill intelligent misrepresentations.

Spatial-transient thinking tests your capacity to mentally picture objects, which is critical to effectively see space and situating ourselves. Numerical thinking encourages us to get, structure, arrange and take care of issues with scientific techniques or equations. Consistent thinking likewise assists with critical thinking aptitudes in that it offers different recommendations by utilizing what we definitely know and what we accept to know and even what we don't have the foggiest idea.

There a lot more instances of when rationale works out, yet before you even start testing yourself and improving your critical thinking abilities, it's imperative to deal with yourself. Make certain to adhere to a decent rest plan, do ordinary physical activities, keep a thought diary to encourage imaginative reasoning, even have a go at doing yoga or a reflective practice. Everything primes your body and mind and improve your critical thinking abilities.

3. Imagination

Imagination—it's not only for specialists. Inventiveness is basically having the option to discover an answer that is novel. This implies not reacting to issues with an automatic response, or some sheltered arrangement that will probably bring unacceptable outcomes.

What imagination calls for is having the option to take a gander at an issue from numerous points of view, not simply the one you're OK with. You've heard the adages: step out of your customary range of familiarity, consider new ideas, redefine known limits. All things considered, there's some reality to these announcements, regardless of whether they've been rehashed to the point of silliness.

Things being what they are, what are imaginative reasoning aptitudes? Conceptualizing for one. It opens the talk to more than your perspective and broadens the focal point to open a more extensive perspective on the scene. Conceptualizing is a kind of joint effort, which is an incredible method to think inventively in light of the fact that it adds more voices to the blend. In any case, don't hang tight for motivation. Keep in mind, you have to get into the everyday practice, so when motivation hits you can misuse it. Have a go at utilizing innovativeness activities to get into the mind-set.

4. Perfect

Before we leave the subject, we should share one critical thinking system you can attempt then next opportunity an issue comes up that you should manage. The IDEAL strategy is an abbreviation that represents Identify (the issue), Define (the snags), Examine (your alternatives), Act (on a concurred game-plan) and Look (how it turns out and whether any progressions are required).

This procedure fuses quite a bit of what has just been examined and gives an unmistakable layout to tending to issues and rapidly settling them. At the point when you identify the issue, get notification from everybody in the group. At that point characterize the obstructions as well as your objectives in settling it. The investigation of potential arrangements should take a gander at if it will work, yet if it's sheltered, sensible, the best arrangement, and so forth. When an answer has been concurred on follow up on it.

What we've not talked about, which is a piece of the IDEAL strategy, is the last advance, Learn. Whatever strategy is taken, it's basic to screen and cover how it functioned or didn't function. If it doesn't work, at that point return to the start and start new. This will likewise educate you on what to do and what not to do whenever a comparable issue occurs.

5. Choosing

It sounds silly, yet one of the boundaries to taking care of an issue is having the option to act and settle on a choice. Research and investigation are significant, obviously, however, if you fall prey to examination loss of motion, at that point the issues endure. Thinking about an issue and talking about how to react to it is ineptitude without settling on something.

Some may state anything is superior to sitting idle, and there's some reality to that, yet the choice must be based on the exploration with the systematic slashes so as to have the impact you need. You should assess what is the best arrangement, and there will be multiple, so you'll need to pick what is most reasonable and sensible.

Would you be able to settle on that choice rapidly? With experience, you'll be progressively ready to act quick. If you don't have a lot of understanding, at that point the examination and systematic abilities are an extraordinary weight to keep you above water and cruising the correct way in the midst of the tempests that issues work up. Overhauling your basic leadership procedure is probably the quickest approach to improve your critical thinking, so know about how and for what reason you're settling on your choices.

6. Research

Research means doing the due steadiness before setting out on executing your venture, and it is the stone on which all your critical thinking sits. Consequently, to not put it down as a fundamental aptitude that all great issue solvers share for all intents and purpose would leave a major opening in your critical thinking abilities.

Issues, as a rule, don't appear without a history, and where there's a history, there's likewise a point of reference for reacting to the issue. To comprehend the manner in which others fixed an issue is to discover an exit from the one you're in now.

Be that as it may, there's additional. The more profound your examination, the more uncertain you'll have an issue in any case. That and the way that your commonality with a procedure will improve you ready to identify an issue before it turns into an issue. Conceptualizing with your group just extends the information base and improves critical thinking, particularly if they're encountered and have leaked that experience into the research of their own.

7. Correspondence

As with nearly everything, there is no hope without the informative aptitudes to convey the answer for the individuals who must purpose it. Interchanges appear to be simple until you attempt to convey. Indeed, even straightforward thoughts are frequently obfuscated by poor talk, also the mess that accompanies attempting to hand-off complex ones and take care of issues.

It's not simply having the option to convey plainly to orders yet realizing the correct channel to impart your message is likewise significant. That message needs to go to the correct individuals and contact them at the earliest opportunity. Finding an answer for an issue is just one connection in a bigger chain. If that arrangement isn't conveyed to the gatherings that need it to fix the issue for the undertaking to push ahead, at that point all is in vain. Attempt our free correspondence plan format to plainly guide out your interchanges.

Not every person is brought into the world an incredible communicator, however, there are approaches to figure out how to impart better. It takes sympathy and undivided attention to create trust and unwaveringness. Without that security between a group, regardless of how expressly you convey your message, it will be misheard or even overlooked.

Chapter 45: Critical Thinking to Improve Problem-Solving and Decision-Making Tips

1. See potential reasons for the issue

It's astounding the amount you don't think about what you don't have a clue. Consequently, in this stage, it's basic to get a contribution from other individuals who notice the issue and who are affected by it.

It's regularly valuable to gather contributions from different people each in turn (in any event from the outset). Something else, individuals will, in general, be hindered about offering their impressions of the genuine reasons for issues.

Record what your sentiments and what you've gotten notification from others.

Concerning you think maybe execution issues related to a worker, it's regularly valuable to look for exhortation from a friend or your boss so as to verify your impression of the issue.

Record a depiction of the reason for the issue and as far as what's going on, where, when, how, with whom and why.

2. Plan the usage of the best option (this is your activity plan)

Cautiously consider "What will the circumstance resemble when the issue is comprehended?"

What steps ought to be taken to execute the best option in contrast to tackling the issue? What frameworks or procedures ought to be changed in your association, for instance, another strategy or technique? Try not to depend on arrangements where somebody is "simply going to invest more energy".

In what manner will you know if the means are being pursued or not? (these are your pointers of the achievement of your arrangement)

What assets will you need as far as individuals, cash, and offices?

What amount of time will you have to execute the arrangement? Compose a calendar that incorporates the beginning and stop times, and when you hope to see certain markers of accomplishment.

Who will fundamentally be answerable for guaranteeing the execution of the arrangement?

Record the responses to the above inquiries and consider this as your activity plan.

Convey the arrangement to the individuals who will be engaged with executing it and, at any rate, to your prompt director.

3. Select a way to deal with determination the issue

When choosing the best approach, consider:

Which approach is the well on the way to take care of the issue as long as possible?

Which approach is the most sensible to achieve for the present? Do you have the assets? Is it true that they are reasonable? Do you have sufficient opportunity to execute the methodology?

What is the degree of hazard related to every option?

4. Identify options for ways to deal with purpose the issue

Now, it's valuable to keep others included (except if you're confronting an individual and additionally worker execution issue). Conceptualize for answers for the issue. Simply put, conceptualizing is gathering whatever number thoughts as could be expected under the circumstances, at that point screening them to locate the best thought. It's basically when gathering the plans to not pass any judgment on the thoughts - simply record them as you hear them. (A superb arrangement of abilities used to identify the basic reason for issues is Systems Thinking.)

Chapter 46: Focus on the Problem You Are Solving

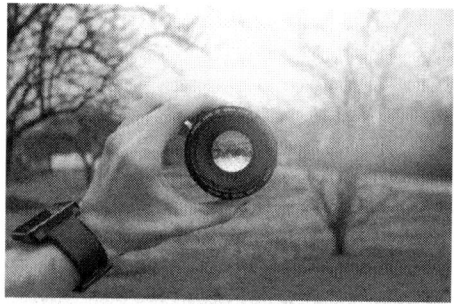

Effective problem-solving skills generally call for you to focus on the actual situation you are trying to deal with. Often, you might get insights regarding other issues that might be related to the task at hand. However, if you allow your attention to dissipate toward other issues, you will be doing yourself a disservice by letting your creative energies distribute unevenly.

When you are able to focus on one issue at a time, you will find that you can solver things a lot more effectively than if your mind was meandering about. Hence, your attention is the most prized commodity in this regard.

Here is one short and effective strategy which can help you: time blocking.

While there are times when you need to think on your feet and make decisions in real-time, often, most issues will allow you enough time to sit down and go over it. Of course, when you are faced with life-or-death problems, you may no choice but to go with your instincts. But the fact of the matter is that most situations can be put off until a better time.

This is where you can block off your time. You can set aside a fixed amount of time to deal with that problem. This may be 30 minutes one morning, it might mean getting up earlier one day to work on it, or it might even mean clearing an entire afternoon. Whatever the time you need, you can try your best to clear it up. That way, you will be able to focus solely on this.

Also, don't be afraid to brainstorm ideas while you are at it. Often, some of the most outrageous ideas end up becoming viable alternatives to problems that you have been struggling to solve. So, take the time to go over your ideas and contemplate the best course of action. Please keep in mind that the more time you are able to devote to an issue, the easier it will become to solve.

Chapter 47: Find Simple Solutions

Have you ever heard of "Occam's Razor"?

Occam's Razor is a philosophical axiom that states: the simplest solution is usually the right one.

While you might be thinking that it is an over-simplistic view of reality, the fact is that the best solution is often simple and low-tech. Sure, solving some of the world's biggest problems has required humankind's cleverest minds. But often, some of the world's biggest issues have been solved with a very mundane solution.

If we translate this to everyday life, your problems, no matter how complex they are, can be boiled down to a simple and effective solution.

For instance, you are struggling financially. So, you are clear about the fact that you need more money. A highly complicated solution would be to become a cyberterrorist and digitally rob a bank.

That seems kind of convoluted, doesn't it?

However, you consider other low-tech solutions. Based on this, you choose to sell t-shirts. While that is hardly the sexiest business out there, it is the kind of business that has been proven to generate revenue. Alternatively, you choose to suck it up and get another job.

Of course, these solutions might not make you rich, but they will be enough to get you out from behind the eight-ball.

The beauty of implementing a low-tech, low-risk, low-complication approach is that it allows you to build layers on the complexity on top of them. So, you can start out by selling t-shirts at a local flea market. As you progress, you can migrate to an online empire. The ultimate point is that you are able to make things more suited to your particular condition as you gain experience.

So, don't be afraid to start off small. After all, how many of the world's largest corporations started out in a garage?

Chapter 48: Make Fact-based decisions

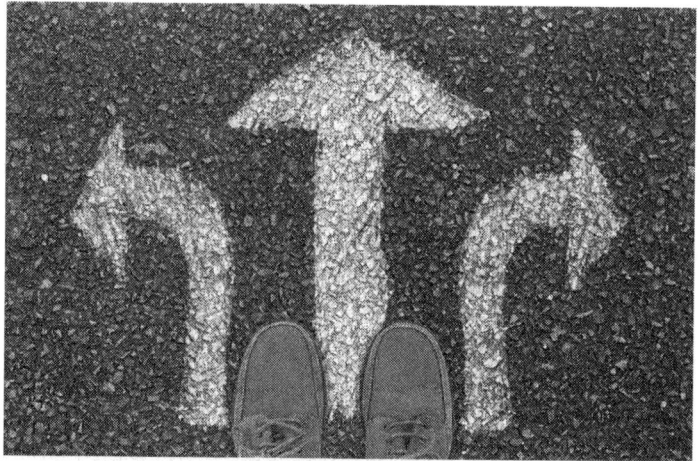

For all the gut an intuition out there, the truth is that making decisions based on fact are always guaranteed to be more effective than those based on assumptions. In fact, some of the world's biggest mistakes have been made when basing decisions on assumptions.

In the financial world, speculation can make investors insanely rich overnight. If they guess right, they can make their retirement with a few keystrokes. However, if they are wrong, they can end up in jail.

That is why savvy investors base their decisions on numbers, financials, and solid technical analysis. If the numbers don't paint the right picture, the savvy investor is prepared to leave a deal on the table.

Now, learning to listen to your gut is important. Yet, listening to your gut is a skill that becomes sharpened with experience. As you learn throughout the course of your life, your instincts tell you when something is on the up and up, or if there is something fishy. It isn't some magical sixth sense; it's your experience telling you what might be a good opportunity from a poor choice.

At the end of the day, your decisions ought to be based on the information you have on hand at any given moment. For instance, if you are planning to make a large purchase and you are betting on a future raise or promotion which may, or may not happen, then you are asking for trouble.

If you base your decision on the information you have available at the time of making a said decision, you will err on the side of caution. So, if you do end up getting that promotion, you won't have to sweat it. You will have extra money to play around with. However, if you bet on getting that promotion, and it doesn't happen, you'll find yourself in a pickle when it comes time to pay up.

So, always base your decisions on fact, not assumptions, and you'll come up a winner each time.

Chapter 49: Stop Overthinking for an Easier and Happier Life

At this point, there is one more thing to be said: overcoming any tendencies to overthink will lead you to a happier and easier life.

How is this possible?

Think about it along these lines: the amount of brainpower that you are freeing up will allow you to focus on the truly productive and truly valuable things in life. You will be able to get ahead in your profession and cherish the moments with your loved ones.

Naturally, everything must come to an end at some point. But if you stop dwelling on the fact that your loved one might leave you one day, and instead opt for treasuring the time they are actually with you, you will find that living a happy and productive life is not nearly as hard as you might have once thought.

You have everything you need to be happy and successful. It's just that we often make the mistake of misallocating your time and energy on fruitless endeavors. When you learn to see such activities for what they are, you will become a much more balanced and centered person.

While overthinking will creep up to you from time to time, the truth is that you shouldn't let it become more important than it ought to be.

So, please look at life's problems in terms of opportunities rather than problems. When you look at life in terms of opportunities, the world magically opens up. Since you are not dwelling on the issue itself, but rather on the solution, you can pick and choose from the worst, and certainly the best, options available to you.

Then, when you are able to solve the problem at hand, you will come out of it a much more experienced and interesting person. You will be able to offer the world the fruits of your efforts.

What could be better than that?

Conclusion

Thank you for making it through to the end of *Overthinking*, let's hope it was informative and able to provide you with all of the tools you need to achieve your goals whatever they may be.

The next step is to put to practice what you have learned.

Strategies to Overcome Stress

Positive Mindset to Stop Negativity
Anxiety and Anger Management Tips

Mindfulness and Neuroplasticity Approach to Reach Mental Health and Live a Longer, Happier Life

By Albert Dales

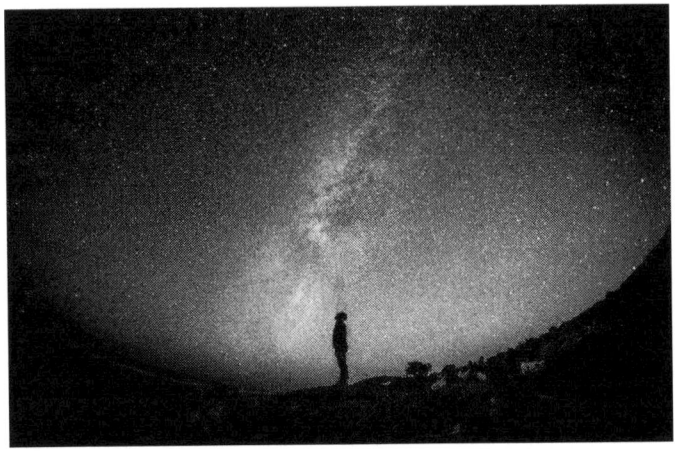

© **Copyright 2019 by Albert Dales - All rights reserved.**

The content contained within this book may not be reproduced, duplicated or transmitted without direct written permission from the author or the publisher.

Under no circumstances will any blame or legal responsibility be held against the publisher, or author, for any damages, reparation, or monetary loss due to the information contained within this book. Either directly or indirectly.

Legal Notice:

This book is copyright protected. This book is only for personal use. You cannot amend, distribute, sell, use, quote or paraphrase any part, or the content within this book, without the consent of the author or publisher.

Disclaimer Notice:

Please note the information contained within this document is for educational and entertainment purposes only. All effort has been executed to present accurate, up to date, and reliable, complete information. No warranties of any kind are declared or implied. Readers acknowledge that the author is not engaging in the rendering of legal, financial, medical or professional advice. The content within this book has been derived from various sources. Please consult a licensed professional before attempting any techniques outlined in this book.

By reading this document, the reader agrees that under no circumstances is the author responsible for any losses, direct or indirect, which are incurred as a result of the use of the information contained within this document, including, but not limited to, — errors, omissions, or inaccuracies.

Table of Contents

Introduction 248
Chapter 1: What Is Stress? 251
The Science Behind Stress 252
Different Types of Stress 253
Acute Stress 254
Episodic Acute Stress 254
Chronic Stress 255
Symptoms of Stress 256
Chapter 2: Causes of Stress 260
External and Internal Stress Factors 260
External Stress Factors 261
Internal Stress Factors 262
Common Causes of Stress 263
Financial Problems 263
Work 264
Personal Relationships 265
Parenting 266
Daily Life 266
Personality 267
Common Triggers of Stress 267
Work-Related Triggers 267
Financial Triggers 268
Health-Related Triggers 269
Relationship Triggers 269
Chapter 3: How to Overcome Stress 271
Tip #1: Identifying Your Stressors 271
Tip #2: Practice Stress Management 272
Tip #3: Get Active 274
Tip #4: Socialize 275
Tip #5: Leisurely Activities 276
Tip #6: Time Management 277
Tip #7: Maintaining Balance 278
Tip #8: Relieving Stress in the Moment 279
Other Important Tips: 279
Chapter 4: Other Mental Health Disorders Related to Stress 280
What Is An Anxiety Disorder? 280
Generalized Anxiety Disorder (GAD) 281
What Are the Different Types of Anxiety Disorders? 282
Social Anxiety 283
Specific Phobias 283
Panic Disorders 284
What Is a Depression Disorder? 286
Types of Depression 287
Mild and Moderate Depression 287
Major Depression 287
Atypical Depression 287
Seasonal Affective Disorder (SAD) 288
What is an Anger Disorder? 288
Anger as a Manifestation of Other Emotions 288
Chapter 5: How to Overcome Mental Health Disorders 290
Lifestyle Changes 290
Psychotherapy 291
Cognitive Behavioral Therapy 292
How does Cognitive Behavioral Therapy Work? 293
Interpersonal Therapy 295
Psychodynamic Therapy 297
Blended Approaches 298
Medical Treatment 298
Chapter 6: Stress and Anger Management Techniques 300
Action-Oriented Approaches 300
Emotion-Oriented Approaches 301
Acceptance-Oriented Approaches 301
Anger Management Techniques 301

Chapter 7: Mindfulness And Meditation Techniques 304
Mindfulness Meditation 304
The Joyful Mind Meditation 305
Chapter 8: Neuroplasticity 310
Factors That Increase Neuroplasticity in Adults 310
Conclusion 312

Introduction

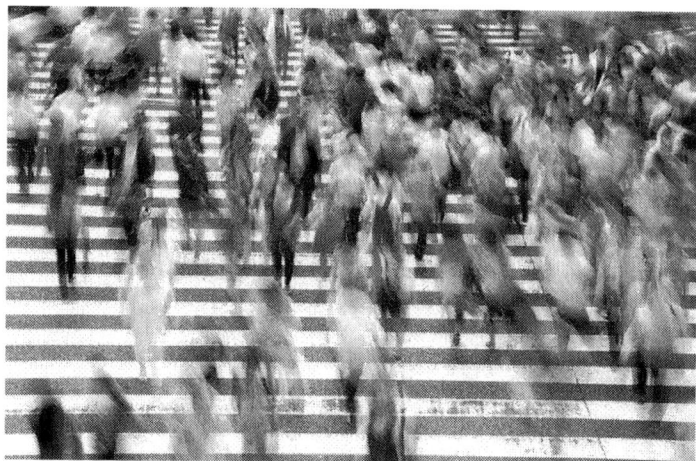

As our modern world becomes increasingly fast-paced, many of us find ourselves overwhelmed with stress on a daily basis. Are you someone that is constantly stressed out about things in the workplace? Or are you someone that's recently going through a hard time? Or maybe you are planning to make a big life change, and there are a lot of factors you need to consider. Regardless of where your stress is coming from, too much of it is never good, and stress could start affecting our mental and physical health. This book will help guide you into learning about what stress is, causes of it, and ways to overcome it. More importantly, stress can affect people so much that they increase their risk of developing other mental disorders such as anxiety, depression, anger disorders, and panic disorders. This book will help explore what those disorders are and techniques to manage and overcome them. We will be learning about techniques that range from lifestyle changes to psychotherapy methods like Cognitive Behavioral Therapy and Medical treatment. Towards the end of this book, we will explore stress and anger management techniques, mindfulness, and meditation, and learn about neuroplasticity.

Before we dive into all of that, what exactly is stress? We have all felt it, experienced it, and dislike it, but have you ever thought about what it actually is? The dictionary definition of sex states that stress is 'the body's reaction to any change that requires an adjustment or response. The body reacts to these changes with physical, mental, and emotional responses.' In simple terms, stress is a reaction that we feel when we are faced with situations that are unpleasant and out of the ordinary. Stress is a normal part of human life and is actually a natural response in our body. Without stress, the human race would not have evolved to the way it is now. Stress is our body's way of warning us from danger or letting us know that our actions will have a negative effect on our mental wellbeing.

From the time that we were cavemen, stress has been very much existent. While humans today stress about having enough money to pay their rent or whether or not their significant other is cheating on them, humans back in the day stressed about hunting and gathering food or whether or not they would make it through the winter with the limited sources that they have. Although circumstances are largely different, the stress we feel is still exactly the same. In the modern world today, stress has become a huge epidemic that affects over 54% of our population. In fact, stress is such an impending epidemic in our world today that the CDC stated that over 110 million die every year as a direct result of stress. So, you must be wondering, why is everyone so stressed? How come people back in the day aren't as stressed compared to us? Well, the simple answer is that the world we live in is many times more fast-paced compared to the world our ancestors lived in. Us humans now are exposed to what we call an 'information overload' through the invention of social media and the internet. We are constantly connected with other people from all over the world and of different life stages. We find ourselves comparing to celebrities with extravagant lifestyles and people we know that seem to have 'everything together' on social media. We constantly feel as if what we have is not enough and we are constantly striving for more. In fact, we live in such a toxic society nowadays that people are being praised for dedicating their entire life to work. People that try to balance their work and personal life are deemed as 'lazy' or they have no ambition. Using your sick days or calling in sick to work when you're feeling under the weather is a negative thing. This type of culture in our world today is one of the leading causes of the significant increase in stress.

Moreover, the society we live in today is expensive. What used to cost $1 now costs $5. Housing prices are on the rise, and it doesn't seem like it's stopping anytime soon. Due to the invention and popularity of credit cards and housing loans, people are burying themselves in significant debt. Life nowadays seems like a constant race in trying to simply catch up. In some ways, society is built against us. All of these reasons are why people are beginning to suffer many mental health disorders due to the overwhelming amount of stress.

When people spend most of their time working only to make ends meet, they begin to get discouraged easily. For instance, housing prices in big cities in the world like New York City, San Francisco, and Toronto are at an all-time high. A one-bedroom apartment that used to cost $1200 now is costing upwards of $2300. Salaries have remained unchanged for the most part. Most adults that make a fair salary of $50,000 can barely afford to live in their own one-bedroom apartment. When people are struggling with financial instability, stress begins to arise more than ever and slowly seeps into other parts of their life. For instance, if you are someone who is constantly struggling to pay rent and have enough money for other life expenses, you likely won't engage in social gatherings, self-care habits and exercise. Your stress remains in the financial realm, so you focus all your energy on making ends meet. By doing that, you are actually neglecting a lot of activities that are crucial for stress reduction. Humans are social creatures and require contact from other people in order to remain content. Exercise is also a natural way for humans to feel good and confident. Due to just one problem of financial insecurity, it begins to affect other parts of a person's life, which increases their overall stress level even more. This book will help guide you in terms of providing you with techniques to prevent extreme stress in the first place and to teach you how to overcome stress when you are confronted with it.

If you haven't gotten the message yet, stress reduction is extremely important, and everybody needs to be aware of the significant and negative effects it has on people. A common misconception about stress is that you can just 'ignore' it, or you are 'weak' for even feeling stressed in the first place. These thoughts are all incorrect. We know that stress is a natural reaction in humans and therefore, we are not 'weak' by feeling it. In fact, humans would've never made it this far if they simply just 'ignored' their feelings of stress. They likely would've been hunted by some sort of predator if they didn't have the instinct to tell them what to do. Other than the fact that reducing stress will help you live a happier and healthier life, it also helps prevent other problems such as mental disorders and bad physical health. Mental disorders such as anxiety and depression are often caused when a person undergoes a huge amount of stress. Although this is not the only factor in having these disorders, stress is one of the biggest ones. Moreover, stress also heavily impacts a person's physical health. Another common misconception is that physical health is entirely related to physical factors like your diet and exercise levels. Stress actually directly impacts a person's physical health due to its huge role in their mental health. Just like how it is hard to have good mental health when a person is in bad physical condition, it is hard to have good physical health when a person is in bad mental condition. There needs to be a healthy balance of maintaining good wellbeing and health at the same time.

You might be thinking that some of this stuff sounds very scary. However, you'd be happy to know that with a few simple techniques and lifestyle changes, you can significantly reduce your stress. By changing certain habits mentally and physically, they both influence each other to give you a healthier mind and body. The ideal way to overcome stress is to prevent it in the first place. This book will provide you with tips and steps on how to do this. You will also be given the opportunity to learn everything you need to know in order to overcome stress when you are facing it head-on. Rather than letting it take over you entirely, this book will help you find ways to cope and to better manage it in order to minimize the effect it has on your health. Let's not waste any time and dive right in!

Chapter 1: What Is Stress?

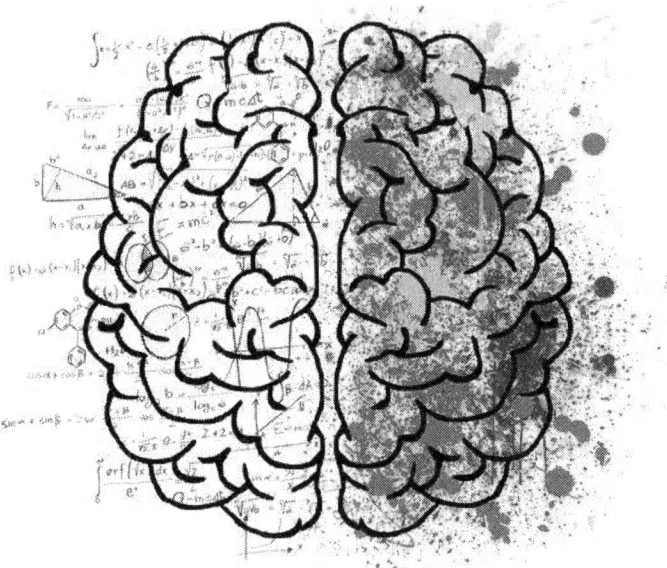

Imagine you are trying to concentrate on a deadline for work that's due in one hour. It's 7 pm at the office, and everyone has left. All you can hear are the overnight cleaning staff that is chatting away in the office and moving things around loudly. You feel your heart rate rising, and you are beginning to grind your teeth. Your stomach begins to feel bothered as well. Your mind starts racing, and you literally start contemplating just quitting and never coming back to this place. That would be better than being unable to finish that deadline looming over you. This is exactly what stress feels like to most people. According to recent statistics, nearly 40% of people reported that their levels of stress have gone up over the last year and almost 45% said their stress had increased significantly over the past 5 years.

Most people that participated in those studies agreed that stress negatively impacted their quality of life. However, although most of these people all agree on understanding the symptoms of stress, more than 30% of these participated were convinced that stress is simply a psychological experience and believed that it did not impact their physical health. Throughout this book, you will slowly find that this is extremely untrue. Let's start looking into the human stress response and see how it physically impacts a person.

Numerous experts across the globe all agree that thinking stress is only a psychological feeling that is a very dangerous misconception. They used an analogy to explain this further. Since the human stress response has evolved over the millions of years, it originally helped our ancestors identify danger and food. This is very natural; without it, humans would be trying to befriend bears rather than gathering berries from forests. There are a lot of threats back in those days that range from avoiding predators to finding food. This is completely natural and without our stress response, we would've never made it this far. However, what isn't natural is how modern life exposes us to milder threats, but the stress we feel is constant. This is due to being overwhelmed with stimulation, juggling too many things, multitasking, and being always on the go. In simpler terms, humans were not designed to run away from predators for 10+ hours per day without any breaks. Essentially, this is what humans are doing in modern-day society.

Many experts have named the common condition of chronic stress in our society as the "superstress". Humans are now being overwhelmed with numerous stressors that we almost take for granted. This includes; inadequate salaries, job dissatisfaction, being overworked, not having enough time for family and friends, lack of time outside, noise pollution, and feeling like their life has no purpose or meaning. The crazy part about all of this is that our body cannot physically differentiate the difference between being attacked by a bear and getting a bad job review. The chemical and biological response in our body is the exact same. Due to this, the body begins to get worn down due to the intensity of the stress.

When people are constantly in a state of stress all day, they are overusing every element of their bodies. The result is a series of stress symptoms. In fact, some people's stress can get so bad that it evolves from simply being 'annoying' into debilitating. Many people can develop other mental disorders when they are under too much stress such as; anxiety and depression. Let's take a look into what is happening with our biochemistry when we are stressed out.

The Science Behind Stress

The stress response that we feel starts within your brain. A stress signal is sent throughout your brain to the hypothalamus, which then messages your nervous system to protect you from the threat. This then influences the nervous system to begin increasing your heart rate to get you ready for fight or flight mode. Due to this, all your blood rushes to your muscles to get you ready to defend yourself which then slows down the other functions of your body. This includes; your digestive secretions, intestines, and your body begins to flood with cortisol. When your body is reacting this way too often, it begins to cause significant physical damage. Whenever there is too much cortisol running through your brain for extended amounts of time, hippocampal brain damage begins to occur. This causes people to have their sleep cycle disturbed, have memory loss, mood swings, and they always feel not 'all there' due to the brain fog.

The pituitary gland also becomes very affected during stress responses. Its responsibility is to regulate bodily functions such as; thyroid activity, urine production, and body temperature. This is why when people are nervous or anxious, they feel like they have to use the bathroom frequently. During times of high stress, cortisol is produced from these glands and pulls fat and glucose from the body into the person's bloodstream for energy. This is why during acute stress that a lot of people feel like they don't have an appetite.

The heart is another organ that is heavily affected during high-stress times. Blood vessels become constricted which makes it difficult for the heart to properly pump blood. People begin to have high blood pressure due to the smaller blood vessels. In addition, your adrenal glands are heavily affected as when your body detects stress. It signals your adrenal glands to release adrenaline and noradrenaline into your body. These hormones are responsible for increasing both blood pressure and heart rate. Due to your blood being pumped into your extremities, it produces a feeling like there are 'butterflies' in your stomach. When this process happens frequently and does not leave you time to recuperate in between, you begin to feel wound up and tired at the same time. Almost like the feeling of drinking coffee but still feeling tired and having a racing heart. When people go through stress too often, the stress wears out the adrenal glands which can lead to exhaustion, depression, physical weakness, immune suppression, skin problems and hormone imbalances in the long term.

As mentioned earlier, a person's stomach and digestive system are heavily affected when under times of stress as the blood is being pulled from there and spread to other parts of your body. When your digestive system is slowed down due to this process, your digestive acids can either be overproduced which will lead to acid reflux or under-produced which means that your stomach has lower digestive power. When a person has too little stomach acid, the food in their belly actually ferments rather than digests, which creates bloating.

Although there are even amounts of people that report stress helped them lose weight and helped them gain weight, research found that having high levels of cortisol encourages weight gain. Cortisol increases a person's appetite for fast energy creating cravings for sugar and carbohydrates. It also puts in extra glucose in a person's body, and when it's not burned off through exercise, the extra glucose gets stored as fat in the body. When a person is under chronic stress, it is the true enemy to overall fitness. People tend to gain weight because their cravings are stronger, and it's making it more likely that you hold onto food as fat, especially in the abdominal area.

The reproductive system is also affected when under stress as the increased production of cortisol causes a lower production of progesterone, which is a hormone for fertility in women. When those amounts are lowered, it leads to possible infertility and low libido. This is why when people are under a lot of stress, they don't want to have sex or engage in sexual activity.

I hope this explanation of the science behind stress helps you understand that stress does indeed play a huge role in the physical wellbeing of someone. It is not simply just a 'psychological' response. When a person is under chronic stress for extended amounts of time, their physical health begins to suffer significantly. This is why millions of people every year have to take time off as a 'stress leave' as their bodies are suffering too much from the reactions. Let's start taking a look at the different types of stress that people feel.

Different Types of Stress

As you may already know, there are different types or levels of stress. The stress that you feel before writing an exam compared to the stress that you feel when you are going through a traumatic experience is very different. The frequency of the stress you feel also plays a huge factor in what type of stress you have. According to the APA (American Psychological

Association), there are 3 different types of stress; acute stress, episodic acute stress, and chronic stress. Within each of these stress types, they each have their own duration, symptoms, characteristics, and treatments. This is why stress management is very complicated. The 3 different types of stress can also be in the form of single, repeated, complicated, or chronic. Due to this, each type requires different levels and types of treatment and management according to that individual's lifestyle, environment, coping resources, personality, and developmental history. Let's take a look into the three different types:

Acute Stress

Acute stress is usually very brief and is the most common stress type out there. It also tends to happen frequently and is caused by reactive thinking. When a person has negative thoughts that dominate their mind in situations that have occurred recently, future situations, or near-future demands. For instance, if a person has been in an argument recently, they may begin to have stress that is related to the negative thoughts that are ongoing in their mind. They may also be having acute stress regarding an upcoming deadline, which is also induced through their thoughts. However, when a person changes those negative thoughts into something more positive or if they reduce the frequency of those negative thoughts, their stress will begin to subside as well. Here are some of the most common symptoms of acute stress:

- Transient stomach problems; heartburn, constipation, diarrhea, flatulence, acid stomach, and any gut and bowel problems
- Transient muscular distress; headache, tension, back pain, jaw pain, neck pain, and other muscular tensions
- Transient emotional distress; a combination of irritability or anger, and anxiety and depression
- Transient hyperarousal; increased heartbeat, rapid pulse, increased blood pressure, dizziness, migraines, sleep problems, shortness of breath, chest pain, heart palpitations, and cold hands/feet

Episodic Acute Stress

People who experience acute stress frequently, or is living a life that is full and frequent with stressors, are more likely to have episodic acute stress. These people who suffer from this tend to live in a life of crisis and chaos. They tend to feel pressured all the time and are always in a rush. They may take on too many responsibilities but struggle with staying organized when there are too many deadlines. There are two main personality types that are more likely to have episodic acute stress. The first type is anyone with "A" type personality, and the second type is the 'worrier'.

People who have 'Type A' personalities tend to be very competitive, abrupt, aggressive, impatient, and have a strong sense of urgency. They also tend to be insecure about their performance and feeling the need to be perfect every time. People with these personality traits often create episodes of stress for themselves frequently. Due to this, scientists have found that people with 'type A' personality tend to be more likely to develop heart disease later on in life.

The worrier type are people that constantly have negative thoughts that negatively cause stress on their mental and physical health. These types of people are always projecting disasters or negatively assuming a catastrophe throughout their lives. They tend to have a strong belief that the world is a dangerous place where something bad will always happen to them. These people have a lot of negative thoughts that make them depressed and anxious. These people are more likely to be diagnosed with GAD (generalized anxiety disorder). Here are some of the symptoms of the episodic effects of acute stress:

- Immune system compromise: Constantly getting allergies, flu, colds, and other types of illnesses related to immune system compromise
- High blood pressure: migraines, rapid heartbeat, dizziness, insomnia, heart disease, heart palpitations, and cold hands/feet
- Stomach: irritable bowel syndrome (IBS), constipation, diarrhea, flatulence, acid stomach, heartburn, bowel problems, and gut problems
- Muscular distress: Ligament problems, tendons, pulled muscles, jaw pain, back pain, headaches, and body tension
- Deterioration of interpersonal relationships: workplace becomes too stressful for them
- Cognitive distress: mental fatigue, compromised new learning abilities, compromised processing speed, compromised attention, and concentration
- Emotional distress: Tenseness, impatience, short-tempered, depression, anxiety, irritability, and anger issues

Chronic Stress

The most harmful type of stress out of all three types is chronic stress. When it is left untreated for an extended amount of time, chronic stress can cause damage that can damage your physical and mental health irreversibly. For instance, poor work environments, long term poverty, unemployment, repeated abuse in any form, dysfunctional family, or an unhappy marriage can cause a person significant chronic stress. When a person feels hopeless and does not see any way out of it and gives up entirely on finding solutions, chronic stress can set in and begin affecting their physical and mental health. When a person continuously lives with chronic stress, their emotional and behavioral actions can become ingrained within them. The wiring of their brain and body begins to change and makes them more prone to the negative effects that stress has on a person's body regardless of what's actually happening to them.

Chronic stress is a grinding type of stress because it wears people down day after day. It negatively impacts the body and mind in a significant way and has the power to change a person forever. Chronic stress can be so dangerous in fact, that it can kill people due to suicide, heart attacks, strokes, and even cancer. There are treatment practices that can help people manage their chronic stress, but it requires them to be actively practicing those techniques throughout their lives. Later on, this book, we will be exploring numerous treatment methods for stress disorders and related disorders that can be caused by stress. If you think you are someone that is suffering from chronic stress, get help right away. Seek professional opinion and get it diagnosed, that will be the first step in discovering what methods are most suitable for your type of stress. In some cases, you may not even have chronic stress and just another type of stress. In that case, different methods and techniques will be pursued in order to properly manage it. Next up in this chapter, we will be looking at the general symptoms of stress. This will help you identify whether or not you feel like you have a stress disorder.

Symptoms of Stress

At this point, you have an understanding of the science behind stress and the different types of stress. In order to further your knowledge in this area, let's take a look at some of the symptoms of stress. Although stress shows itself in different ways depending on the individual, there are a few common symptoms that most people experience. By understanding the symptoms related to stress, you will be able to identify when you are experiencing it. An important part of stress management is identifying triggers and stressors, in order to be able to do this, you need to know what symptoms you show when you're stressed and figure out when they occur. Let's take a look at the most common symptoms of stress:

- **Acne**

One of the most visible ways that stress shows itself in a person is through acne. When people are under a lot of stress, they have the tendency to touch their faces with their hands frequently, which causes bacteria spreading into their pores, which develops cane. Scientific studies have also confirmed that high levels of stress causes a higher risk of acne. To be specific, one of these studies measured a group of people's level of acne before and during a school exam. At the end of the study, they found that when people had increased levels of stress, they developed more severe acne. A similar study focused on teenagers found that worse acne was also associated with stress levels, particularly in boys. Although these studies show a strong association between stress levels and acne, it doesn't take into account other factors that may be playing a role. More research in this area is needed in order to further prove the connection. Besides stress, acne can be caused by; blocked pores, excess oil production, bacteria, and hormonal shifts.

- **Headaches**

Just like acne, many scientific studies have found a relationship between high levels of stress and headaches. This includes pain that is in the head or neck region. One scientific study that tested this relationship consisted of around 250 people that were suffering from chronic headaches. The scientists found that within those people, 45% of them had recently endured a stressful event. A similar but larger study found that the increased number of headaches that occurred over a one-month span was associated with an increase in stress intensity. If that's not enough evidence, another similar study focused on 150 military professionals at a clinic specialized for headaches. They found that nearly 70% of those who had headaches said that they are stress-induced. This makes stress the second most common trigger for headaches. Lastly, other common triggers of headaches can include dehydration, alcohol consumption, and lack of sleep.

- **Chronic Pain**

People commonly report that they have an increased amount of pains and aches in their bodies when they are under a lot of stress. One study that focused on this relationship consisted of about 40 people that had sickle cell disease. They found that when they had increased levels of stress on a daily basis that they also felt an increase in pain as well. Another study focused on studying cortisol, the stress hormone, and how it is also associated with chronic pain when it's levels are increased. For instance, there was a study that consisted of 16 people who reported to have chronic back pain. When they studied them further, they found that these people had high levels of cortisol. Another similar study found that people who reported to have chronic pain had higher levels of cortisol within their hair. This is an indicator of someone who has been under prolonged stress. Again, bear in mind that these studies have shown relationships between stress and chronic pain, but we still have to consider other factors that could be playing a role as well. Moreover, it is still unsure whether chronic pain causes stress or if stress causes chronic pain. This is something that still needs to be further studied. There are several other factors that could be playing a role in increasing chronic pain, such as nerve damage, poor posture, injuries, and age.

- **Frequent Sickness**

If you are someone that feels like you are always sick, or always battling allergies or a case of sniffles, stress can be the culprit. Stress takes a huge toll on people's immune systems, which will put you at a higher risk of infections. In a recent study, a group of 60 adults were given the flu vaccine. They found that the people who had a weakened response to that vaccine indicated that stress is related to decreased immunity. In a similar study, over 200 adults were selected and split into two groups; low stress and high stress. Throughout a 6-month period of time, 70% of the people that were in the high-stress group experienced respiratory infections. They also had 60% more symptoms of the illness compared to the low-stress group. In addition to this study, another similar study showed that a person's increased susceptibility to developing a respiratory illness was linked to increased levels of stress. Again, more of these relationships still require further research as the connection between stress and immunity is a complex one. Although stress is related to a person's immune health, it can also be caused by other factors such as multiple myeloma, leukemia, physical inactivity, and a poor diet.

- **Insomnia And Decreased Energy**

When a person is under high levels of prolonged stress, they can begin to feel that they have decreased levels of energy and chronic fatigue. For instance, a study of over 2000 participants reported that tiredness and constant fatigue was in fact, associated with high-stress levels. Stress also affects a person's sleep cycle and could cause conditions like insomnia, which could be the cause of fatigue. A small study found that people who had high levels of stress-related to work were associated with restlessness before bed and increased sleepiness throughout the day. Another study that also consisted of over 2000 2000 participants found that people who experienced higher numbers of stressful events were associated with an increased risk of insomnia. Similar to other symptoms, these studies show a relationship, but they may not be accounting for other factors that may be causing the symptom. More research in this area is required in order to directly define the relationship between stress and fatigue. Other factors that can cause fatigue include; underactive thyroid, a poor diet, low blood sugar, and dehydration.

- **Decreased Libido**

Numerous people experience a change in their sex drive when they are going through a stressful time. A small study that focused on a group of 30 women evaluated their stress levels and then had them watch an erotic film to measure their arousal. The women that had higher levels of stress reported less arousal compared to those that were less stressed. A similar study that was larger consisted of about 100 women that found that high levels of stress were directly associated with their lower levels of sexual satisfaction and activity. In addition, a similar study focused on over 300 participants and found that the people who reported that they had high levels of stress found that their sexual satisfaction, arousal, and desire were negatively impacted. Again, you must also consider other factors that may be contributing to a person's changing libido. This could include psychological causes, fatigue, and hormonal changes.

- **Digestive Issues**

When people are experiencing higher levels of stress, they tend to have problems with their digestive system, such as constipation and diarrhea. In one study, they had nearly 3000 children that participated, and they found that when they were exposed to stressful events, they had an increased risk of constipation. Stress also affects people who already have digestive disorders such as inflammatory bowel disease (IBD) or irritable bowel syndrome (IBS). These two disorders share traits such as constipation, diarrhea, bloating and stomach pain. In another study of almost 200 women, they found that high daily levels of stress were linked to an increase in their digestive distress. In addition, an overall analysis that focused on 18 different studies that explored the relationship between stress and digestive diseases, found that almost 75% of these studies have found a relationship between a person's digestive system and stress levels. We have to keep in mind that although these studies show a strong association, more studies are required in order to look at how stress impacts a person's digestive system. Other factors can also cause digestive issues such as; medications, infections, physical activity levels, dehydration, and diet.

- **Appetite Changes**

One of the most commonly reported symptoms of stress is a change in a person's appetite. When people are feeling stressed out, they often are showcasing two extremes; they're either raiding their fridge in the middle of the night, or they have no appetite or desire to eat at all. A scientific study that focused on students in college found that around 80% found that they had appetite changes when they were under high stress. Out of this population of students, nearly 40% experienced a decrease in appetite while around 60% reported an increase in appetite. In a similar study of around 100 people, they found that these people, when under stress, exhibited behaviors like eating even when they are not hungry. A person's change in appetite can also be caused by weight fluctuations during high-stress times. For instance, a study of over 1000 people found that weight gain in overweight adults was associated with stress. Although these studies show a strong association between the change in a person's appetite and stress levels and weight, more studies are required in order to further understand what other factors could be involved. Other factors include; psychological conditions, hormonal shifts, drugs, or certain medications.

- **Depression**

Certain studies suggest that the development of depression is related to chronic stress. One study that consisted of around 800 women that had depression found that the beginning stages of their depression were heavily associated with them having chronic or acute stress. Another study discovered that higher levels of depressive symptoms were associated with increased levels of stress. This study consisted of around 200 adolescents. In another study, a study of around 40 people that had major depression found that their depressive episodes were related to stressful life events. Keep in mind that these studies have shown associations between depression and stress, but it does not mean that every case of depression is caused by it. A lot more research is required on this topic in order to 100% confirm the role that stress plays as it relates to depression. Other factors that aren't stress that contribute to depression include; certain medications, environmental factors, hormone levels, and family history.

- ***Rapid Heartbeat***

Symptoms of high-stress levels often include an increased heart rate or a fast heartbeat. One study that found an association between stress and rapid heartbeats discovered that a person's heart rate is much higher when they are going through a stressful situation. Another similar study focused on about 100 teenagers, and they discovered that an increase in heart rate was caused by undergoing a stressful task. In addition, another similar study exposed about 90 students to stressful tasks and found that they had increased blood pressure and heart rates. Interestingly, however, they found that playing relaxing and soothing music during that task prevented a rapid heartbeat. An increased heartbeat can also be caused by other factors such as drinking alcohol, caffeine, heart conditions, thyroid disease, and high blood pressure.

- ***Sweating***

When a person is under a lot of stress, it can cause them to sweat excessively. A small study that consisted of 20 participants that had a condition that caused them to have excessive sweating in their palms. This study monitored their sweating rate throughout the day using a scale of 0-10. They found that stress and exercise both increased the sweating rate significantly by 2 to 5 points. Another study discovered that when a person is exposed to stress, it also resulted in more sweating and odor within 40 teenage participants. Other factors that can cause excessive sweating include; medications, thyroid conditions, heat exhaustion, and anxiety.

Chapter 2: Causes of Stress

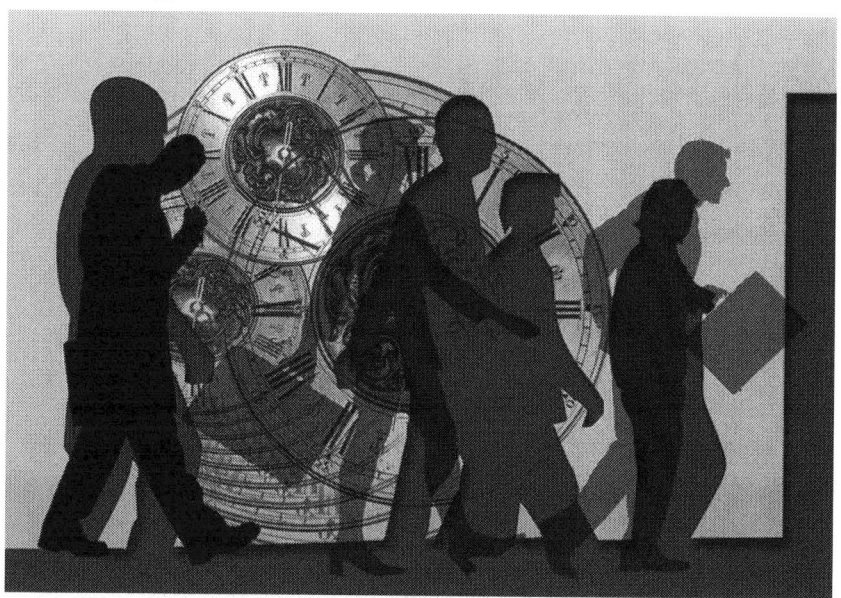

In order to properly manage your specific stressors, you must know what exactly causes your stress in the first place. Some people have a higher tolerance for stress compared to others, but people often share the same causes of stress. Just like back in the ancient days, most people shared the same stressor of being hunted by a stronger predator, like a bear. Nowadays, people likely share the same stressor of not being able to financially support themselves and ending up in an impoverished situation. When a person is able to identify which situations are causing their stress, they can then learn how to either manage those stressors or prevent them in the first place. In this chapter, we will be learning about external and internal stress factors, the common causes of stress, common triggers of stress, and the importance of understanding what your stress triggers are. Let's dive right in.

External and Internal Stress Factors

In order to effectively manage one's stress, it begins with being able to identify what your sources of stress are and then developing the proper strategies to manage them. An effective way to do this is to simply make a list of challenges, concerns, or situations that triggers your stress response. If you can think of a few of these situations off of the top of your head, take a moment to write them down in order to identify what your top issues are right now. You may notice that some of your stressors are events that happen to you outside of your control or while others seem to happen within oneself. Let's take a look at external factors first.

External Stress Factors

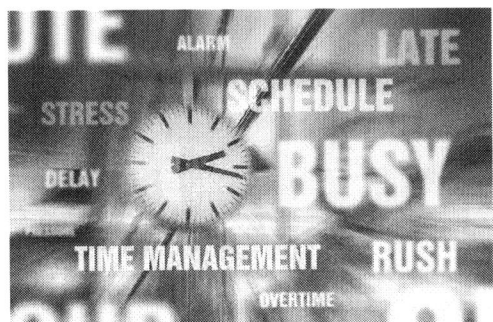

Keep in mind that external stress factors are situations or events that happen to you. Most of the time, these situations are out of your control unless you take active measures to prevent them. External factors include:

Social: Relationships tend to be a huge source of stress for most people. This could range from meeting new people to going on a blind date or even just having a night out with your friends. When you are in a relationship or in close contact with your family, stress tends to spawn from those places. Think about the last fight you had with your significant other, how stressed did you feel?

Workplace: Workplaces tend to be a huge source of stress for many people. Common stressors within the workplace include; sales targets, urgent deadlines, a demanding boss, endless emails, and an impossible workload. Toxic work environments make it very hard for people to not take their work home with them.

Unpredictable events: Events that happen out of the blue like getting into a fender bender or your basement flooding during a storm can cause you to have high levels of stress. These are events that are hard to prevent but unfortunately happens to all of us.

Environment: The environment of the world around us can be a big source of stress. Imagine being stuck in traffic for a few hours a day to get to work or having to prepare for an incoming snowstorm. Other factors like sudden noises from animals (barking dogs) can easily influence your stress levels and mood.

Major life changes: Although a lot of life changes can be positive such as a job promotion, a new home, a planned pregnancy, and a new marriage, some can be negative. Major life changes that are negative, like a divorce or the death of a loved one, can cause high levels of stress for most people.

There are many strategies that you can use to manage external stress factors. We will learn more of these later on in the book, but common strategies that are effective include; getting enough sleep, being physically active and eating a healthy diet. Utilizing others for help can also be helpful. Other factors like learning to be assertive, increasing your problem-solving skills, and managing your time more effectively have also reported to be effective for people that are looking to manage their stress. Like I mentioned earlier, start by writing a list of possible causes of stress. By identifying what those are, you can slowly determine which strategies would be efficient in managing it.

Internal Stress Factors

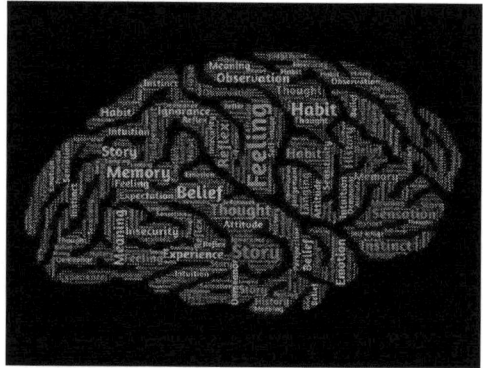

Not all stress is caused by external things happening to you. In fact, most people's stress is actually due to internal factors. Feelings and thoughts that pop into your head that cause you to feel stressed are known as internal stress factors. For instance, if there is a deadline at work looming and you begin to have negative thoughts like 'I'm going to get fired if I don't finish this on time', then that is an internal stress factor. This is why people who have anxiety disorders tend to feel more stressed frequently because they are constantly having anxious thoughts and a negative pattern of thinking. Having constant negative thoughts causes stress levels to rise. Here are some examples of internal stress factors:

> **Beliefs:** Beliefs can be a person's expectations, opinions or attitudes, or a combination of all three. Most people don't really think about how their beliefs shape their experiences, but having preset thought processes tends to cause stress with people. For instance, the expectations you have for yourself to advance your career or simply the expectations you have to create the perfect holiday party for your family and friends.
> **Uncertainty and lack of control:** Not many people enjoy not having control or not knowing what's about to happen. This can often cause stress when a person is faced with the fear of the unknown. For instance, think about how you may feel when you're awaiting the test results from a medical check-up.
> **Fears:** Everyone has fears; some people have more than others. Common fears that people have are flying, public speaking, and fear of failure.

The upside to all of this is that people have the ability to change and control their own thoughts. The downside is, however, that people's fears, expectations, and attitudes have been drilled into their brains for a very long time, and it will often take a lot of time and effort to rewire them. Later on, in this book, we will be learning about techniques that work effectively to help a person change their old and unhelpful thinking processes. Cognitive Behavioral Therapy is a type of speaking therapy that has proven to be extremely effective over the last few years. We will be learning more about it later.

Common Causes of Stress

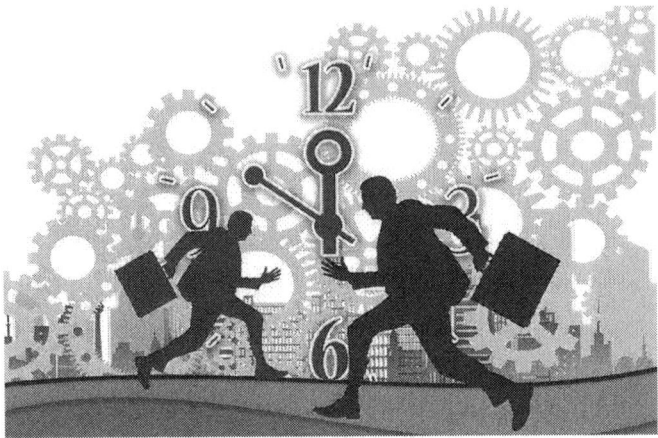

Although stress is a normal human reaction and is one that we need to survive, too much of it can cause us serious harm. Despite stress being something that everyone has experienced and continues to experience, it can manifest and be caused by different things from person to person. For example, one person may become very stressed and overwhelmed when they are stuck in a traffic jam, and they have some other place to be, while another person may be in the same situation but feel indifferent. Some people might be bothered all day if they had an argument with their significant other while another person may not be bothered by it at all! Some people may already aware of what exactly causes them to feel stressed. However, since preventing and overcoming extreme stress is crucial to having a happy and healthy life, it is definitely worth learning about what factors may be causing you stress specifically. Just because someone else gets stressed out about certain things, it may not apply to you! By learning specifically about what your stressors are, you can build a stress-reduction plan that is catered to you as an individual. Let's take a look at some of the most common causes of stress.

Financial Problems

Statistics-wise, money is the number one cause of stress in the United States. According to a survey conducted in 2015, it was reported that approximately 70% of Americans were stressed out about money in a recent time frame (less than one month). More than half of the people who participated in this study reported that money is the biggest cause of their stress with nearly 80% of these people feeling anxious about their finances. Although financial stress is a huge category, different people may experience different versions of it. Some people may be stressed about not having enough money for expendable income and may worry about not being able to go out to the bar with their friends on Friday nights while other people may be stressed about not having their electricity cut off since they weren't able to pay their bill for the fourth month in a row. Although these experiences are drastically different, both people still feel high levels of stress and need to find their own individual ways to overcome it and prevent it. Here are some signs of what financial stress may feel like:

- Being afraid to check their bank account balance, open their mail, or answer any phone calls
- Feeling guilty about spending money on items that are 'non-essential.'
- Having arguments with family and friends about money
- Feelings of worry and anxiety regarding money

Financial stress can take a long time to get out of. We're talking about months and years. Since financial stress is a type of long-term stress, it may cause extended health effects that are physical and psychological. Long-term effects of financial stress include; high blood pressure, stomach problems, headaches and migraines, insomnia, chest pains and a general feeling of unhealthiness. Through extended studies in the area of financial stress, it has been linked to a series of health issues. These include; anxiety, depression, arthritis, diabetes, and skin problems. If you think you are someone that is suffering from long-term financial stress, it may be time to put an action plan together to recover from whatever financial situations you are dealing with. This may be easier said than done, but avoiding financial problems only make it worse. Seek guidance from a financial advisor or a debt recovery service in order to explore your options.

Work

According to recent statistics, Americans now spend nearly 10% more time working compared to the working hours 20 years ago. Nearly 13% of people have to work a second job on top of their full-time job. It was also reported that 40% of people say their jobs are stressful, and nearly 30% of people report feeling burned out from working their job. There are multiple different things that can contribute to someone feeling work stress. This includes; job insecurity, too much work, dissatisfaction with their job or career, and conflicts with colleagues or bosses. Work stress can be caused in so many different ways. One person may be worried about a specific deadline at work that they are trying to meet, or they could be feeling like they are being treated unfairly, or they may be feeling stressed because they heard rumors about lay-offs while the holiday season is coming up. Often times, when people put their job ahead of other important things like family and relationships, it may begin to impact other aspects of their lives, such as their physical health, mental health, and personal relationships. There are also factors outside of work itself that could cause a person to have work stress; this could be their general health or how much emotional support they have away from the workplace. People who work stressful jobs but have a good support system of loved ones tend to be able to manage their stress better than those who don't. Here are some signs that point to work-related stress; it can be both physical and psychological:

- Difficulty making decisions or concentrating
- Mood swings
- Depression
- Anxiety
- Heart palpitations
- Stomach problems
- Muscle pains/tensions
- Headaches

- Fatigue

When people struggle to cope with their work stress and are feeling overwhelmed, it can impact not only their working behavior but their personal behavior as well. Here are some effects that work stress may have on people:
- Isolation
- Disinterest
- Increased levels of frustration and lower levels of patience
- Diminished initiative and creativity
- Problems with personal relationships
- Decreased work performance
- Increased number of sick days

Although work stress is normal when it comes to regulated amounts, too much of it can impact other parts of people's lives and may even increase stress in other areas. In order to keep work stress to a minimum, it is important to not bring your work home with you. Otherwise, people begin to feel like their entire lives are only about work and can cause feelings of resentment and depression. For most people, changing jobs may help greatly in reducing stress, while some may only require a change of mindset when they get home. Regardless, it is crucial to figure out not only if you have work stress but what part of the work it's coming from.

Personal Relationships

Stress can also be caused by the people in our lives. A family member, friend, coworker, or your significant other may be giving you a hard time which is causing your stress. It is impossible to not encounter any toxic people as you live your life and the stress caused by these people or maintaining a relationship with them can affect a person's mental and physical health. There are many causes of stress in romantic relationships, especially if the couple is under a lot of pressure or if there is a risk of their relationship ending. Although romantic relationships are the first type of relationship stress to come to mind, more common forms of relationship stress are actually from familial relationships. It could be the holidays coming up, and all family members are planning a get-together and you're feeling stressed about having to see a family member that you don't get along with. Here are some of the common relationship stressors:
- The relationship has abuse or a control problem
- Your partner and yourself are considering a divorce
- You and your partner are having too much alcohol or drug consumption
- There are serious communication problems between you and your partner
- Sex and intimacy have become infrequent due to health problems, busy-ness, or any other reasons
- Being too busy to have time to spend with one another and to distribute responsibilities evenly

Signs of stress that are caused by relationships are very similar to the symptoms of general stress. It can include a range of physical and mental health problems, especially when it comes to sleep. Often, you may find yourself avoiding the person you have conflict with or feeling agitated and irritated when they are near you. Nowadays, people can experience relationship stress through social media. Platforms like Instagram and Facebook encourage and make it easy for people to compare themselves with others. This can lead to feelings of inadequacy and also increases the chance of cyberbullying. Due to the technology in our society, you may not even need to know people directly in order to have relationship stress generated. You may simply be feeling stressed by looking at other people's pictures on social media and comparing what they have versus what you have.

Parenting

Parents are likely the most stressed people out of all of us. They are often juggling numerous things at once, like; working a full-time job, raising children, household duties and many other life duties. Numerous demands at the same time can cause a person a lot of stress if they are struggling to balance numerous important things at once. When a person is under a high level of parenting stress, it can cause them to be negative, harsh and have authoritarian-like interactions with their children. When a parent is under a lot of parenting stress, it can negatively impact the relationship between the parent and the child. For instance, a parent who is constantly in a bad mood and only focuses on lecturing their children rather than connecting with them may cause their child to not come to you for advice and may cause arguments often.

Causes of parenting stress can include single parenting, working long hours, lower-income, relationship, or marital problems, or raising a child who has a disability or has been diagnosed with behavioral disorders. In fact, parents with children who have health disorders or developmental delays actually are at the highest risk for increased parenting stress. In fact, many studies have shown that parents of autistic children report having higher parenting stress compared to parents with children that don't have those conditions.

Daily Life

Daily inconveniences are the causes of daily life stressors. For instance, running late to work, misplacing your wallet, or forgetting to bring an important document to a meeting with you are examples of how stress can be caused by day to day activities. Although these types of setbacks are minor, if they begin to happen frequently, they grow into a source of anxiety, which negatively impacts a person's psychological and/or physical health. Due to modern life growing increasingly busier for people, people are starting to have less and less time to pursue their own hobbies and leisurely activities. This creates a lot of stress for many people. Sadly, most of the time a person's busy-ness is created out of complete necessity in order to make ends meet. A common example of this is getting a second or even a third job in order to make enough money to get by. In other cases, some people may be making themselves busier due to agreeing to do things for/with other people in order to not want to disappoint people. People who struggle with assertiveness and being able to say 'no' are often the ones who end up having minimal time for themselves to do their own thing or even just attending to their basic needs. Have you ever heard of the saying 'you can't pour from a glass that's empty'?

That's exactly the case here. In order to spend time with others or to live a happy life, a person must take care of themselves; otherwise, they are at risk of a 'burnout'.

Personality

Lastly, personality is a huge part of determining how much stress a person feels and its effects on them. A person's personality traits affect all the other causes of stress above and can also be an independent source. People who classify as 'extroverts' tend to experience stress less often compared to others due to having more social resources, which act as a support system and buffer against stress. However, people who are 'perfectionists' may create more stress for themselves due to their high standards and often struggle with more physical and mental effects of stress. People that are opposite of perfectionists and are under-achievers are easily satisfied with their work as long as the job is done, these people are often under less stress as they don't hold a high expectation for themselves. Moreover, people who have the 'type A' personality not only stress themselves out, they can also stress out the people that are around them. These people tend to perfectionists but also are control freaks, so they want to make sure they are minimizing every risk possible in their lives. Money can also reduce stress as a person may be able to hire people in order to delegate stressful tasks. This is a resource that can help people reduce stress but can also cause people more stress if they don't have enough of it.

Common Triggers of Stress

After reading the last subchapter, you should have a general idea of what causes your stress specifically. You could be someone that doesn't get stressed at work, but if you are having an argument with a loved one, it may cause you extreme stress. By knowing what the general cause of stress is, you can look even more deeply into yourself and identify what exactly triggers your feelings of stress. For instance, if your main cause of stress is work then why are you feeling stressed about work on the weekends? The answer may be that you got an email or a work phone call on a Saturday morning that triggered your work stress. Or maybe your cause of stress is relationship problems, but all your relationships are doing fine at the moment, so why are you suddenly feeling stressed? Maybe you encountered a couple having an argument next to you when you were in line at the coffee shop, and it triggered feelings of stress related to relationships of your own. I hope this is starting to make sense to you because although you are not feeling stressed out due to your common causes of stress, factors around you can trigger feelings of stress. Keep in mind that stress triggers are different from stress causes. One can be triggered into feeling stressed, even if they have no reason to be.

Work-Related Triggers

If one of your main causes of stress is work-related, then work-related things or situations may trigger you into feeling stressed. For instance, if you were working hard all week to meet a deadline for the end of the day on Friday, you may be feeling a bit burnt out by the time the weekend rolls along. If you suddenly get an email on Saturday morning that is related to the project you just delivered, you may feel stressed and begin to think that there is something wrong with the project you delivered. Due to this, you may begin to panic. However, you may find that when you opened the email related to your work, it may just be a coworker saying 'great job!'.

Work-related triggers could range from emails, phone calls, or working relationships. For example, you may have agreed to go shopping with one of your coworkers on the weekend, but you may be feeling a bit apprehensive because you know you will end up talking about work, which would stress you out. Although working itself isn't actively stressing you out, the thought of conversation about work is. Here are some work-related triggers that you can look out for:

- Emails on off-hours
- Phone calls on off-hours
- Meeting up with coworkers outside of the workplace
- Being in the same vicinity as your workplace during off-work hours

If you identify with some of these triggers, there are active steps you can take in order to minimize your work-related stress. For starters, turn off all emails and work phone calls during the times you are not working. This will prevent you from being distracted from your leisurely time. Next, if you can avoid it, try not to be in the same vicinity as your workplace when you are not working. This may bring up feelings of stress as your brain automatically associates stress with a physical place. Lastly, unless necessary, avoid meeting up with coworkers outside of the workplace if that is a stress trigger for you. Oftentimes, hanging out with coworkers will cause conversations regarding work, which can easily bring up feelings of stress.

Financial Triggers

If one of the main causes of stress for you is money, then you may need to look deeper and figure out what exactly triggers that stress. It could be an upcoming bill payment or a phone call for debt collection, or it could be having to tell someone you can't go to dinner with them because you don't have any money. Regardless of what it is, when you identify what exactly your financial triggers are, then you can begin to manage your stress. For instance, if debt collection calls are the main sources of stress for you and you normally just ignore those calls or don't pick up when you see an unknown number, it may be time to tackle it, so these calls don't happen as frequently. You could pick up and work out some sort of payment plan with them even if it's in small amounts, that way, you are tackling your problem, and they won't call you as often if you make a plan with them. Here are some common financial triggers that cause people stress:

- Incoming debt collection calls
- A letter/bill for an overdue payment
- Overdraft warnings in your bank account
- Credit card promotions that you don't qualify for
- Not qualifying for a loan for something you need (e.g., a car, a mortgage)

If you identify with some of these triggers, it may help to seek advice from financial advisors or debt recovery professionals. There are options to settle your debt through consumer proposals or filing for bankruptcy. The positive effects of this type of debt recovery outweigh the downsides. When a person can start again at 0 with their finances, it often takes away a huge amount of stress and will cause some of their financial triggers to diminish. For instance, if they filed for bankruptcy and legally have no more debt, they will not get any more debt collection calls or mail about overdue payments.

Health-Related Triggers

If one of the main causes of your stress is due to health-related problems, then things that remind you of health issues can be your triggers. For instance, you may be feeling perfectly healthy, but you may have just read an article about how using Bluetooth earphones can cause brain cancer. This can cause you to become stressed since you use your Bluetooth headphones often. By identifying what your health triggers are, you can either make an effort to prevent being exposed to them, or you can seek therapy in this particular field to help heal from it. Here are some health-related triggers:

- Feeling like you're about to get sick
- Reading about health issues and thinking that you are affected by it
- Getting a medical check-up and awaiting the results
- Someone else around you is sick, and you're afraid they're contagious

If you relate to some of these triggers, then it may be time to find ways to prevent them. Typically, when people feel healthier, they feel that they are less likely to get sick. Making the proper lifestyle changes like eating a healthy diet and exercising frequently can help reduce some health-related stress. Frequent medical check-ups may help prevent nervousness around them if you constantly hear that your health is in order. A person's health and physical feeling are important in reducing stress. The healthier you feel, the bigger the buffer is to stress.

Relationship Triggers

If one of the main causes of your stress is due to your relationships, then you must identify what exactly those triggers are. For instance, if you had a history of verbal abuse from your family members, experiencing that happening to someone else may be enough to cause you stress even though it is not directly happening to you. Since relationships can be romantic, familial, friendship or professional, there can be a range of different triggers that cause you stress. Here are some examples of triggers related to relationships that could affect your stress:

- Witnessing an argument with other people
- Seeing an ex-significant other
- Contact from a person that you no longer speak with
- Seeing someone on social media
- Conversation about someone that you have a history with

If you can relate to some of these triggers, then it is important to find ways to prevent these situations or to manage them. Oftentimes, if you have very strong feelings about someone, it may be caused by PTSD. Certain therapies and stress management techniques may help to mitigate some of the stress you feel when encountered in one of those situations.

It is extremely important to understand what your specific stress triggers or stressors are. Minimizing the chances of you encountering your stress triggers will prevent you from experience stress often. Although you can't avoid and prevent every single stress trigger, even cutting them down by a certain percentage is better than letting it continuously affect you. Before we move on to the next chapter, think deeply about what normally causes you stress and specifically the triggers that do so. Are you feeling stressed out because of work emails flooding in on the weekend? Or are you feeling stressed out because you ran into someone that you're no longer friends with? These two examples require two different techniques to manage, so by identifying what your triggers are, you can find the right ways to overcome your stress.

Chapter 3: How to Overcome Stress

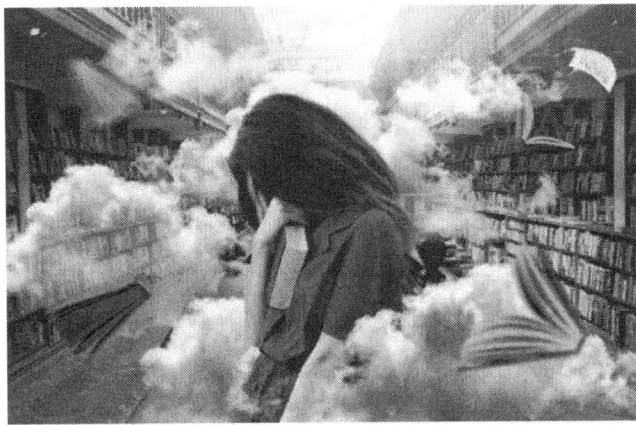

Earlier in this book, you learned about all the negative symptoms of stress that can deeply affect someone's physical and mental health. In order to prevent serious health problems, people must get their stress under control. Although most people think that stress is just a psychological feeling and they can overcome it just by 'pushing through' or ignoring it, they are very wrong. Thoughts directly affect a person's brain chemistry, and the effects of stress are very physical. This is why learning to overcome stress is important in maintaining a healthy and balanced life. There are various ways to do it that range from stress prevention to stress management to therapy. In this chapter, we will be focusing on tips that you can use in day to day life to help overcome stress. Later on, in this book, we will be learning about more specific techniques that combat more serious stress problems such as anxiety and depression. Let's take a look at 8 tips to overcome stress:

Tip #1: Identifying Your Stressors

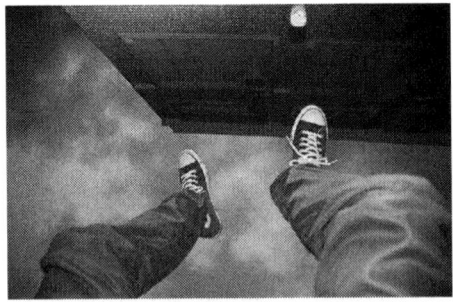

Overcoming and managing stress all starts with identifying the causes of it in your life. Although it sounds easy, it really isn't as straightforward as you'd think. It's easy to identify huge stressors such as moving homes, changing your job, or if you are going through a divorce, but finding out other sources of stress is much harder. When you are used to dealing with a certain kind of stress, it is easy to overlook the thoughts and feelings that you have about it. You may know that you are always worrying about deadlines at work, but maybe it's your procrastination that is causing your stress, not the job itself. In order to help you identify your main causes of stress, you must take a close look at your excuses, habits, and attitude:

- Do you normally blame your stress on external events like people or situations? Do you view your stress as 'normal' and no different from others?
- Do you think that your stress is a part of your work and personal life? E.g. 'Things are always crazy at work' or 'I'm just an anxious person!'
- Do you define your stress as 'temporary'? E.g. 'I'm just super busy right now!', even though you don't remember the last time you weren't stressed?

The first step to overcoming your stress is to accept responsibility for the role that you play in maintaining or creating it. Until then, your stress level won't be something you can control.

Tip #2: Practice Stress Management

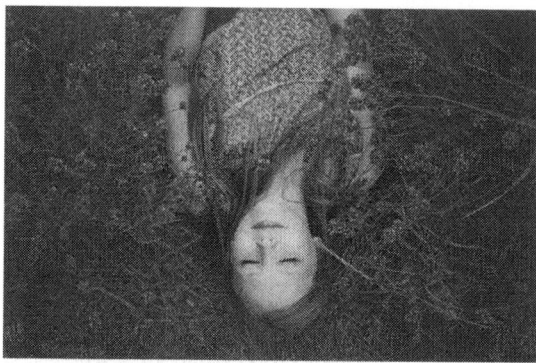

Stress may be an automatic response created by our bodies. Some stressors can come up at very predictable times. For instance, a meeting with your manager, your commute to work, or family gatherings during the holidays. When you are faced with predictable stressors, you can either change the situation altogether or change the way you react to it. When you are deciding to either change the situation or the reaction, think about the Four A's: avoid, alter, adapt to accept. This may help you identify a solution to your stress the quickest.

- **Avoid unnecessary stress:** Although it isn't healthy to constantly be avoiding situations that need to be addressed, you can still eliminate a lot of stressors by avoiding them. Here are a few tips:
    - Learn to say 'no'. Know what your boundaries are and stick to them. This is relevant in your personal and professional life. When you take on too many things, you are creating stress for yourself. Be able to distinguish the difference between your 'musts' and 'shoulds'. Learn to say no when you know you are taking on too much.

- Avoid people who cause stress. If there is a certain someone who tends to cause you stress, either end the relationship or limit how much time you spend with them.
- Control your environment. If watching the news stressed you out, turn it off. If driving in traffic stresses you out, consider a different method of travel. If Christmas shopping at a busy mall is stressful for you, consider doing your shopping online this year.
- Minimize your to-do list. Prioritize the things you REALLY need to do and analyze your current schedule. If you have too many things on the go at the moment, let go of the tasks that aren't 100% necessary.

- **Alter the situation:** If a stressful situation isn't avoidable, try to change it instead. This may involve changing your communication style or how you operate in your everyday life.
  - Express your feelings and emotions instead of hiding them. If there is something bothering you, whether it's a situation or it's a person, learn to be assertive and communicate your feelings in a diplomatic way. If you have an upcoming exam that you need to study for and your chatty sister had just gotten home, tell her directly, but nicely, that you only have 5 minutes to chat before you have to get back to studying. If you don't communicate your feelings, stress, and resentment will increase.
  - Be open to compromise. If you are asking someone to change the way they behave, be open to making some changes yourself too. If both people are willing to take one step back, you'll have a much better shot of finding a happy middle ground.
  - Create a balanced schedule. If you are only working and not doing leisurely activities, you are setting yourself up for burnout. Try to find the perfect balance between your professional and personal life.

- **Adapt to the stressor:** If you aren't able to change the stressor, change yourself instead. People are adaptable creatures. You can find a way to adapt to situations that are stressful and regain control.
  - Look at your problems in a different way. Try to look at situations that are stressful from a more positive light. For instance, rather than being upset about being stuck in traffic, try to think of it as an opportunity to listen to some music or your favorite podcast.
  - Take a step back and look at the big picture. Try to get some perspective on whatever stressful situation you are feeling at the moment. Ask yourself how important this one stressful situation will be to you in the future. Focus your time and energy on things that will matter in the future.
  - Being a perfectionist is a big source of stress. Change your standards and stop stressing yourself out from holding such high standards. Set more reasonable standards for yourself and learn to be comfortable with who you are.

- o   Practice gratitude frequently. When you are feeling extremely stressed out, take some time to think about all the things in your life that you appreciate. This includes materialistic things and your own positive qualities. This strategy is simple and helps give people a better perspective.

- **Accept things that can't be changed:** In some cases, stress is unavoidable. For instance, you can't change big stressors like a death of a family member or having a serious illness. In these cases, the best way to cope with your stress is to accept things for the way they are. Although acceptance may be hard at first, it is beneficial in the long run to not fight it so hard.
    - o   Don't try to control things that you can't. There are tons of things in life that are beyond our control, especially in regards to other people. Rather than being stressed because of someone else's actions, focus on things that are in your control, such as how you react to stressful situations.
    - o   Be optimistic. When you are faced with a big obstacle, try to look at it as an opportunity for growth rather than a setback. If it was your own choices that led you to this stressful circumstance, reflect on those decisions and learn to make better ones in the future.
    - o   Practice forgiveness. Accept the fact that nobody is perfect in this world and that everyone will make mistakes. Let go of negative feelings like resentment and anger. Allow yourself to be free from negative energy by forgiving and moving on.
    - o   Express your feelings. Expressing the things that you are going through can be challenging. However, a problem shared is a problem halved. Talk to a friend or a loved one for some support.

Tip #3: Get Active

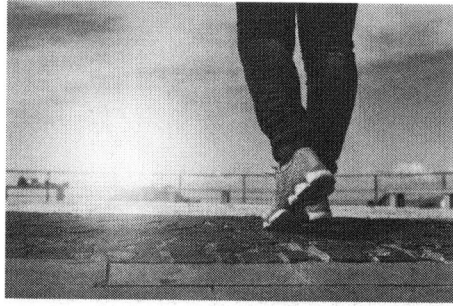

Often times, when people are feeling stressed, they likely do not want to get up and do something physical. However, exercising is a great way to relieve stress, you don't have to spend hours at the gym to reap the benefits, you can simply do a light exercise or just go for a quick walk for your brain to release the endorphins that make you feel good. People get the most benefit from exercise if they do it for at least 30 minutes per day. Small exercise activities

will add up over the course of a day. Here are some suggestions that you can try to incorporate into your schedule:
- Play an active game with your family/friends (e.g., ping pong, Wii)
- Find an exercise partner and hold each other accountable
- Parking your car as far as you can and get yourself to walk to wherever you're going
- Walk to do your errands instead of driving
- If you have a dog, take him/her out for a walk
- Play some music and dance around

Tip #4: Socialize

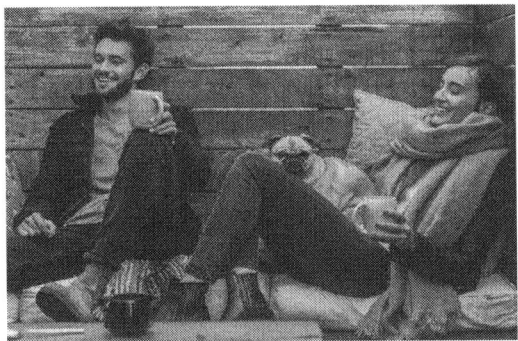

Spending quality time with other people gives us a sense of calming and makes us feel understood and safe. In-person interactions actually counteract our bodies' fight or flight mechanism and is a natural stress reliever. So, make an effort to go out and socialize regularly with family and friends. Keep in mind that the people you choose to hang out with don't need to be able to help with your stress. Simply being a good listener is enough for you to get some weight off of your shoulders. People who care about you will be happy that you are comfortable with opening up to them and will strengthen your relationship with them. Although it's not always realistic to have someone close by that you can talk to about your feelings, building a close circle of friends that you can talk to can improve your resilience to the stresses of life. Here are some relationship building suggestions:
- Talk to your colleagues at work
- Meet up with a friend for lunch or coffee
- Help out others by volunteering
- Call to chat with an old friend
- Confide in someone you trust like a teacher or your sold sports coach

Tip #5: Leisurely Activities

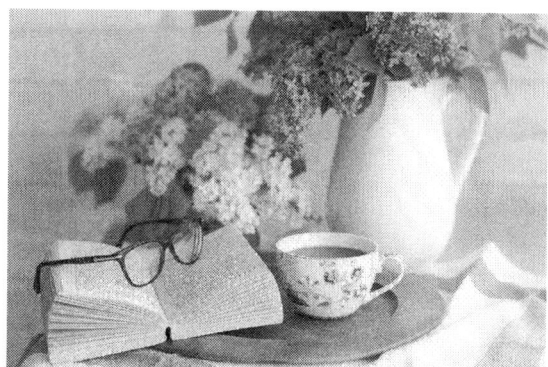

Besides changing your attitudes regarding stressful events, you can lower the stress you feel in everyday life by making sure you are getting enough 'me' time. Don't forget about leisurely activities when you're caught up in the busy-ness of life. Take care of your own needs first. Make time for relaxation and fun events, and you'll be in a much better spot to handle your stress. Here are some things you could do:

- **Practice relaxation:** Take up some relaxation practice through meditation, breathing exercises, or yoga. This helps activate a person's relaxation response and promotes a state of restfulness. As you learn these techniques, you will notice that your stress levels have lowered, and your mind and body will function in a more relaxed manner.
- **Use your sense of humor:** Learn the ability to laugh at yourself and don't take life so seriously. Laughing more often helps fight off stress.
- **Do something that you like every day:** Schedule time for activities that make you happy; this could be playing videogames or working on your custom motorcycle.
- **Set aside time for leisure:** Make sure to make time for relaxation in your everyday schedule. Don't let other obligations take over your leisurely time. Take a break to recharge so you can feel energized.

Tip #6: Time Management

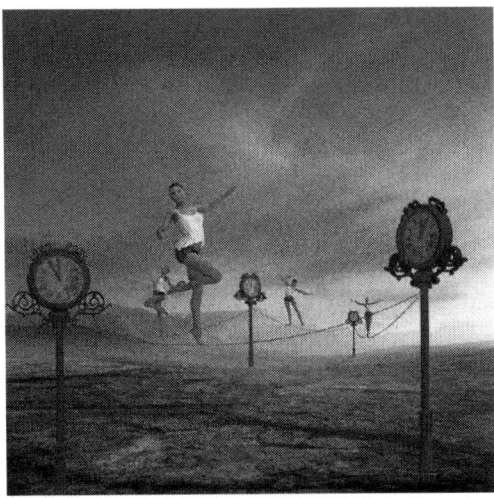

When you are bad at managing your time, this can create a lot of stress. This could either be in the form of not having enough time to get the necessities done, or it could be not scheduling enough time for self-care. When a person is stretched too thin, it is hard to stay relaxed and calm. You will also be more likely to cut back on the healthy living activities that you should be doing in order to better maintain your stress. This includes getting enough sleep or exercising. There are a few things that you can do in order to achieve a better work-life balance:

- **Delegate responsibility:** You don't have to do everything yourself all the time. Other people can help you with tasks, and they are likely very willing to help! Let go of the idea of needing to control every step of the way. By doing this, you are letting go of unnecessary stress.
- **Break tasks into smaller ones:** One large task seems overwhelming, but breaking it down into manageable steps will lift a lot of stress from your shoulders. Focus on one step at a time, and you'll slowly start to feel a sense of accomplishment that will motivate you into doing more steps.
- **Prioritize your tasks:** Make a list of things you need to do and do them in order of importance. Finish your most important things first, and suddenly you'll feel a lot better.
- **Don't overcommit:** Avoid over scheduling things such as back to back engagements or trying to fit too many activities in one day. We often underestimate how long it actually takes to do something, so if you're overscheduled, you'll likely begin to feel stressed out.

Tip #7: Maintaining Balance

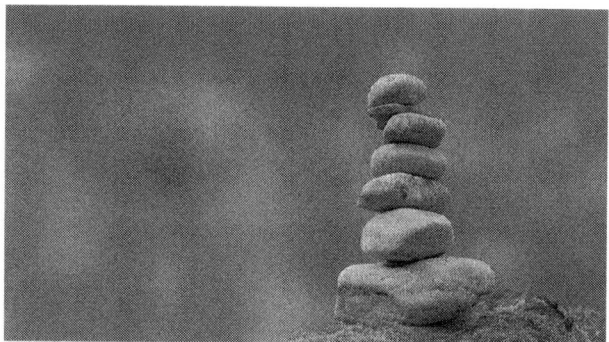

On top of increasing your activity levels through exercising, make sure you are also eating a healthy diet. Having the proper nutrients helps increase people's resistance to stress. Here are some tips:

- **Get enough sleep:** Adults need 7 – 9 hours of sleep every night. Getting enough sleep helps keep our mind healthy. Feeling tired and sluggish will only make your stress worse.
- **Limit consumption of alcohol, drugs, or cigarettes:** Self-medicating through the use of drugs or alcohol may provide temporary relief from stress, but it may cause you to become reliant on it. Rather than avoiding the problem, deal with it head-on so that it doesn't re-occur.
- **Reduce the intake of sugar and caffeine:** Although sugar and caffeine may boost your energy for a period of time, it always ends in a crash in both your energy and your mood. When you reduce your coffee and sugar intake, you will begin to feel more relaxed and be able to get better sleep.
- **Eat a healthy diet:** Healthy bodies are much better at dealing with stress, so pay attention to what you're eating. Start your day by eating a healthy breakfast in order to boost your energy and help you have a clearer mind throughout the day.

Tip #8: Relieving Stress in the Moment

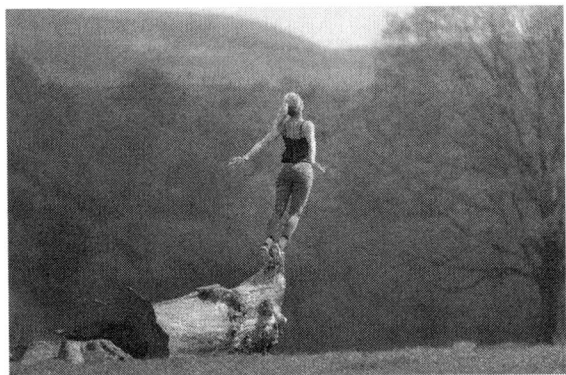

When you are stressed, the best way to deal with it is not to ignore it. It is to overcome it as it is happening. If you are frustrated by the traffic jam during your morning commute, find a way to manage your stress levels. You can reduce stress the fastest by practicing breathing exercises and mindfulness. Pay attention to the things going on around you such as what you hear, feel, see, and taste. You can listen to relaxing sounds like the flow of a river or ocean waves. Find out what sort of sounds and experiences relaxes you the most and make sure you have access to it at all times in order to use it during moments of high stress.

Other Important Tips:

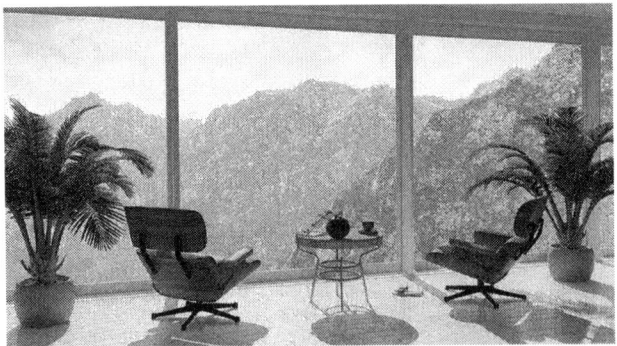

Besides these eight tips, people can lower stress by creating a more organized and positive environment. You can do this by keeping your home, and your office organized and de-cluttered. When things are all over the place, and you are struggling to find items that you need, this is just another avenue for stress to be created. By keeping the environments that you frequently clean and tidy, you are promoting a healthier space and productivity. In addition, having a more positive mindset is a great way to repel stress. You can do this by changing your thinking habits through the use of Cognitive Behavioral Therapy. You will have the opportunity to learn more about this therapy method later on in this book.

Chapter 4: Other Mental Health Disorders Related to Stress

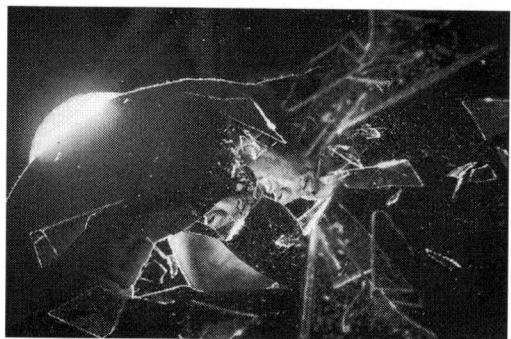

When a person is under a lot of stress for an extended amount of time, it increases their risk of developing other mental disorders. Common disorders that can be caused by high-stress include; anxiety, depression, anger disorders, and panic disorders. In this chapter, we will be taking a deeper look into each of these disorders and what different forms they come in. This is important if you are someone who is under high-stress, as learning what these disorders are may help you identify it or learn to cope with it.

What Is An Anxiety Disorder?

So, what exactly is anxiety? A lot of the times, when people use the term 'anxiety' they are referring to generalized anxiety. Anxiety is a basic feeling and experience that literally all species of animals experience. Although anxiety is not a pleasant feeling, it is not dangerous. Actually, anxiety is helpful for us in certain situations. Some people wish to get rid of anxiety completely, but that goal isn't possible or realistic! When it comes to Cognitive Behavioral Therapy, the approach is to help you build the skills required to help you manage and understand your anxiety as opposed to getting rid of it altogether (again, not possible).

We all have to keep in mind that anxiety is a normal emotion and that it is not dangerous. The symptoms of anxiety actually serve a function. Anxiety is actually a natural reaction to a perceived threat and helps us humans respond to it. However, if you have excessive anxiety, it can also be a problem.

Since anxiety is a normal response to a threat, when a person perceives that they are in a threatening situation, their fight or flight instinct is triggered which its sole purpose is to protect itself by fighting or fleeing from danger. When somebody is feeling threatened, their brain sends messages to your autonomic nervous system (this is a section of your nerves). When this nervous system reacts, adrenalin and noradrenalin are released from your brain, which then triggers the anxiety response and automatically prepares us for danger. This nervous system is eventually stopped when these chemicals are destroyed by our bodies in an attempt to calm the body down.

This fact is extremely important to remember because those who suffer from anxiety disorders are convinced that their anxiety will go on forever. However, biologically, this cannot happen since anxiety is limited by time. Although it may feel that the anxiety is going on forever, it has a limited lifespan. After some time, your body will determine that it has had enough with the fight or flight instinct and restore the body to its neutral feeling. Anxiety cannot continue endlessly or damage your body. Although highly uncomfortable, this whole cycle is perfectly harmless and natural. In fact, this behavior is an instinct to us because, in the wild, it is necessary for our bodies to reactive this response because we know that danger can return.

Overall, the fight or flight response activates the entire body's metabolism. This is what makes someone feel hot, flushed, and tired afterward because the entire process uses up a lot of energy. After a strong anxiety experience, most people feel drained, tired, and completely washed out.

Now that you know what anxiety is and how it is a natural emotion that we feel for protection - what is an anxiety disorder? An anxiety disorder is a medical condition where the individual feels symptoms of extreme anxiety or panic. In other words, an anxiety disorder is when the individual is feeling severe anxiety or panic and is unable to manage their symptoms.

We will be going through all the different types of anxiety disorders in the next subchapter, but in this one, we will be talking about the most common ones that people face nowadays. The most common anxiety disorder that people face in present-day is Generalized Anxiety disorder.

Generalized Anxiety Disorder (GAD)

Generalized anxiety is the susceptibility to engage in excessive panic, worry, or anxiety regarding numerous events or situations. Usually, the person has major difficulty controlling their feelings of worry and is associated with other symptoms such as fatigue, restlessness, concentration difficulties, sleep disturbance, irritability, and muscle tension. The feeling of worry is actually defined as a process where it is focused on the uncertainty of the outcome regarding future events. It is actually not an emotion itself, but it leads to feeling the emotion of anxiety. The main and most obvious symptom of generalized anxiety disorder is the "what if" thoughts that begin to occur. These "what if" thoughts work hand in hand with worrying, and it often feels like it is uncontrollable. In addition, the process of worry is often associated with physical symptoms that are related to the flight or fight response. It happens often that the individual will think of the future in a negative light and have thoughts that are followed by feelings of anxiety.

People with GAD often feel worried and anxious most of the time and not just in specific situations that are stressful. The worries that they have been constant, intense, and interferes with their daily routine. Their worries are typically multiple aspects and not only one. It may include work, health, finance, family, or just everyday life things. Trivial tasks such as household chores or being late for a meeting can lead to extreme anxiety, which then leads to the feeling of doom.

Most people are diagnosed with GAD if they showcase some of the symptoms for 6 months or more:

- You feel extremely worried about numerous activities or events
- You struggle to stop worrying
- You are finding that your anxiety has made it very hard for you to do your daily routine (e.g., studying, working, hanging out with friends)
- You feel constantly restless or on edge
- You are always/easily tired
- You struggle with concentration
- You are easily irritable
- You have tension in your muscles (e.g., neck or sore jaw)
- You struggle with sleeping (e.g., difficulty staying asleep or falling asleep)

The most common treatment for GAD is Cognitive Behavioral Therapy. Medication will be used if psychological treatments are ineffective. We will be diving into the details in the later chapters on why and how CBT is an extremely effective treatment for those who have GAD.

What Are the Different Types of Anxiety Disorders?

Now that we have learned about the most common anxiety disorder, generalized anxiety disorder (GAD), and the largest component that leads to it (worry), we will move on to learning about other types of anxiety disorders that people suffer from. The other types of anxiety disorders that we will learn about are:

- Social Anxiety
- Specific Phobias
- Panic Disorder
- Obsessive-Compulsive Disorder (OCD)
- Post-traumatic Stress Disorder (PTSD)

Social Anxiety

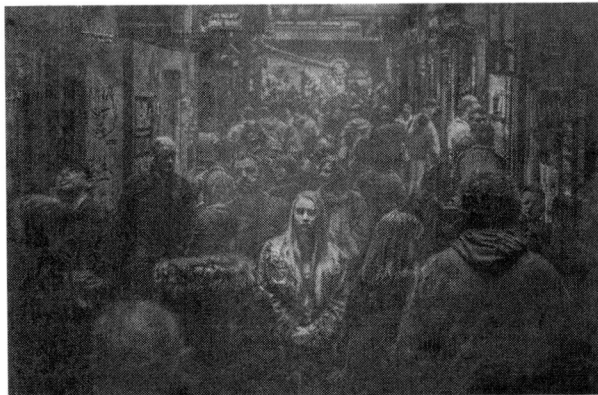

Although it is very normal to feel a certain level of nervousness in social situations, it is not normal to feel an overwhelming amount of anxiety. Situations such as attending formal events, public speaking and doing presentations are likely events in which you feel some nervousness and anxiety. However, for those who suffer from social anxiety (or otherwise known as social phobia), speaking, or performing in front of other people and general social situations can lead to extreme anxiety. This usually stems from the fear of being criticized, judged, humiliated, or laughed at in front of other people. A lot of the times, they are afraid of trivial and ordinary matters. For example, those who suffer from social anxiety may feel that eating at a restaurant around other people can be extremely daunting.

Social anxiety usually occurs during the lead up to performance events (e.g., having to give a speech or working while they are being watched) and situations where social interaction is involved (e.g., having lunch with coworkers or normal small talk). Social anxiety also occurs during the actual event, as well as the lead-up. Moreover, this type of phobia can also be very specific where the individual has a fear of a specific situation. For example, they can be fearful of having to be assertive during work meetings.

The symptoms of social anxiety include psychological and physical symptoms. People with social phobia find it very distressing when they experience physical symptoms. These physical symptoms include:

- Excessive perspiration
- Nausea/Diarrhea
- Trembling
- Stammering, stuttering, or blushing when speaking

Specific Phobias

Phobias are probably one of the most well-known disorders that we hear about in present-day society. You probably see people on TV and movies that have phobias of clowns, spiders, or heights. Fear or concern regarding certain situations is common, but that does not mean you have a phobia. Feeling anxious when you come across a spider, or being in a high place is fairly normal. Fear is actually a rational and natural response when we are in situations where we feel threatened.

However, some people have a huge reaction when it comes to certain activities, situations, or objects due to them imagining and exaggerating the danger. The feelings of terror, panic, or fear that someone may feel due to a threat are completely out of proportion. In a lot of cases, even a thought of the phobic stimulus or seeing it on TV is enough to cause a reaction in these individuals. These types of extreme reactions could indicate a specific phobia disorder.

Although a lot of the times, people are not self-aware of where their anxiety is coming from, people who suffer from phobias are usually aware that their fears are irrational and extreme. However, they do feel that their reactions are automatic and cannot be controlled. Sometimes, specific phobias lead to panic attacks. During these panic attacks, the individual finds themselves overwhelmed with undesirable physical sensations. These sensations include nausea, heart racing, choking, chest pain, dizziness, faintness, and hot/cold flashes.

The symptoms of specific phobia are as follows:

- You have a constant, extreme, and irrational fear of a situation, activity, or object. For example, fear of heights, clowns, or spiders.
- You are constantly avoiding situations where there is a possibility that you have to face your phobia. For example, not going outside because you may encounter a spider. If the situation is something that is difficult to avoid, you may start to feel high levels of distress.
- You find that your avoidance and anxiety of certain situations where your phobia might exist makes it hard for you to go about your daily routine. For example, it begins to interfere with your work, school, or social life.
- You find that your avoidance and anxiety are constant, and you have been struggling with it for over 6 months.

Panic Disorders

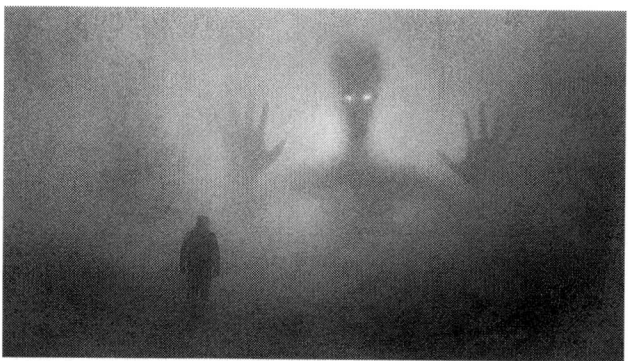

Panic disorders, or more commonly known as 'panic attacks' is the term used to describe when these attacks are recurring and disabling. Usually, panic disorders are defined by:

- Unexpected and recurring panic attacks.
- Worrying for a long duration (1 month+) after having a panic attack that you will have another one.
- Worrying about the effects or consequences after that panic attack. A lot of people will think that a panic attack is a symptom of an undiagnosed medical issue. For instance, individuals may do repeated medical tests due to these worries, and although nothing shows up, they still are afraid of being in poor health.
- Having significant behavior changes that are linked to the panic attacks. For example, avoiding exercise because your heart rate will increase.

Usually, during a panic attack, you become overwhelmed with the physical feelings described above. The peak of the panic attack is usually 10 minutes in and will last up to 30 minutes and leave you exhausted afterward. They can occur up to numerous times a day or a few times per year. They can happen when someone is sleeping which will wake them up during the attack. Many people have actually experienced a panic attack at least one time in their lives. Up to 40% of the human population has experienced a panic attack at some point in their lives. This does not mean you have a panic disorder. Here are the common symptoms and signs of a panic attack:

- A feeling of overwhelming fear or panic
- Having the thought that you are choking, dying, or 'going crazy.'
- Heart rate increases
- Having difficulty breathing (e.g., hyperventilating)
- Feeling like you are choking or your lungs aren't working
- Perspiring excessively
- Light-headedness, dizziness, or faintness

What Is a Depression Disorder?

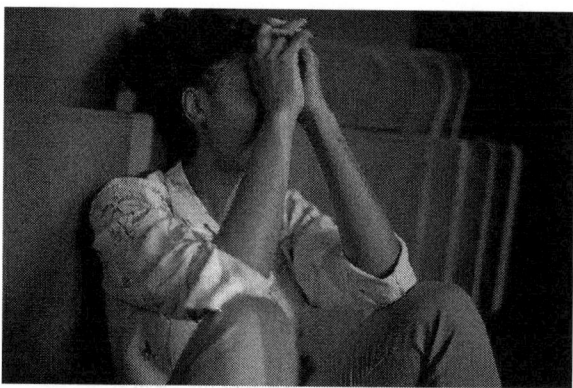

The dictionary definition of depression is 'feelings of severe despondency and dejection'. However, we have to keep in mind to not get mix depression up with feelings of sadness or grief. The death of a loved one or the ending of a relationship are both very difficult experiences for a person to experience and endure. During these hard times, it is completely normal for feelings of sadness and grief to arise in response to those situations. People who are experiencing an event of a loss might often describe themselves as being 'depressed'.

With that said, being sad is not the same as having the disorder of depression. A person's grieving process is unique to every individual, but it does share a lot of the same feelings that a depression disorder brings. Both depression and feelings of grief involve the feelings of sadness and withdrawal from a person's usual activities. Here are a few important ways of why they are different:

- When a person is feeling emotions of grief, their painful feelings often come in waves. They are usually mixed with positive memories about the person who's passed. When a person is feeling intense grief, their interest and mood are decreased for around two weeks.
- When a person is in grief, their self-esteem usually does not change much. When a person has depression, they have constant feelings of self-loathing and worthlessness.
- For most people, the death of a loved one can cause major depression. For other people, it could be losing their job or being a victim of physical assault. When depression and grief are co-existing, the grief is usually the more severe feeling and lasts longer than grief without depression. There is some overlap between depression and grief, but despite this, they are still different. Helping a person distinguish between grief and depression is necessary in order to help them get help, support, or treatment.

Types of Depression

As we mentioned earlier, depression is different for everyone, and therefore, different people require different treatment methods. Depression isn't just one size fits all; it is a disorder that comes in many shapes and forms. When people get diagnosed with depression, doctors will define the severity of it by determining where it is mild, moderate, or major. Determining this can be a complicated task but knowing what type of depression you have can help you manage your symptoms and help you find the most effective depression to your specific type of depression. Let's learn about a few different types:

Mild and Moderate Depression

The most common types of depression are mild and moderate depression. This type of depression is more than just feeling 'sad' or 'blue' the symptoms of this type of depression often interferes with people's lives by robbing them of motivation and joy. These symptoms can feel amplified in moderate depression and often leads to lowering a person's self-esteem and self-confidence.

A type of 'low-grade' depression is called dysthymia. When a person has dysthymia, they feel mildly to moderately depressed more often than not, but these people do have brief periods of feeling a normal mood. Here are some defining traits of dysthymia:

- Symptoms of dysthymia are not as severe or strong as the symptoms of major depression, but they do have a tendency to last for a long time (minimum of 2 years)
- Some people report that they experience intense depressive episodes on top of having dysthymia, this is a condition called 'double depression'
- When a person is suffering from dysthymia, they may feel like they have always been depressed for their whole lives. They may think that their consistent low mood is 'just the way they are'

Major Depression

Major depression is a less common form of mild or moderate depression. It is characterized by symptoms that are severe and relentless. Here are two characteristics of major depression:

- If major depression is left untreated, it usually lasts for about 6 months
- Although some people only experience one depressive episode in their life, major depression can be a disorder that is recurring throughout their life

Atypical Depression

Atypical depression is a subtype of major depression that is very common that has specific symptom patterns. It has a better response with some medications and therapies compared to others, identifying this type of depression is very helpful when it comes to prescribing treatment. Here are a few traits to describe it further:

- People who have atypical depression usually experience a temporary increase in mood in response to positive events. This includes hanging out with friends or receiving some sort of good news.
- Atypical depression includes increased appetite, weight gain, sleeping excessively, sensitivity to rejection, and a 'heavy feeling' in their arms and legs.

Seasonal Affective Disorder (SAD)

Although a lot of people think this type of depression is just a myth, it is a real condition. Some people, when they experience reduced daylight hours during winter, can cause them to form a type of depression called seasonal affective disorder (SAD). Although this is not a popular type of depression, SAD affects 1% - 2% of the general population, predominantly in young people and women. SAD can make a person feel completely different from the person they are in the summer. People tend to feel stressed, sad, hopeless, tense and have little interest in friends or activities that they normally enjoy. SAD usually begins during Autumn or Winter, where the days are short and remains until brighter days of Spring come along.

What is an Anger Disorder?

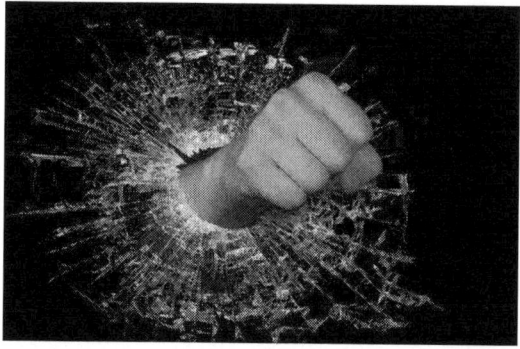

Anger is a very complicated emotion, and looking into it in more depth is extremely helpful when it comes to stress and other mental disorders. When negative feelings are constantly repressed and not expressed in a healthy manner, a person may become subject to an anger disorder. Let's take a look at how different feelings can cause someone to have anger problems.

Anger as a Manifestation of Other Emotions

Anger is an emotion that is said to be a manifestation of many other types of emotions. What this means is that when a person feels anger, they are actually feeling something different, or a combination of other emotions. This school of thought says that anger itself is not a genuine emotion. The reasoning behind this is that anger is a type of fuel that helps a person get things done or take action to remedy a situation, while sadness or disappointment are emotions that could be debilitating and leave you wanting to do nothing but lie in bed and cry. When we feel this way, sometimes we may feel anger instead of sadness, for example, because then we approach whatever it is that is making us feel this way with aggression and energy. When you are feeling anger, this would be one of those times to look deeper and deeper in order to find out what you are really feeling. Below, we will look at the other emotions that could manifest themselves as anger.

Another reason that anger is often a manifestation of other emotions is that people often use it to cover up the vulnerability that comes with other emotions such as sadness or fear. When a person is angry or acting out in anger, they appear strong or intimidating, and the majority of people would choose this over appearing "weak" or vulnerable. Sometimes intense feelings of any emotion will quickly be converted to feelings of anger in an effort to hide or disguise the genuine feelings. This may happen so quickly and automatically that the person themselves does not even recognize it. Nonviolent communication requires a person to work on themselves in many ways, and this is one of them. It is often not as easy as just glancing inside to see what emotion you are feeling but challenging yourself to look deeper and be vulnerable.

Anger is seen as one of the most primal human emotions, as it dates back to the beginning of humans. Anger is actually present in our emotional range in order to protect us from perceived threats. This results from the time that humans were hunters and needed to protect their families and their land in times of war and other tribes. Anger is strongly related to the fight or flight response, so this can tell us why we feel the need to take immediate action when we feel intense anger. "fight" from the fight or flight response does not need to involve a physical altercation but can involve fighting with words as well. Knowing that anger is there to protect you can help you when trying to manage it, as you can stop and recognize that you do not need to react as there is no threat to survival as there would be if it was the year 30000BC.

Chapter 5: How to Overcome Mental Health Disorders

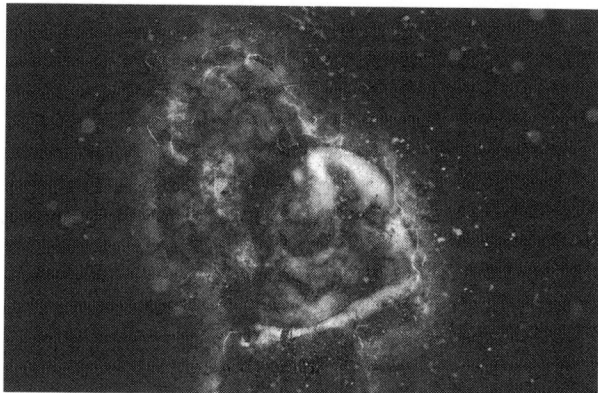

By now, if you have made it this far in the book, you should have an excellent understanding of what stress is, the science behind it, symptoms and causes, and the risk factors that come with leaving stress untreated. In this chapter, we will begin to discuss some practical techniques that can be used to treat mental disorders that are caused by stress. Keep in mind that a technique that works for you doesn't necessarily work for someone else. Often times, people are prescribed treatment plans that contain multiple methods. This could include lifestyle changes, medication, and therapy. Since depression manifests in a different way with each individual person, doctors often have to prescribe treatment through the use of trial and error.

In this chapter, we will be focusing on learning multiple different techniques that a person can try in terms of treatment. There are numerous elements here that a person can attempt, but the ideal case is seeking professional treatment in order for a doctor to properly assess you. However, I want this chapter to be useful to you in a way where you are well educated with all the options of techniques that you can use to treat common mental disorders like anxiety and depression if you or someone you know is faced with it. The techniques in this chapter range from simple lifestyle changes all the way to psychotherapy and medication.

Lifestyle Changes

Lifestyle changes may be seemingly simple, but they are actually very powerful tools when it comes to treating depression and anxiety. In some people's cases, a lifestyle change is all they may need to recover from depression and anxiety. In the case that a person needs other treatment as well, making good lifestyle changes can help cure depression even faster and prevent it from happening again. Here are a few changes that people can try:

- **Exercise:** Researchers have found that regularly exercising can be just as effective as medication when it comes to treating depression and anxiety. Exercises boost the 'feel-good' brain chemicals in the brain such as serotonin and endorphins. These chemicals also trigger the growth of new brain cells and connections similar to what antidepressants do. The best part about exercise is that you don't need to do it intensely in order to have the benefits. Even a simple 30-minute walk can make a huge difference in a person's brain activity. For the best results, people should aim to do 30 – 60 minutes of aerobic activity every day or on most days.

- **Social Support:** Just like I mentioned earlier, having a strong social network reduces isolation, which is a huge risk factor in depression and anxiety. Make an effort to keep in regular contact with family and friends (ideally on a daily basis) and consider joining a support group or class. You can also opt to do some volunteering where you can get the social support you need while helping others as well.
- **Nutrition:** The ability to eating properly is imperative for everyone's mental and physical health. By eating smalls meals that are well-balanced throughout the day, you can minimize your mood swings and keep energy levels up. Although you may crave sugary foods due to the quick boost of energy that it can bring, complex carbohydrates are much more nutritious. Instead, complex carbohydrates can provide you with an energy boost without a crash at the end.
- **Sleep:** A person's sleep cycle has strong effects on mood. When a person does not get enough sleep, their symptoms of depression or anxiety may get worse. Sleep deprivation causes other negative symptoms like sadness, fatigue, moodiness, and irritability. Not many people can function well with less than seven hours of sleep per night. A healthy adult should be aiming for 7 – 9 hours of sleep every night.
- **Stress reduction:** When a person is suffering from a lot of stress, it intensifies their depression or anxiety and increases their risk of developing more serious depression or anxiety disorders. Try to make changes in your life that can help you reduce or manage stress. Identify which aspects of your life creates the most stress, such as unhealthy relationships or work overload and find ways to minimize their impact and the stress it brings.

Psychotherapy

Once a person has ruled out that they do not have an underlying medical cause for their depression or anxiety symptoms, then talking therapies are very effective treatments. The things that people learn in therapy gives them insight and skills in order to feel better and also prevents depression and anxiety from coming back in the future. In terms of psychotherapy, there are multiple types available to treat depression or anxiety. The most common and effective type of therapy is cognitive-behavioral therapy. We will be spending a whole chapter on learning about this type of therapy and how it can help with treating depression or anxiety. There are also other common types of therapy that include psychodynamic therapy and interpersonal therapy. The most common approach is to use a blended treatment.

Therapies like CBT teaches a person practical technique on reframing their negative thinking or their automatic negative thought processes in order to change their behavior to combat depression and anxiety. Therapy can also be effective by helping a person work to the root of their depression or anxiety in order to help them understand why they feel certain ways and what their depression or anxiety triggers are. They also learn how they can utilize this information to help them stay healthy.

One of the main symptoms of depression and anxiety that people speak about is the feelings of overwhelmed and their inability to focus. Therapy helps people take a step back and look at the 'big picture' to identify what aspects may be contributing to their depression and anxiety and what changes they need to make in order to change their situation. Here are some themes that therapy can help a person with:

- **Relationships:** When a person begins to understand the patterns of their relationships, they can begin to improve current relationships or start building better ones. This will help them reduce isolation and building a better social network, which is crucial in treating and preventing depression and anxiety.
- **Setting healthy boundaries:** If a person is feeling overwhelmed and stressed, they are at higher risks of depression and anxiety. Setting healthy boundaries in relationships, whether it's personal or at work, can be a huge help in relieving stress. Therapy helps people not only identify the boundaries that you need but to validate them as well.
- **Managing general life problems:** Simply speaking to a therapist that you trust can help you get some suitable opinions on better ways to handle the problems that life throws at us.

Cognitive Behavioral Therapy

As we discussed at the very beginning of this book, Cognitive Behavioral Therapy is a type of talking therapy that is used to treat people with mental disorders. The fundamentals of CBT are based on three components; cognition (thought), emotion, and behavior. All three components interact with each other, which leads to the theory that our thoughts determine our feelings and emotions which then determines or behavior.

How does Cognitive Behavioral Therapy Work?

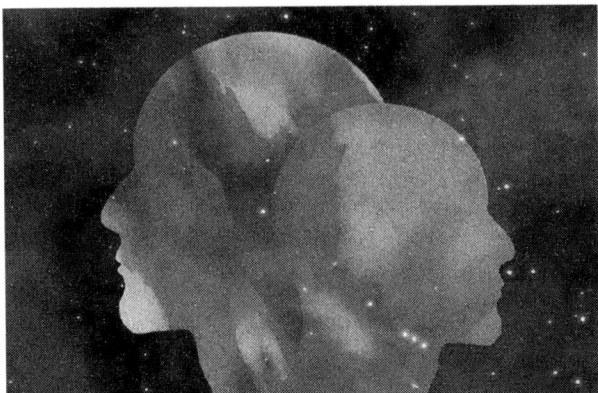

Cognitive Behavioral Therapy works by emphasizing the relationship between our thoughts, feelings, and behaviors. When you begin to change any of these components, you start to initiate change in the others. The goal of CBT is to help lower the amount you worry and stress and increase the overall quality of your life. Here are the 8 basic principles of how Cognitive Behavioral Therapy works:

1. **CBT will help provide a new perspective of understanding your problems.**

A lot of the times, when an individual has been living with a problem for a long time in their life, they may have developed unique ways of understanding it and dealing with it. Usually, this just maintains the problem or makes it worse. CBT is effective in helping you look at your problem from a new perspective, and this will help you learn other ways of understanding your problem and learning a new way of dealing with it.

2. **CBT will help you generate new skills to work out your problem.**

You probably know that understanding a problem is one matter, and dealing with it is entirely another can of worms. To help start changing your problem, you will need to develop new skills that will help you change your thoughts, behaviors, and emotions that are affecting your anxiety and mental health. For instance, CBT will help you achieve new ideas about your problem and begin to use and test them in your daily life. Therefore, you will be more capable of making up your own mind regarding the root issue that is causing these negative symptoms.

3. **CBT relies on teamwork and collaboration between the client and therapist (or program).**

CBT will require you to be actively involved in the entire process, and your thoughts and ideas are extremely valuable right from the beginning of the therapy. You are the expert when it comes to your thoughts and problems. The therapist is the expert when it comes to acknowledging the emotional issues. By working as a team, you will be able to identify your problems and have your therapist better address them. Historically, the more the therapy advances, the more the client takes the lead in finding techniques to deal with the symptoms.

4. The goal of CBT is to help the client become their own therapist.

Therapy is expensive; we all know that. One of the goals of CBT is to not have you become overly dependent on your therapist because it is not feasible to have therapy forever. When therapy comes to an end, and you do not become your own therapist, you will be at high risk for a relapse. However, if you are able to become your own therapist, you will be in a good spot to face the hurdles that life throws at you. In addition, it is proven that having confidence in your own ability to face hardship is one of the best predictors of maintaining the valuable information you got from therapy. By playing an active role during your sessions, you will be able to gain the confidence needed to face your problems when the sessions are over.

5. CBT is succinct and time-limited.

As a rule of thumb, CBT therapy sessions typically last over the course of 10 to 20 sessions. Statistically, when therapy goes on for many months, there is a higher risk of the client becoming dependent on the therapist. Once you have gained a new perspective and understanding of your problem, and are equipped with the right skills, you are able to use them to solve future problems. It is crucial in CBT for you to try out your new skills in the real world. By actually dealing with your own problem hands-on without the security of recurring therapy sessions, you will be able to build confidence in your ability to become your own therapist.

6. CBT is direction based and structured.

CBT typically relies on a fundamental strategy called 'guided recovery'. By setting up some experiments with your therapist, you will be able to experiment with new ideas to see if they reflect your reality accurately. In other words, your therapist is your guide while you are making discoveries in CBT. The therapist will not tell you whether you are right or wrong, but instead, they will help develop ideas and experiments to help you test these ideas.

7. CBT is based on the present, "here and now".

Although we know that our childhood and developmental history play a big role in who we are today, one of the principles of CBT actually distinguishes between what caused the problem and what is maintaining the problem presently. In a lot of cases, the reasons that maintain a problem are different than the ones that originally caused it. For example, if you fall off while riding a horse, you may become afraid of horses. Your fear will continue to be maintained if you begin to start avoiding all horses and refuse to ride one again. In this example, the fear was called by the fall, but by avoiding your fear, you are continuing to maintain it. Unfortunately, you cannot change the fact that you had fallen off the horse, but you can change your behaviors when it comes to avoidance. CBT primarily focuses on the factors that are maintaining the problem because these factors are susceptible to change.

8. Worksheet exercises are significant elements of CBT therapy.

Unfortunately, reading about CBT or going to one session of therapy a week is not enough to change our ingrained patterns of thinking and behaving. During CBT, the client is always encouraged to apply their new skills into their daily lives. Although most people find CBT therapy sessions to be very intriguing, it does not lead to change in reality if you do not exercise the skills you have learned.

Interpersonal Therapy

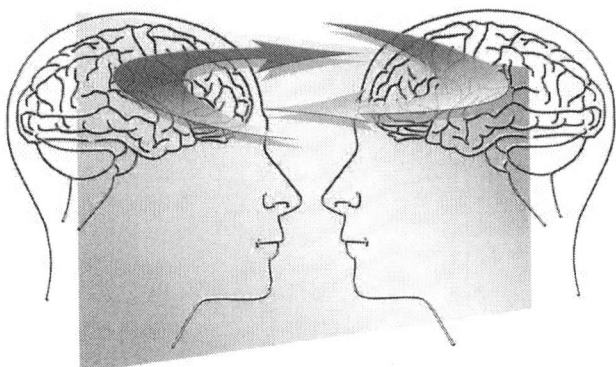

Interpersonal psychotherapy (IPT) is an evidence-based, focused and time-limited approach to treat mental disorders like depression and anxiety. The primary goal of IPT is to improve the quality of a person's social functioning and interpersonal relationships in order to reduce their distress in those situations. There are four main areas that IPT helps the client with. Firstly, it focuses on addressing interpersonal deficits such as involvement in unfulfilling relationships and social isolation. Secondly, IPT helps clients manage their unresolved grief especially if the reason for their distress is related to the loss of a close person in their lives either in the past or recently. Thirdly, IPT can also help with challenging life changes such as moving to another city, divorce, or retirement. Lastly, IPT is also recommended for people that are dealing with conflict-related to relationships such as with coworkers, family members, close friends, or partners.

IPT was initially developed in order to treat major depressive disorders (MDD). It is also effectively used to treat perinatal depression, eating disorders, drug, and alcohol abuse, dysthymia, and other mood disorders such as bipolar disorder (BPD). IPT is different from the traditional types of therapy by focusing on the present rather than past relationships or upbringing. This practice is different from CBT because it speaks to maladaptive thoughts and behaviors only with how they are applied to relationships. The goal of IPT is to change a person's relationship patterns and not their depressive symptoms and also target relationship struggles that exacerbate the symptoms. IPT is less structured compared to CBT as it focuses on the areas that the client has specified without focusing on their personality traits.

Treatment using IPT usually is in the form of individual therapy sessions and group work that is completed anywhere from 12 weeks to 16 weeks. Its methodology is structured on a daily basis and includes assessments throughout the treatment, interviews with the therapist, and homework exercises. The first stage of IPT requires the therapist to assess the client's social history and depressive symptoms within the first three sessions. They examine the client's social history in-depth, making note of any changes in the patterns of their relationships. After that, the therapist and client will work as a team in order to implement the treatment strategies that were chosen specifically to areas that they have the most problems with. As treatment develops, they may change their targeted problem area. Group sessions are similar to the individual ones in the sense that they are semi-structured, focused on interpersonal dynamics and are time-limited. Group therapies provide clients a safe and supportive environment to practice their interpersonal skills. Pre, mid, and post-treatment are also included in group therapy in order to review the client's individual progress, goals, and strategies.

IPT has been developed over 20 years ago and originally had the purpose of being a time-structured treatment for people who had severe depression or anxiety. In recent years, it gained a lot of popularity. IPT practitioners believe that changing a person's social environment is an important factor in treating depression or anxiety and preventing it. IPT was originally developed for adults, but it has been modified in recent years, so adolescents and elderly people can benefit from it as well.

Psychodynamic Therapy

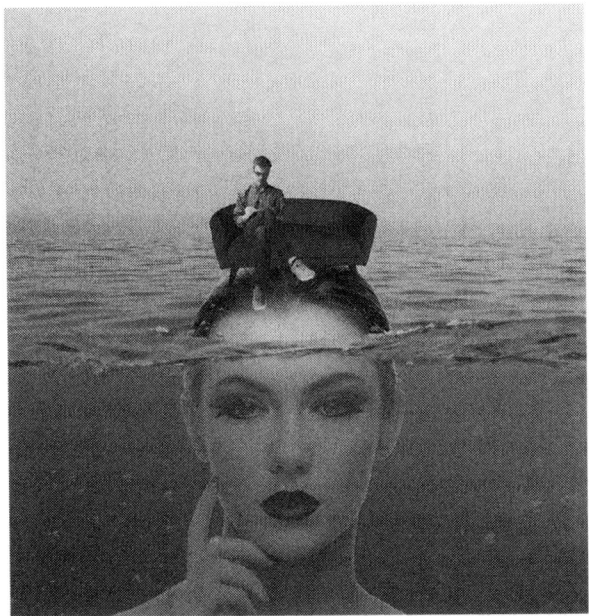

Psychodynamic therapy is similar to psychoanalytic therapy in a way that is an in-depth form of talking therapy based on psychoanalysis principles and theories. However, psychodynamic therapy is not as focused on the relationship between the client and therapist but is more focused on the client's relationship with their external world. Usually, psychodynamic therapy is not as long as psychoanalytic therapy when it comes to the number of sessions and frequency; however, this differs case by case.

Psychodynamic therapy is mainly used to treat depression or anxiety and other severe psychological disorders. It focuses especially on the people who may have lost meaning in their lives and struggle with maintaining and forming personal relationships. Studies have found that people who suffer from eating disorders, addiction, and social anxiety disorders benefit from psychodynamic therapy. During psychodynamic therapy, the client is encouraged to speak about anything that comes to mind including dreams, desires, fantasies, current issues, through the help of the therapist. The goal of this therapy is for the client to experience a reduction of their depression or anxiety systems but also achieve other benefits such as better use of their own abilities and talents, increasing self-esteem, and an improved ability to develop and maintain better relationships. The client may continue to experience the benefits even after this therapy has ended. Some patients may find that short-term therapy (less than one year) is sufficient; some other patients may require long-term therapy in order to gain lasting effects.

Psychodynamic therapy's theories and techniques distinguishes itself from other forms of therapy by focusing on acknowledging, recognizing, expressing, understanding, and overcoming contradictory and negative feelings and repressed emotions in order to help the client improve their interpersonal relationships and experiences. This includes helping the client understand how their previous repressed emotions affect their current behavior, relationships, and decision-making. This type of therapy also aims to help the client who may be aware of their social difficulties but don't have the tools or skills to overcome this problem by themselves. During this therapy, the clients will learn to analyze and resolve their current issues and then change their behavior in their current relationships through the use of deep exploration and analysis of their past experiences and emotions.

Blended Approaches

We talked about the three main types of psychotherapy which is CBT, IPT, and psychodynamic therapy. There is another common approach that is either a blend of a few different types of psychotherapy, or it could be one psychotherapy with integrated talking therapies with digital content. For instance, while a person is going through CBT, they may be given homework through educational modules or using apps that can monitor their sleep or mood. This usually helps the therapist have reflective conversations with the client.

Blended approaches of psychotherapy haven't been fully integrated into mental health services at the grand scale. Researchers are still studying the best methods to integrate digital content with the traditional face to face therapy, as well as how they can collect evidence on the effectiveness of it all. In a general sense, identifying barriers and facilitators for these digital methods has been a distinguishing line of work over recent years as this method is growing in popularity. For instance, some people may not have the means to pay for a therapist so they can opt for CBT programs online or through a self-help book in order to self-direct their therapy and learning. This is a great area of opportunity for researchers to study.

Medical Treatment

When it comes to antidepressants, it is the most advertised treatment for depression and anxiety, but it doesn't necessarily mean that it is the most effective. Depression is about chemical imbalances in the brain, but it does not mean that it is only that. Medication often can help relieve the symptoms of moderate to severe depression, but it does not solve the underlying problem and is not a long-term solution. Like we learned previously, antidepressants come with side effects, and if a person is not weaned off properly, they can suffer from withdrawal.

In order for you to make the right treatment decision for yourself, we will be exploring antidepressants more in-depth in this subchapter. Antidepressants are a range of medications that are used to treat depression or other mental disorders. They are the most commonly prescribed medications these days. Antidepressants include SSRIs (serotonin reuptake inhibitors), SNRIs (serotonin-norepinephrine reuptake inhibitors, TCAs (tricyclic antidepressants), atypical antidepressants and MAOIs (monoamine oxidase inhibitors).

Antidepressants are designed to adjust the neurotransmitters in the brain to help correct the balance of chemicals. When a person is in the trenches of torment depression's pain and anguish, simply taking a pill can seem like a method of relief that is simple and convenient. However, it is important to keep in mind that the imbalance of brain chemicals isn't the only cause of depression. Instead, it is a combination of that and other psychological, biological, and social factors that include coping skills, relationships, and lifestyle, all of which medication would not be able to address. However, does not mean the antidepressants are not effective. When a person's depression is on a severe level, antidepressants can be lifesaving or very helpful. Although medication can help people relive some of their symptoms, antidepressants do not cure depression and is not a recommended long-term solution. However, as more time goes by, people who originally had found antidepressants to be useful can fall back into depression, this goes the same for the people who stop taking the medication. In addition, antidepressants also come with undesirable side effects, so it is important for people to consider the pros and cons when they are considering taking depression medication.

Chapter 6: Stress and Anger Management Techniques

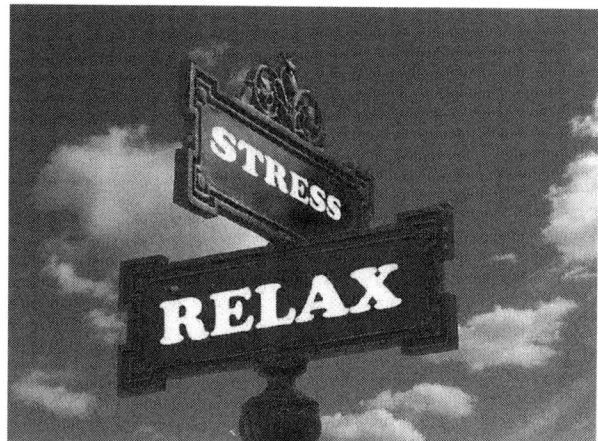

In our earlier chapters, we learned about some tips and tricks to help prevent and manage stress when you are faced with it. In this chapter, we will be focusing on three specific techniques of stress management; Action-Oriented approaches, Emotion-Oriented Approaches, and Acceptance-Oriented Approaches. Without further ado, let's jump right in.

Action-Oriented Approaches

Approaches that are action-oriented allows you to take action by yourself to change the stressful situation you are in. Let's take a look at some simple steps to do this.

1. Assertiveness

Being assertive allows us to express what we need and have people listen and accommodate your needs. The important part of being assertive is doing it in a fair and firm manner while also considering other people's feelings. This way, you're not being abrasive but just firm on what you're asking.

2. Reduce Distractions

We may think that distracting ourselves with the internet or Netflix may help us de-stress; in fact, it just clutters our mind even further. Switch off your technology or other stimuli for a few moments and let your mind take a break. Assess how much time you are spending with these technologies and see if it helps to cut down some screen time.

3. Manage Your Time

If we don't manage our time properly, we'll either spend too much time working or too much time relaxing. To create a less stressful environment, schedule your time properly to achieve a balance. This will help bring down stress levels when you know that you have a pre-made plan.

Emotion-Oriented Approaches

Emotion-oriented approaches are used to change our minds rather than our actions. It helps up gain a different perspective on the stressful situation at hand. Let's take a look at how we can do this.

1. Imagery and Affirmations

Positive imagery and affirmations are a very powerful tool and have been proven by scientists all over the world to positively impact a person's emotions. When a person is thinking of a positive experience, the human brain thinks it is actually reality. By replacing negative and stressful thoughts with positive ones, you can change the way you see and feel.

2. Cognitive Restructuring

Cognitive restructuring is the modern-day Cognitive Behavioral Therapy. The basis behind this is teaching a person to change their thoughts and thinking patterns to one that is more positive than negative. Since our thoughts directly affect our emotions, changing our thoughts will change our emotions and then our behavior.

Acceptance-Oriented Approaches

Acceptance-oriented approaches are most helpful in situations that you cannot control. For instance, if there was a recent death in the family, you cannot change this, but you can learn ways to accept it.

1. Diet and Exercise

We talked about this briefly in the earlier chapters, taking care of your physical body will affect your mental health and vice versa. Simple changes like reducing consumption of alcohol and sugars will do wonders to make you feel better.

2. Meditation

Techniques such as guided visualizations, deep breathing, and yoga are effective ways to calm your body and induce deep relaxation. You will have the opportunity to learn more about meditation later on in this book.

Anger Management Techniques

In this chapter, I am going to present several anger management techniques that will help you in those times where you are feeling angry, and all you want to do is act out in anger. If you are a person who tends to act on your feelings of anger with aggression, verbal outbursts or even physical violence, these techniques will prove quite useful in your journey to employ nonviolent communication.

1. Counting

When you feel the anger inside you that is making your blood boil, count up to ten or fifty, depending on your level of anger. If you are furious, make it 100. This technique is helpful in giving you time to calm yourself physically. Your heart rate will slow down to a normal level, and your adrenaline responses will subside as well. This allows you to take a step back and think more clearly.

2. Breathing

When you are angry, your breathing becomes shallow and short. When you are feeling angry, focus on your breathing by slowing it down and making yourself take long and deep breaths. Inhale through your nose and exhale through your mouth. By focusing on your breathing, it helps you calm yourself and gives your brain the oxygen it needs to think clearly.

3. Mantra

Having a mantra may seem a little airy-fairy if you are not usually one to use this type of thing, but it proves quite helpful in times of intense emotion. A mantra is a word or a phrase that you repeat, which is designed to help you concentrate on meditation. In day to day life, though, it helps bring your consciousness back to the moment, just like meditation does. Your mantra can be anything, such as "relax," "you're safe," or anything that helps you to calm yourself in the moment. Decide on your mantra in a moment of calm and quiet so that it is there in the back of your mind when you need it in a moment of anger.

4. Stretching

Stretching is a good practice for moments of intense anger because it helps to bring you back down to earth. It reconnects you with your body and your muscles, which will help bring you to the moment and will help with your blood flow. Any stretches are good, neck rolls, leg stretches, or shoulder rolls are great.

5. Visualizing

This is a great tool for when it is difficult to control your anger. Go somewhere quiet and get comfortable. Close your eyes and visualize your ideal relaxing scene. Imagine you are there. Imagine the sights, smells, sounds, and feelings that you would be experiencing. By doing this, you are tricking your brain into thinking you are in this scene, which will bring you feelings of relaxation, joy, and comfort.

6. Stopping

If you are having an outburst or yelling out everything that you would not have said had you not been so angry, make yourself stop talking. Glue your lips together, and do not allow yourself to open them for a few minutes. This time where you cannot allow yourself to spit out a slew of words that you do not mean will give you some time to think before you decide what you want to say or do.

7. Exercising

Exercise does great things for your body, especially in times of intense anger. The positive feelings of "runner's high" that you get after doing exercise will help to dispel some of your anger. Also, putting your anger into the gym will help you to harness and take your anger out in a healthy way.

8. *Writing*

There are likely many things that you want to say, but that you know would do more harm than good, especially if you say them in a time of anger. Write these things down. This way, you are still expressing yourself and your anger, but you are not hurting anyone or your relationships by doing so. This helps you process your emotions and can help you to examine them from afar in order to decide the best course of action.

9. *Ranting*

Ranting to someone who is not involved in the situation can help you to express yourself without offending someone who is involved and risking damaging your relationship. Healthy ranting to a third party is helpful in allowing you to express yourself and process the situation as well as your feelings about it.

10. *Laughing*

Laughing can actually help to diffuse your anger. Laughing is a strong medicine, so making yourself laugh when feeling intense feelings of anger can help you to relax a little and take a step back. Watching a funny show, talking to a friend who makes you laugh, or scrolling the internet for funny content are all ways of doing this.

Chapter 7: Mindfulness And Meditation Techniques

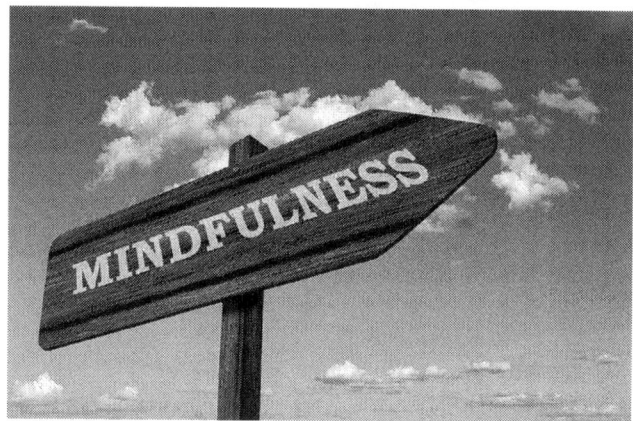

The most commonly practiced meditation is mindfulness meditation. Mindfulness meditation is a type of mental training practice that involves you focusing your mind on your own thoughts and sensations in the present moment. This includes your current emotions, physical sensations, and passing thoughts. Mindfulness meditation usually involves breathing practice, mental imagery, awareness of your mind and body, and muscle and body relaxation. It is typically easier for beginners to follow a guided meditation directing them throughout the whole process. It is extremely easy to drift away or fall asleep while in meditation if there is nobody guiding you. Once you become more skilled in mindfulness meditation, you are able to do it without a vocal guide, but this requires strong mental capabilities.

Mindfulness Meditation

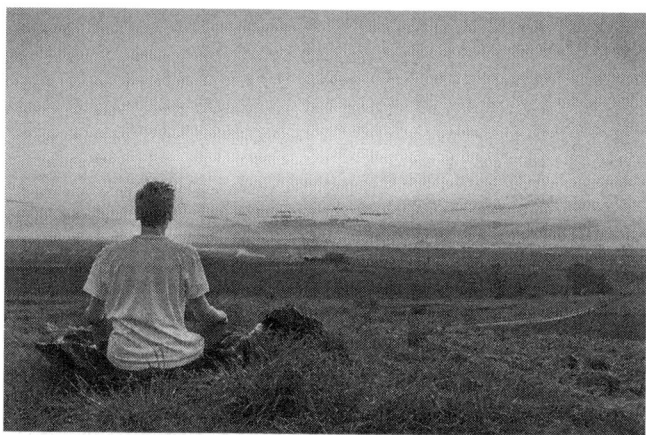

Next, we are going to discuss how to practice mindfulness meditation. One of the original and standardized programs for this type of meditation is called the Mindfulness-Based Stress Reduction (MSBR) program. This program was developed by Jon-Kabat-Zinn, Ph.D., who used to be a student of a Buddhist monk; Thich Nhat Hanh. This particular standardized program focuses on your own awareness and bringing your attention to the present. This method has actually been increasingly incorporated into medical settings to treat many health conditions including stress, pain, and insomnia. This method is fairly straight forward; however, it is recommended that a teacher or program can help guide you as you start. Most people do it for at least ten minutes a day but even a couple minutes every single day can make a difference in your wellbeing. This is the basic technique that will help you get started:

1. Find a quiet place that you feel comfortable in. Ideally, your home or someone where you feel safe. Sit in a chair or on the floor. Make sure your head and back are straight but are not tense.
2. Try to sort your thoughts and put aside those that are of the past and future. Stick to the thoughts about the present.
3. Bring your awareness to your breath. Make sure to focus on the feeling and sensation of air moving through your body as you inhale and exhale. Feel the way your belly rises and falls. Feel the air enter through your nostrils and leave through your mouth. Make sure to pay attention to the differences in each breath.
4. Watch every thought come and go. Act as if you are watching the clouds, letting them pass by you as you watch each one. Whether your thought is a worry, fear, anxiety, or hope - when these thoughts come up, don't ignore them or try to suppress them. Simply acknowledge them, remain calm, and anchor yourself with your breathing.
5. You may find yourself getting carried away in your thoughts. If this happens, observe where your mind went off to, and without making a judgment, simply return to your breathing. Keep in mind that this happens a lot with beginners. Try not to be too hard on yourself when this happens. Always use your breathing as an anchor again.
6. As we near the end of the 10-minute session, sit for a minute or two and become aware of where you physically are. Get up gradually.

The Joyful Mind Meditation

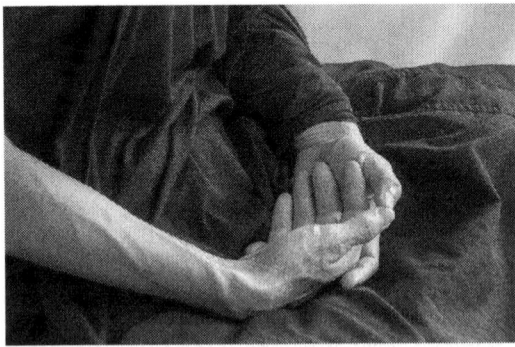

This meditation can be used for a time of stress and anxiety. It will help guide you into a more relaxed state where you can focus on the present and find inner peace. Please use this meditation method when you find your mind racing. This can also be used if you feel like you are about to have an anxiety or panic attack.

"Welcome to the joyful mind, guided meditation.

Please find yourself in a quiet area to sit and dim the lighting.
Make sure you are comfortable. Sit with your back straight and shoulders relaxed. Loosen any tight clothing that may be restricting you.

Let your hands lie loosely and relaxed into your lap. Close your eyes and take a deep breath. Now, relax.

Now that your eyes are closed, you may begin to connect with your inner self of thoughts and feelings.

Gradually, let the outside world fade from your awareness.

For the next few minutes, allow yourself to enjoy and submerge into this relaxing experience.

You are free from all your responsibilities during this meditation. Any thoughts, tasks, or concerns that you may have do not require your immediate attention. Tuck those thoughts away and focus on your inner thoughts.

You may find that your mind will begin to wander during this meditation. This is okay, and this is normal. Simply bring your awareness back to the present and to the sound of my voice. I will guide you into a place of inner peace and deep relaxation.

Remember that you are always in control of yourself. If you wish to end this meditation, you can do so by opening your eyes.

Begin to take a slow, long, and deep breath in through your nose. Release that breath through your mouth.

Find your inner self begin to relax.

Begin to take another deep breath in, and exhale.
Notice how calming this type of breathing is. Be aware of the feelings of relaxation starting to spread throughout your body. Starting from your lungs, all the way down to your toes.

Continue to breathe deeply, slowly, and gentle. Try not to breathe too quickly.

With each inhale and exhale, your thoughts start to become lighter.

You may start to feel a sense of spaciousness inside of you. It will open up slowly.

Keep relaxing.

Allow the soft movement of your breath to guide you into an even more relaxed state of being.

Breathe in. Breathe out. Deeper you go into this state of relaxation.

Breathe in. Breathe out. Let your mind gradually slow down. Breathe in. Breathe out. Let it slow down some more.

Breathe in. Breathe out.

You are now in a state of relaxation. You may now begin to enjoy a guided journey into your inner place of joy and serenity.

Allow images and visualizations to form in your mind naturally, as I speak. Do so at your own pace.

If visualizations and mental pictures aren't coming easily to you, simple sense your imaginary surroundings instead of visualizing them.

Begin to let your expectations drift away from you. Let them go. Allow yourself to experience this meditation journey in whatever form comes naturally to you.

Begin to imagine that you are standing in a green and beautiful grassy field. The field stretches on for miles. You can feel the heat of the sun on your face, slowly warming your body.

You feel the soft and lush green grass, cushioning your bare feet. You can smell the nature all around you.

You can hear the sounds of nature around you. You hear the rustling of the blowing grass. Birds are singing. The rustling of leaves in the distance.

You feel very much at home in this serene place.

You have all the time in the world.

You are safe and happy here.

Take a moment to appreciate your surroundings.

You notice a large luscious tree growing close by.

You begin to walk towards that tree.

Take your time walking. There is no rush whatsoever. Stay in the moment and appreciate the feeling of each step.

As you walk towards the tree, you feel yourself falling more deeply into a state of relaxation.

You are now standing under the tree. It's long branches, and large leaves hang right above your head.

You notice that the tree holds many delicious fruits in all shapes, sizes, and colors.

This is not just an ordinary tree. Its fruits carry special powers.

Reach your arm up and take a piece of fruit from the branches. Watch it for a moment. Notice the color of this fruit, the texture, and the weight. It's quite heavy in your hand.

Take a bite of this fruit.

As you swallow the fruit, it slides down your throat and into your belly. You begin to feel something wonderful happen.

A feeling of happiness and peace begins to glow inside of your body.

The sensation starts in your abdomen, and it spreads to your chest and into your heart.

Let go of thinking, and begin to bring all your attention on feeling. Embellish in the sensation of joy, love, and peace. Feel your body gently glowing with these feelings.

Take another bite of the magical fruit. Taste it. Savor every bite.

This wonderful feeling begins to intensify even more.
Feel yourself begin to radiate this beautiful sensation to love and happiness.

Take another bite of the fruit. Take as many bites as you'd like.

Relax and let yourself drown in this enchanting feeling. Instead of trying, just let it effortlessly take over. Break down any walls that you feel comfortable breaking and let it surround you as much as you like.

Stay with these joyful and peaceful feelings. Enjoy this time of meditation.

You may remain in this relaxed state of meditation for as long as you please. Don't feel rushed to leave."

When you are ready, you may finish this meditation. Simple open your eyes to leave. Take a deep breath and give yourself a few moments to adjust before standing up.

Chapter 8: Neuroplasticity

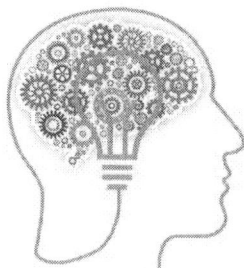

In the last chapter of this book, we are going to be learning about Neuroplasticity. This may sound like a complicated term, but it really isn't. Neuroplasticity is the 'muscle building' part of our brains. It is what determines what skills we grow stronger at with practice and what skills begin to fade away if we don't use them often. This explanation is based on the theory that doing an action or thinking a thought over and over again increases its power. When you do this for an extended period of time, it becomes 'muscle' memory in your brain and will be hard to forget or lose. Since our brain is the most important organ that helps us think and do actions, if we are able to harness neuroplasticity, then we can improve on all the things we want to do and think. Let's take a look at some factors that help increase neuroplasticity in adults.

Factors That Increase Neuroplasticity in Adults

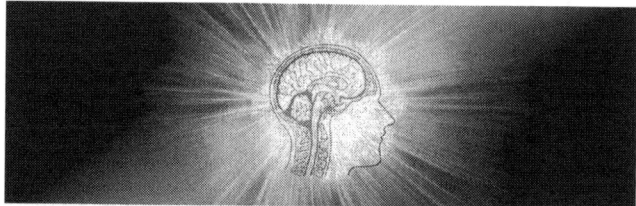

Neuroplasticity is extremely important as it is what helps a person recover if their brain becomes injured or is damaged by illness. Your brain has the capability to reorganize its physical structure and the wiring of it based on what environment you're in. Recent discoveries of the human brain found evidence that it is not a 'fixed' organ, as some people used to think. It has been proven that the human brain has the ability to rewire and repair itself. The benefit of this is that your brain can use its neuroplasticity to recover from a brain injury, but you can also use it to build better habits and prevent mental disorders like stress, anxiety, and depression. Let's take a look at 5 factors that help increase neuroplasticity.

1. Getting Quality Sleep

The human brain requires good quality sleep in order to reset the connections that are crucial for learning and memory. Even just one night of bad sleep or no sleep at all heavily impacts the brain's ability to reset those connections, which impacts a person's memory. For adults, the standard amount of sleep required is between 7 – 9 hours per night.

2. Continue Learning

When a person uses their brain to learn something, it improves their neuroplasticity. It has been proven that learning new languages strengthens brain functions. Not only is mental exercise good for the human brain, but physical exercise, especially cardiovascular exercises, also helps with boosting oxygen supplies into the brain which increases the brain volume.

3. Reduce Stress

Stress is the brain's silent killer; not only does it have a ton of negative physical and mental effects on your body; it also diminishes neuroplasticity. As we mentioned throughout this book, if you can't lower the number of stressors in your life, then you must learn to change how you perceive it or respond to it.

4. Find a purpose

It has been proven that if you are motivated and alert, your brain functions will change more significantly. If you have a strong purpose behind a reason for learning something, you naturally will be able to focus harder and longer. This has been proven to improve a person's neuroplasticity.

5. Read Books

Reading has been a proven source of improving brain connectivity. It helps stimulate it to get juices flowing and helps with initiating some of your learning functions as well. Plus, it's a great stress reliever and is much better for you than surfing the web or watching TV.

Conclusion

First of all, I'd like to congratulate you for reading until the end of this book. Your determination and motivation to learn more about stress and how to overcome it is extremely respectable. By understanding what stress is and how it works, you should have a much better idea of why the methods suggested in this book will work to help you overcome it. In order to be able to tackle your stress, you first have to identify what the causes of your stress are and the triggers as well. By knowing exactly what they are and when they tend to happen, you will be able to either avoid it or make a plan to tackle it, so it does not catch you by surprise.

Remember, stress reduction is extremely important in day to day life. Most people think stress is something they can 'just get over' or that if they acknowledge it, people will think that they are 'weak'. These are all unhealthy misconceptions that you need to let go of. Although it is true that stress is a part of life, too much of it can cause a lot of harm to a person's mental and physical health. Just like how changing your physical health can greatly affect your mental health, changing your mental health can affect your physical health. Be sure to keep looking out for symptoms of stress and keep track of them. You don't want high-stress levels to manifest into other disorders like anxiety and depression. Luckily, there are numerous proven treatments that have helped millions of people significantly to treat common mental disorders.

Let's take a look at everything that we learned in this book and help you to apply it in real life. We started off this book by learning about what stress was, the different types of it, and the symptoms. With this knowledge, you should be able to identify what your type of stress is and what symptoms you are experiencing. This will help you determine the level of stress you have (acute, episodic, chronic). Next, we learned about the most common causes of stress. Is your stress caused by mostly external factors or internal factors? This makes a huge difference because the solutions to this are drastically different. We then learned about the common triggers of stress to help you identify the exact moment or situations that your stress gets triggered. Next, we learned several tips on how to overcome stress. These tips are ones that you can apply to your everyday life without the help of a therapist. Towards the meat of this book, we learned about other mental disorders that are related to stress, such as; anxiety, depression, and panic disorders. We then proceeded to learn about different techniques to overcome them; this includes lifestyle changes, psychotherapy (cognitive behavioral therapy) and medical treatment. We then proceeded to learn more techniques to manage stress and anger. Towards the end of this book, we studied meditation and mindfulness techniques that can help you learn how to practice deep relaxation. This not only helps reduce stress, but it is also a great way to prevent other disorders like GAD. In the last chapter, we studied neuroplasticity and learned about how it plays a big role in the health of a person's brain. We studied the different factors that we can look at in order to increase a person's neuroplasticity, so they are more resilient and have a better ability to heal from trauma and illnesses.

Remember, the only way for these techniques to work is for you to test them out in real life. Just because your friends and family said a certain technique worked for them, it doesn't mean it will work for you. Everybody is different. Try out each technique for at least 2-3 weeks before trying something new. Remember to incorporate different techniques that help different parts of your body. For instance, make sure you are combining techniques that are focused on restructuring your cognitive functions and techniques that are focused on increasing your physical health (like exercising). Most people find that the best treatment plan is one that is a combination of both mental therapy and physical therapy. Remember, stress isn't something that will just go away if you ignore it. It is one of the most silent killers in today's world. In order to live a healthy and fulfilling life, you have to actively practice stress prevention and management techniques until they are part of your routine.

Meal Prep Cookbook for Beginners

Useful Weekly Plans Simple, Healthy Keto Recipes

Ready-To-Go Meals for Kids and Busy Family
Easy Cooking Steps to Save Time, Money, Lose Weight and Feel Better

By Alan Dieter

© Copyright 2019 by Alan Dieter - All rights reserved.

The content contained within this book may not be reproduced, duplicated or transmitted without direct written permission from the author or the publisher.

Under no circumstances will any blame or legal responsibility be held against the publisher, or author, for any damages, reparation, or monetary loss due to the information contained within this book. Either directly or indirectly.

Legal Notice:

This book is copyright protected. This book is only for personal use. You cannot amend, distribute, sell, use, quote or paraphrase any part, or the content within this book, without the consent of the author or publisher.

Disclaimer Notice:

Please note the information contained within this document is for educational and entertainment purposes only. All effort has been executed to present accurate, up to date, and reliable, complete information. No warranties of any kind are declared or implied. Readers acknowledge that the author is not engaging in the rendering of legal, financial, medical or professional advice. The content within this book has been derived from various sources. Please consult a licensed professional before attempting any techniques outlined in this book.

By reading this document, the reader agrees that under no circumstances is the author responsible for any losses, direct or indirect, which are incurred as a result of the use of the information contained within this document, including, but not limited to, — errors, omissions, or inaccuracies.

Table of Contents

Introduction 318
Chapter 1: Meal Prep Principles 320
   Meal Prep – Storage & Reheating 321
   Correct Refrigerator Organization 322
   Equip the Kitchen 323
   Preparation – Useful Items 324
   Purchase or Prepare the Containers You Want to Use 325
   Popsicle Molds or Push-Up Pop for Smoothies 326
Chapter 2: Multitasking Skills Using Time Organization 326
   Consider These Additional Tips 327
Chapter 3: Simple Meal Prep 331
   Week 1 331
   Day 1 331
   Day 2 336
   Day 3 340
   Day 4 345
   Day 5 350
   Day 6 355
   Day 7 361
   Week 2 366
   Day 8 366
   Day 9 371
   Day 10 377
   Day 11 382
   Day 12 388
   Day 13 394
   Day 14 399
Chapter 4: Keto Diet 405
   What Is the Keto Diet? 405
   Variations of the Ketogenic Diet Plan 406
   Benefits of the Keto Diet 407
   Week 1 408
   Day 1 408
   Day 2 413
   Day 3 418
   Day 4 424
   Day 5 431
   Day 6 437
   Day 7 443
   Week 2 449
   Day 8 449
   Day 9 455
   Day 10 461
   Day 11 466
   Day 12 470
   Day 13 476
   Day 14 481
Chapter 5: Meal Prep for Kids 485
   Week 1 486
   Day 1 486
   Day 2 491
   Day 3 497
   Day 4 502
   Day 5 507
   Day 6 512
   Day 7 516
   Week 2 521
   Day 8 521
   Day 9 526
   Day 10 530

Day 11 535
Day 12 540
Day 13 544
Day 14 549
Chapter 6: Delicious Snacks Dips & Spreads **554**
    Dips & Spreads 566
Conclusion **572**

Introduction

Congratulations on purchasing your copy of the *Meal Prep Cookbook for Beginners,* and thank you for doing so. There is a wealth of information to get you started. We will discuss how to perform meal prep and better understand you are setting your unique methods using these suggestions. As you begin your nutritional journey, it's vital to understand better the healthy eating pyramid is simply an elaborate grocery list.

The food pyramid is a triangular diagram introduced initially in Sweden in 1974. The *Food Guide Pyramid* was developed in 1992 by the United States Department of Agriculture (USDA) to display food groups according to their values. The plan was updated to *My Plate* in 2011. The guidelines are divided into four categories comprised of these food items:

- Vegetables are 40%
- Grains are 30%
- Fruits are 10%
- Proteins are 20%

Know What Your Body Is Craving

To maintain a healthier body, you need to take care of its needs and know what it's craving. These are a few suggestions to consider:

Soda: You may have a calcium deficiency if all you want is the delicious taste of soda pop. Try eating, kale, broccoli, sesame seeds, mustard greens, or legumes to help remove the urge.

Sugary Foods: Several things can trigger the desire for sugar, but typically phosphorous, and tryptophan are the culprits. Have some chicken, beef, lamb, liver, cheese, cauliflower, or broccoli.

Chocolate: The carbon, magnesium, and chromium levels are beckoning a portion of spinach, nuts, and seeds, or some broccoli and cheese.

Salty Foods: It is possible that you may have a chloride deficiency. Enjoy a few olives, celery, tomatoes, or add some sea salt to your diet.

Cheese: You may be lacking the essential fatty acids deficiency. Help remedy the craving with some walnuts, ground flaxseeds, chia seeds, sesame seeds, flax oil, legumes, broccoli, kale, or mustard greens.

Fatty or Oily Foods: The levels of calcium and chloride need repair with a serving of spinach, broccoli, cheese, or fish.

You will have an array of meal plans to choose from consisting of simple preps, Keto diet preps, and kid-friendly preparation lists.

Chapter 1: Meal Prep Principles

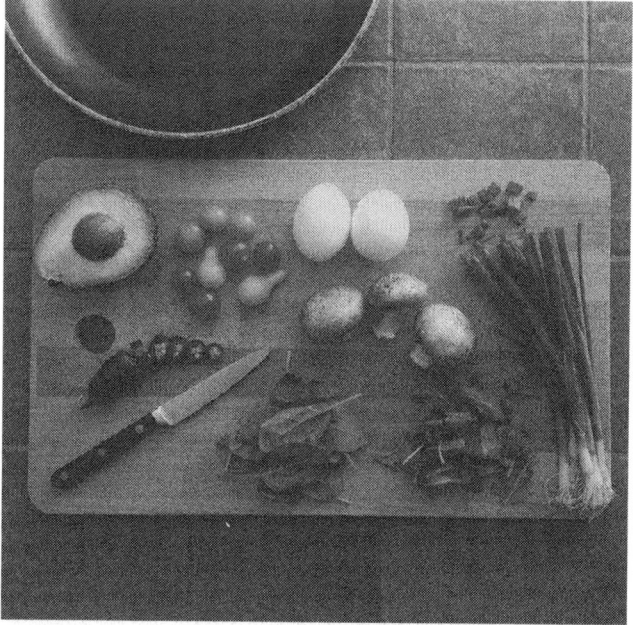

Save a Ton of Effort and Time: All it takes is a few tasty recipes and a little bit of your valuable time. In most of thecases, these recipes are geared towards a fast lifestyle and will be ready with just a few simple steps. After some time and practice, you will know which ones will be your favorites.

Use Your Freezer: Purchase meat when it's on sale and buy it in bulk. Freeze it for later. Assemble your meals in zipper-type bags and defrost when you want a quick and easy meal.

Mix & Match: If you have a busy lifestyle, purchase veggies and fruits pre-chopped and peeled and create an omelet or a stir-fry dinner. Use divided containers and prep into them.

Use Batch Cooking: Use a big pot on the stovetop or a slow cooker to prepare a batch of soup, chili, curry, or other delicious meals. By using sheet pan meals and dump dinners, you can save a ton of time and have a variety of meals.

By using these suggestions and the additional ones provided in your new cookbook, you will derive so many more benefits, including eating healthier, dropping a few unwanted pounds, and saving money since you will eliminate wasted food. It all comes down to your organization and multitasking skills. It can begin by choosing one strategy each week to improve your meal prepping skills.

Meal Prep – Storage & Reheating

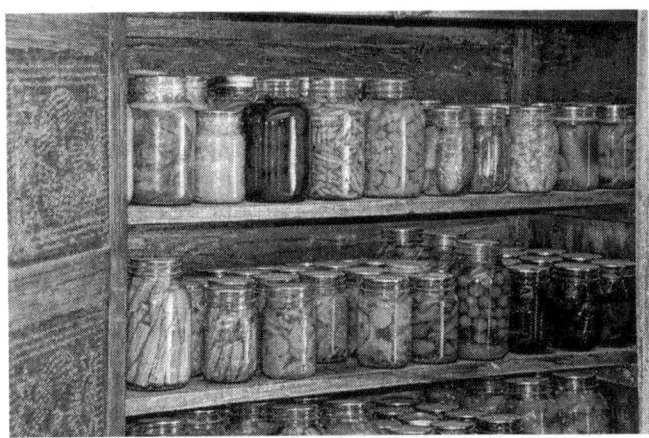

Don't store hot food in the fridge: Keep your refrigerator set at an adequate temperature (below 40° Fahrenheit). If your refrigerator is warmer than this, it promotes the growth of bacteria. Any drastic temperature changes will cause condensation to form on the food items. You need to let your prepared food cool down in the open air - before putting it in a container and closing the lid. The increased moisture levels can open the door to bacteria growth.

Label the Containers: There are some other things you have to consider when freezing your meals. You should always label your container with the date that you put it in the freezer. You also need to double-check that your bottles, jars, or bags are each sealed tightly. If your containers aren't air-tight, your food will become freezer burnt and need to be trashed.

Meat Cooking – Internal Temps

- **Poultry** - should reach a minimum of 165° Fahrenheit.
- **Whole cuts of lamb, pork, and beef** - a minimum of 145° Fahrenheit.
- **Ground veal, pork, lamb, and beef** - a minimum of 160° Fahrenheit.

Correct Refrigerator Organization

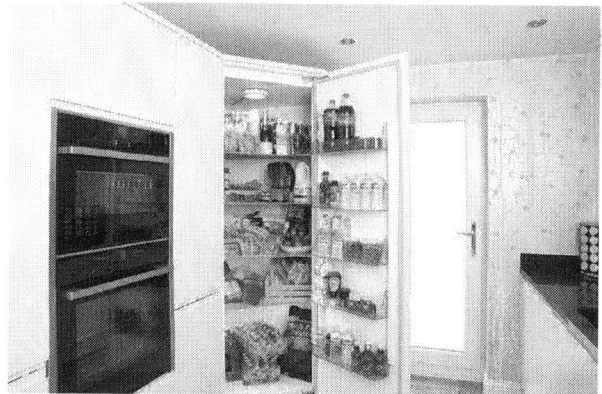

Since you are taking the incentive to understand meal prep better, you also have to consider the proper storage of your valuable products. You have several compartments in the refrigerator to store your prepared foods. You must understand which foods store best in each location.

- **Lower Shelves:** This is generally the coldest section of the refrigerator, making it an ideal space for dairy, eggs, and raw meat. Your unit may have individual drawers for these items to ensure a consistent temperature.

- **Top Shelves:** Once you have prepared your meals or smoothies, it's recommended to place them on the upper shelves since these are items used most often. They also have the most consistent temperature settings.

- **Sealed Drawers:** Fruits and veggies should get stored in this space while avoiding the mixing of meat, fruits, and vegetables. Storing these foods together can create a risk of cross-contamination.

- **Doors:** Many refrigerators have a door to access frequently retrieved food items - available as pullout drawers without opening the main door. Non-perishable items such as drinks, some condiments, water, and other items that don't quickly spoil could be placed here.

- **Top:** Don't place bread or baked products on top of the refrigerator. The heat from the fridge could cause it to spoil more quickly.

Equip the Kitchen

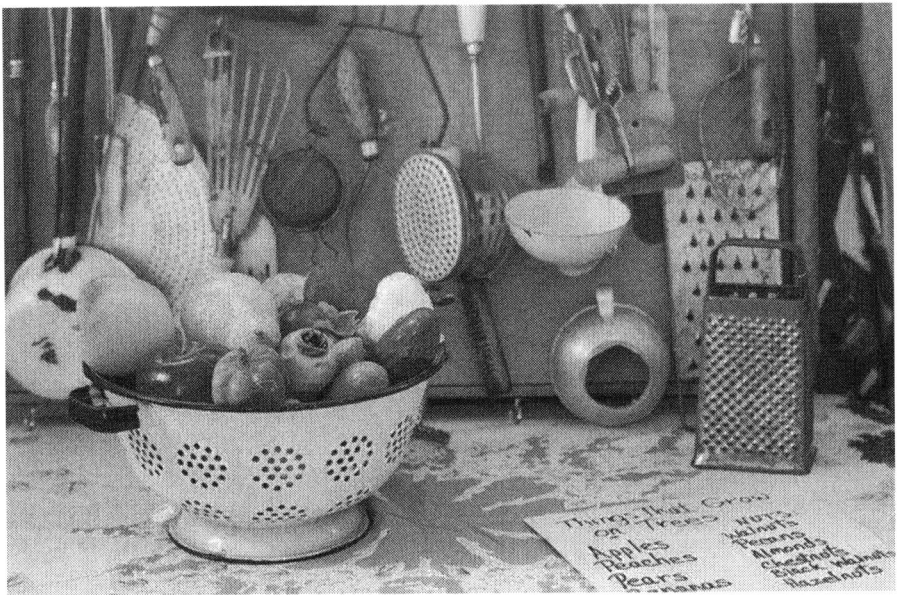

A Good Set of Scales: Portion control is essential for baking bread. You want a scale that will accommodate your needs. Consider these options:

- ***Seek a Conversion Button:*** You need to know how to convert measurements into grams since not all recipes have them listed. The grams keep the system in complete harmony.

- ***Removable Plate:*** Keep the germs off of the scale by removing the plate. Be sure it will come off to eliminate the bacterial buildup.

- ***The Tare Function:*** When you set a bowl on the scale, the feature will allow you to reset the weight back to zero (0).

Accurate Measuring Tools: A measuring cup and spoon system that shows both the Metric and US standards of weight is essential, so there is no confusion during food prep.

Sifter: Purchase a good sifter for under $10, and you will be ensured a more accurate measurement for your baking needs.

Immersion or Regular Blender & Food Processor: These are useful in many stages of meal preparation at the restaurant level as well as in your kitchen.

Buy a Spiralizer or a Sharp Knife & Paring Knife: You can prepare zoodles, which are noodles cut from zucchini easily.

Preparation – Useful Items

An unglazed terra cotta tile at the bottom of a clean oven or a baking stone might be a good investment if you are planning on doing a lot of baking at home. You can also purchase an upgraded stand mixer with a dough hook. It's a good idea to have a few different sized loaf pans.

You should also invest in several mixing bowls to use.

A bench knife, better known as a dough scraper, can be used to clean surfaces, divide the dough, and to pre-shape the loaves of bread. Some even use it to dice veggies and apples.

- ***Sheet Pans/Rimmed Baking Sheets:*** (2) 12x18-inch pans.
- ***Skillets:*** Choose from a cast-iron skillet or a 10-12-inch nonstick skillet with a lid.
- ***4-Quart Saucepan:*** Prepare veggies using this type of pan, for example.
- **8-quart covered stockpot:** Prepare your favorite stews and soups.
- ***Meat Thermometer:*** To ensure proper cooking.
- ***Garlic Press or Spice mill:*** These two utensils add additional flavor to your food and reduce the temptation of using a shaker of salt.
- ***Vegetable Steamer:*** This is essential because it will make the preparation of healthy vegetables much simpler without the use of oil or butter.
- ***Cutting Boards:*** Purchase individual boards for produce and meat/fish/poultry. You can also purchase plastic cutting 'boards' which are easily cleaned

These are a few additional items that will assist you with the baking process:

- Measuring cups for liquid and dry ingredients
- Measuring spoons
- Rolling pin

- Medium to large-sized saucepan

- Rubber spatula

- Wire cooling rack

- Bread cutting board

- Electric mixer

- Plastic wrap – damp tea towel

- Parchment paper will be used for most of the recipes. The baking pans are lined with the paper, and the baked goods do not stick. For most baking needs, you can omit the oils if you choose the paper instead. However, some recipes use paper and oils.

Purchase or Prepare the Containers You Want to Use

These are some guidelines for those:

- Mason Jars – Pint or quart-sized
- Ziploc-type freezer bags
- Rubbermaid Stackable - Glad Containers

- Freezer Safe
- Microwavable
- BPA Free
- Reusable
- Stackable

Popsicle Molds or Push-Up Pop for Smoothies

You can purchase ice-pop clear pouches for <u>one-time</u> use or use a <u>mold</u> to reuse many times. Save money by using freezer bags to avoid using freezer space with a quart-sized freezer-safe Mason jar.

Chapter 2: Multitasking Skills UsingTime Organization

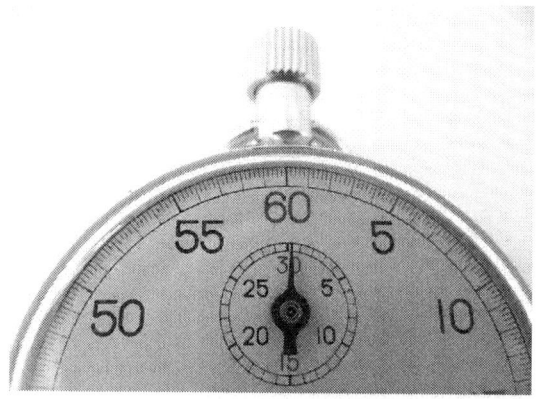

Meal prep might seem a bit challenging at first, but remember— you don't need to prep all of your meals at one time. You can begin with the meats one evening, and veggies the next; it's all up to you!

- *Time Selection:* Choose a time to do your meal prep, so you do not have any interruptions

- *Take Advantage of Your Crockpot & Slow Cooker:* You will find the crockpot a must if you have a busy lifestyle. These are just a couple of ways you can benefit from its use:

  - *Get Ahead of the Meal:* Preparing food with a slow cooker can put you ahead of the game. You can prepare the cooker the night before if you have a busy day planned. All it takes is a few minutes of preparation. Just add all of the fixings into the pot and place it in the fridge—overnight. The next morning, transfer to the counter to become room temperature. Turn it on as you head out of the house.

- *Take A Physical Inventory of the Pantry and Other Food Storage Areas:*

Purchase your food items in bulk to save money. Therefore, you are saving money while on the ketogenic diet is vital. Purchasing your items in bulk can make a severe impact. Shop around and explore your areas for stores such as Walmart, Costco, or Sam's Club. These stores generally have bargain prices. Check your area for local farms that raise their animals on pasture feeding or a local market for fresh produce. After you find a good deal, stock up and purchase pantry items such as seasonings and flour. You can freeze many things and save a bundle of cash.

- *Choose the Menu Plan:* Gather your favorite recipes or try some new ones.
  - *Decide How to Prep:* Do you want to prepare all of the chicken, pork, or other meal selections one night and the veggies the next night? Or: Do you want to cook each meal individually but in bulk? No worries, either way, since each of the recipes has instructions for individual prep tips as well.

Consider These Additional Tips

- Chop your veggies in advance. Make veggie packs to use for tacos, pasta, and stir-fries. You can also use them for snacks.
- Prep starches in advance, including rice and quinoa on a Sunday, and use

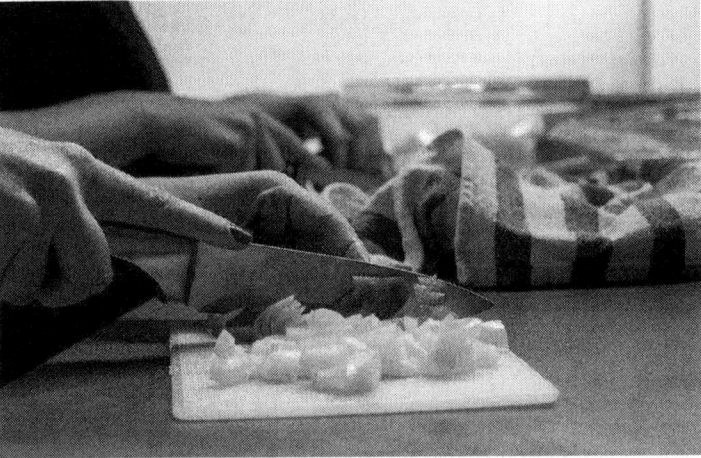

them for the week.
- Prepare and freeze plenty of healthy fruits and yogurt into a delicious smoothie for the entire week. Enjoy one for breakfast or any time you have the craving.
- Purchase foods in bulk to be used for taco meats, breakfast burritos, fajita fillings, soups, egg muffins, and so much more.
- As you prep, include lean proteins for the weekends in a

container for a quick grab 'n' go snack or luncheon for a weekend journey.

- See where your recipe ingredients overlap for different meals. For example, onions and peppers are often used.
- Prepare and freeze the freshly prepared chicken in different marinades so you can have a quick and healthy meal option.

- Consider freezing your meals even if it is just one portion, for those emergencies when nothing else will do!
- Prepare a batch of breakfast options ahead of time. Think about some of the recipes included in your new cookbook, such as overnight oatmeal in a jar if you are on-the-go.
- Prepare batches of dressings and sauces ahead of time, so you always have a delicious option to spice up your meals.

Guidelines for Dairy – Meats & Veggies

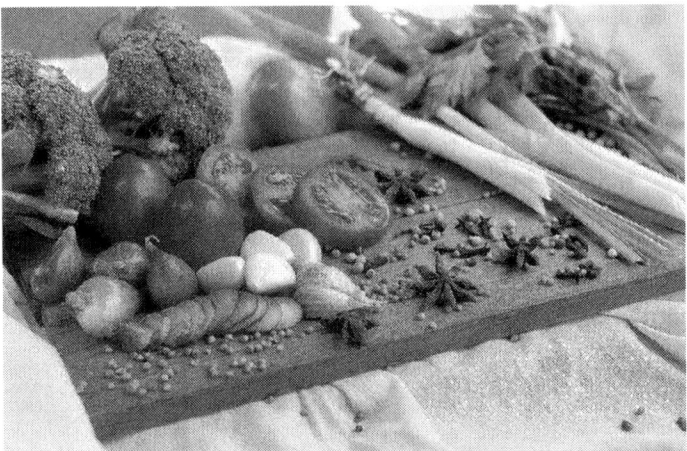

- *Choose fresh meats and dairy when possible:* Try to find meat and dairy that has an expiration date for as far in the future as possible. These choices will tend to remain fresh and last longer. This also applies to the "sell by" dates. The further in the future, either of these dates is, the surer you can bet that the food is going to last the week.

- *Purchase Whole – Not Chopped Meats & Veggies:* You can save big by chopping or slicing your own meats and vegetables. You will pay for the person that is doing the cutting for your convenience.

- *How to Freeze & Reheat Your Meats:* For meals that are scheduled to be eaten at least three days after cooking, freezing is a great option. Freezing food is safe and convenient, but it doesn't work for every type of meal. You can also freeze the ingredients for a slow cooker meal, and then dump out the container into the slow cooker and leave it there. This saves a lot of time and means you can pre-prep meals up to 1-2 months in advance.

The last food safety consideration you need to make with regards to meal prepping is how you reheat food. Most people opt to microwave their meals for warming, but you can use any other conventional heating source in your kitchen as well. The reason people love the microwave for heating their meal prep meals is that it's quick and convenient.

However, you have to be careful with microwaving because over- cooking can cause food to taste bad. To combat this, cook your food in one-minute intervals and check on it between each minute. You can also help your food cook more evenly and quickly but keeping your meat cut into small pieces when you cook it. You should never put food directly from the freezer into the microwave. Let your frozen food thaw first.

Food reheating and prep safety will become second nature over time. Meal prep can be overwhelming and require a lot of thought and patience, but it becomes a lot easier once you get used to it. Many of the mistakes are easy to avoid.

However, mistakes do happen, and as such, it's best to cook for short periods rather than longer ones, so you have less of a risk of making a mistake and needing to scrap everything you have prepared for that substantial period of time. While it is a lot and seems complicated, meal prepping is the best way to set yourself up for success.

Chapter 3: Simple Meal Prep

Week 1

Day 1

Breakfast: Avocado & Egg Breakfast

Yields Provided: 4

Ingredients for Prep:

- Brown rice (.5 cup)
- Large eggs (6)
- Olive oil (2 tbsp.)
- Minced garlic (2 cloves)
- Chopped kale (4 cups)
- Freshly grated parmesan (.25 cup)
- Sliced avocado (1)

Method of Prep:

1. Prepare a pot of boiling water (1 cup) and prepare the rice of choice according to the directions provided.
2. Arrange the eggs in another pan with 1-inch of cold water. Once it's boiling, let it simmer for one minute. Cover and transfer the pan from the burner to rest for 8 to 10 minutes. Use a colander to drain the eggs and peel.
3. Use the medium heat setting to warm the oil. Toss in the pepper flakes and garlic. Sauté for one to two minutes. Fold in the kale, stirring until wilted (5-6 min.)
4. Shake in the parmesan.

Tips for Meal Prep:
1. Let the fixings cool thoroughly.
2. Use a divided container to store the eggs, rice, kale, and avocado.

Lunch: Beef Soup

Yields Provided: 4

Ingredients for Prep:

- Ground beef sirloin (1 lb.)
- Olive oil (1 tbsp.)
- Low-sodium beef stock (32 oz.)
- Whole wheat flour (.33 cup)
- Yellow onion (1)
- Mixed celery & carrots (1 lb.)

Method of Prep:
1. Prepare a soup pot using the oil (med-high heat setting) until it's hot.
2. Add the beef and flour. Simmer for about 5 minutes.
3. Chop and toss in the celery, carrots, and onions. Pour in the stock and stir. Lower the heat setting to medium.
4. Continue cooking the soup for about 15 minutes.

Tips for Meal Prep:
1. Cool thoroughly before ladling into four mugs or other storage containers.
2. Securely close the tops if using a plastic container.
3. Freeze for longer storage. Date the package and use it within several months.

Dinner: Mediterranean Whitefish

Yields Provided: 4

Ingredients for Prep:

- Raw white fish fillets - cod, tilapia, sole, etc. (4 - 4 oz.)
- Olive oil (4 tsp.)
- Mediterranean spice mix or chopped fresh oregano
- Optional: Fresh lemon (as desired)

Mediterranean Spice Mix:

- Dried onion flakes (4 tsp.)
- Dried oregano (1 tsp.)
- Crushed dried parsley (4 tbsp.)
- Ground thyme (1 tsp.)
- Crushed dried basil (2 tsp.)
- Garlic powder (1 tsp.)
- Sea salt (1 tsp.)
- Ground black pepper (.25 tsp.)

Method of Prep:

1. Warm the oven broiler to high.
2. Drizzle the fish with oil. Season using the Mediterranean spice mix.
3. Broil the fish until it's opaque and flakes easily when tested with a fork (3-5 min.).

Tips for Meal Prep:

1. Arrange the cooked fish in a shallow pan or baking sheet and pop into the freezer for quick freezing.
2. Wrap the fish in a moisture-resistant paper or freezer bag. It will store well for up to one month.
3. To thaw, just pop the bag into a pot of boiling water for about five minutes.
4. Spritz to your liking using fresh lemon juice before serving.

Snack: Avocado Hummus Snack Jars

Yields Provided: 4 jars

Ingredients for Prep:

- Chickpeas (1 can)
- Tahini (.5 cup)
- Avocado (1)
- Garlic (2 cloves)

- Lemon juice (1 tbsp.)
- Salt (.5 tsp.)
- Water (.25 cup)
- *Optional Fixings*:
- Sliced sun-dried tomatoes or antipasto
- Celery, carrot, or cucumber sticks
- Assorted chips, crackers, etc.
- Suggested: Vitamix
- Also needed: 4 salad mason jars/other containers

Method of Prep:
1. Rinse and drain the chickpeas. Mince the cloves and dice the avocado.
2. Combine all of the fixings (omit the optional fixings).
3. Remove the lid and stir as needed until fully mixed (5 min.)
4. Scoop the mixture into the jars and top with the desired toppings.

Tips for Meal Prep:
1. Store in the fridge for a quick and healthy snack.
2. Enjoy within the first two or three days for the best results.

Day 2

Breakfast: Broccoli Cheddar Egg Muffins

Yields Provided: 6

Ingredients for Prep:

- Whole eggs (8)
- Egg whites (4)
- Optional: Dijon mustard (.5 tbsp.)
- Broccoli (2 cups **)
- Shredded cheddar cheese (.75 cups)
- Pepper and salt (as desired)
- Diced green onions (2)

Method of Prep:
1. Set the oven at 350° Fahrenheit.
2. Prepare six muffin tins with paper liners or cooking spray.
3. Whisk all of the eggs, salt, pepper, and mustard. Blend in the green onions, broccoli, and cheese.
4. Divide the batter into the tins and bake for 12-14 minutes.
5. ** Use either fresh and steamed or defrosted and frozen broccoli.

Tips for Meal Prep:
1. Transfer the muffins to the countertop to cool.
2. Store in the fridge to use for a quick breakfast.
3. Serve when they are puffy and thoroughly cooked.

Lunch: Apples with Almonds & Figs Salad

Yields Provided: 6

Ingredients for Prep:

- Dried figs (6)
- Large red apples (2)
- Celery (2 ribs)
- Fat-free lemon yogurt (.5 cup)
- Slivered almonds (2 tbsp.)
- Carrots (2)

Method of Prep:
1. Chop the figs and celery. Peel and grate the carrots. Core and dice the apples.
2. Mix the fixings, beginning with the celery, apples, and figs.
3. Prep the carrots and almonds and store them in individual dishes if desired.

Tips for Meal Prep:
1. Store the fixings in the fridge using either individual salad dishes or in one large bowl. Be sure the salad is covered.
2. Stir and blend in the yogurt when it's mealtime.
3. Garnish with the carrots and almonds.

Dinner: Pork Chops with Creamy Sauce

Yields Provided: 4

Ingredients for Prep:

- Black pepper and salt (.5 tsp. each)
- Onion powder (.5 tsp.)
- Center-cut pork loin chops (4 - Approx. 4 oz. each)
- Non-fat Half & Half (.33 cup)
- Fat-free chicken stock (.33 cup)
- Dijon mustard (1.5 tbsp.)
- Dried thyme (A pinch)

Method of Prep:
1. Shake the salt, pepper, and onion powder over the chops.
2. Using the med-high heat setting on the stovetop, prepare a large skillet with cooking spray.
3. After the pan is heated, arrange the chops in it and fry for three to four minutes per side. The internal temperature should reach a minimum temperature on a meat thermometer of 145° Fahrenheit.

Tips for Meal Prep:
1. At this point, place the prepared chops in a container with a lid to cool.
2. Measure and add the chicken stock into the pan and deglaze the browned bits. Stir in the mustard and Half & Half.

3. Lower the temperature setting to medium and continue cooking for about 7 minutes. When the sauce has thickened, add the thyme.
4. Set the sauce aside to cool. Freeze if you won't be using the sauce within one day.
5. Wrap the chops well and store them in the fridge until time to eat. Serve with the sauce and your favorite side dish.

Snack: Bacon Cheddar Cheese Crisps

Yields Provided: 3

Ingredients for Prep:

- Cooked bacon (3 strips)
- Shredded cheddar cheese (1 cup)

Method of Prep:
1. Set the oven ahead of time to 350° Fahrenheit.
2. Prepare a baking tin with a sheet of parchment paper.
3. Pour about one tablespoon of the cheese onto the tray for each serving. Break the bacon to bits and add to the piles of cheese.
4. Bake for 5 to 8 minutes and let cool.

Tips for Meal Prep:
1. Blot the grease away with a paper towel.
2. Fully cool and store in a container in the refrigerator until the desired time to serve.

Day 3

Breakfast: Gluten-Free Roasted Grapes & Greek Yogurt Parfait

Yields Provided: 4

Ingredients for Prep:

- Seedless grapes (1.5 lb./4 cups)
- 2% plain Greek yogurt (2 cups
- Olive oil (1 tbsp.)
- Honey (4 tsp.)
- Chopped walnuts (.5 cup)

Method of Prep:

1. Warm the oven to reach 450° Fahrenheit and place the pan inside.
2. Discard the stems from the grapes and rinse them. Wipe using a towel and toss into a mixing container.
3. Wipe with a towel and put it in a bowl. Spritz with oil and toss to coat and bake for 20 to 23 minutes. They will look slightly shriveled. Stir about halfway through the cooking process.
4. Take the pan from the oven. Cool for five minutes.
5. Meanwhile, assemble the parfaits by adding the yogurt to the glass.

6. Once the grapes are cooled, garnish the yogurt with a teaspoon of honey, two tablespoons of the walnuts, and a portion of the grapes.

Tips for Meal Prep:
1. Prepare each of the four servings into individual dishes.
2. Keep the parfait in the refrigerator for up to three days.

Lunch: Tomato & Olive Salad

Yields Provided: 10

Ingredients for Prep:

- Cucumbers (5)
- Red or purple onion (half of 1)
- Green olives (2.25 oz. can/jar)
- Black olives (5 oz. can or jar)
- Tomatoes (5 large)
- Crumbled feta cheese (4 oz.)
- Red wine vinegar (.25 cup)

Method of Prep:
1. Chop the olives, cucumbers, and tomatoes. Crumble the feta.
2. Combine all of the fixings except the vinegar.

Tips for Meal Prep:
1. Store the dressing and salad fixings in individual containers.
2. Pop it into the fridge until it's time to eat.
3. Drizzle the dressing on top of the salad and serve.

Dinner: Chicken & Asparagus Pan Dinner

Yields Provided: 8

Ingredients for Prep:

- Chicken breasts (4 lbs.)
- Avocado oil (1 tbsp.)
- Trimmed asparagus (1 lb.)
- Sun-dried tomatoes -(4)
- Thick-cut bacon (4 slices)
- Salt (1 tsp.)
- Pepper (.25 tsp.)
- Provolone cheese (8 slices)
- Also Needed: 1 baking pan

Method of Prep:
1. Slice the chicken into 8 thin pieces. Chop the bacon and tomatoes into one-inch pieces.
2. Heat the oven to reach 400° Fahrenheit.
3. Add oil to the baking pan with the chicken and asparagus. Top it off with the tomatoes, bacon, pepper, and salt.

4. Bake until the chicken reaches 160° Fahrenheit internally - or about 25 minutes.
5. Toss in the asparagus and cheese.
6. Garnish with the bacon and tomatoes. Bake another three to four minutes until the cheese has melted.

Tips for Meal Prep:
1. Simply prepare the chicken and store it in the fridge for several days.
2. Place it into plastic bins or freezer bags until ready to use.
3. Prepare the asparagus when ready to eat and combine with the cheese. Garnish and serve.

Snack: Bacon Knots

Yields Provided: 4

Ingredients for Prep:

- Raw bacon (16 slices)
- Shredded parmesan (.25 cup)
- Minced garlic (4 cloves)
- Minced parsley (1 tbsp.)
- Pepper & Salt (to your liking)

Method of Prep:
1. Straighten one slice of bacon. Tie it into a knot.
2. Take another slice, and tie another knot around the first one. Continue until done.
3. Place the chain on a parchment-lined baking tin.

4. Warm up the oven to reach 400° Fahrenheit.
5. Sprinkle the bacon with the garlic and bake for 15 minutes.

Tips for Meal Prep:
1. When crispy, remove from the pan and chill in the refrigerator until mealtime.
2. When it's time to serve, heat the oven to 400° Fahrenheit. Sprinkle using the parsley and cheese.
3. Bake for one or two minutes until hot. Break apart and serve.

Day 4

Breakfast: Spinach Muffins

Yields Provided: 6

Ingredients for Prep:

- Nonfat milk (.5 cup)
- Eggs (6)
- Crumbled low-fat cheese (1 cup)
- Spinach (4 oz.)
- Chopped roasted red pepper (.5 cups)
- Chopped prosciutto (2 oz.)

Method of Prep:
1. Set the oven temperature at 350° Fahrenheit.
2. Combine the eggs, milk, spinach, cheese, prosciutto, and red peppers. Whisk well.
3. Lightly spritz a muffin tray with a cooking oil spray.
4. Dump the batter into the muffin tins and bake until browned (30 minutes).

Tips for Meal Prep:
1. Cool thoroughly on a wire rack.
2. Arrange in a plastic container or freeze to enjoy later.

Lunch: Arugula Salad

Yields Provided: 4

Ingredients for Prep:

- Arugula leaves (4 cups)
- Cherry tomatoes (1 cup)
- Pine nuts (.25 cup)
- Pepper & salt (as desired)
- Grated parmesan cheese (.25 cup)
- Large avocado (1 sliced)
- Rice vinegar (1 tbsp.)
- Olive/Grapeseed oil (2 tbsp.)

Method of Prep:
1. Rinse and dry the leaves of arugula.
2. Slice the cherry tomatoes into halves and grate the cheese.
3. Slice the avocado.

Tips for Meal Prep:
1. Combine the arugula, tomatoes, pine nuts, and cheese into four salad containers.
2. Either place the slices to the side in another container or a divided container for storage.
3. When it is time to serve, add the oil and vinegar with a shake of pepper and salt.

Dinner: Jalapeno Popper Burgers

Yields Provided: 4

Ingredients for Prep:

- Ground beef (1.33 lb.)
- Finely chopped jalapeno (1)
- Cream cheese - reduced-fat (2 tbsp.)
- Mustard (2 tsp.)
- Worcestershire sauce (2 tsp.)
- Shredded cheddar cheese (.5 cup)
- Kosher salt - divided (.5 tsp.)

Method of Prep:
1. Combine all of the burger fixings. Divide into six patties and wait about 10 minutes before cooking for the flavors to mix.
2. Grill to your liking (four to six min. per side suggested). If you prefer, use a frying pan, and cook for five to six minutes for each side.

Tips for Meal Prep:
1. Let the burgers thoroughly cool. Store in the fridge for about three days.
2. When ready to eat, warm the burgers and serve with the desired garnishes.
3. Freeze in plastic containers with other meal items (veggies) or freeze individually in freezer bags.
4. *Note*: You can also use ground turkey.

Snack: Peanut Butter Power Granola

Yields Provided: 12

Ingredients for Prep:

- Pecans (1.5 cups)
- Almonds (1.5 cups)
- Sunflower seeds (.25 cup)
- Almond flour or Shredded coconut (1 cup)
- Swerve sweetener (.33 cup)
- Vanilla whey protein powder (.33 cup)
- Butter (.25 cup)
- Peanut butter (.33 cup)
- Water (.25 cup)

Method of Prep:
1. Set the oven at 300° Fahrenheit.
2. Prepare a rimmed baking tin with a layer of parchment paper.
3. Process the almonds and pecans in a food processor and add to a large bowl.
4. Fold in the sunflower seeds, sweetener, shredded coconut, and protein powder.
5. Place the butter and peanut butter in the microwave to melt. Pour over the nut mixture. Toss lightly. Mix in the water.
6. Spread the mixture evenly onto the baking sheet.
7. Bake for 30 minutes. Stir about halfway through the cycle.

Tips for Meal Prep:
1. Cool before storing in an airtight container.
2. Serve anytime.

Day 5

Breakfast: Greek Yogurt Pancakes

Yields Provided: 14 (5-inch pancakes)

Ingredients for Prep:

- Nonfat plain Greek yogurt (2 cups)
- Baking soda (2 tsp.)
- All-purpose flour (1 cup)
- Slightly beaten eggs (4)
- Salt (1 tsp.)
- 1% Low-fat milk (.5 cup)
- Vanilla (1 tsp.)

Method of Prep:
1. Use an electric mixer stand and scoop the yogurt and remainder of the dry fixings into the mixing dish, blending until just incorporated.
2. Whisk the milk, vanilla, and eggs. Combine everything.
3. Prepare the batter in a griddle pan or sprayed skillet until golden. When the bubbles begin, it's time to flip. Serve and enjoy.

Tips for Meal Prep:
1. Prepare the pancakes and cool them completely.

2. Store in the fridge if you are using them within a day. Otherwise, it's best to freeze them in closed containers or zipper-type freezer bags.
3. Begin by placing two pancakes on a microwave-safe plate. Microwave at 100% power or high power for 1 to 1.5 minutes or until warm, turning once.
4. Add butter and syrup, and breakfast is served!

Lunch: Tomato Soup

Yields Provided: 4

Ingredients for Prep:

- Olive oil (1 tbsp.)
- Onion (1)
- Garlic (3 cloves)
- Carrots (3)
- Roasted tomatoes (15 oz.)
- Tomato paste (1 tbsp.)
- Veggie stock (1 cup)
- Tomato sauce (15 oz.)
- Dried basil (1 tbsp.)
- Black pepper (1 pinch)
- Dried oregano (.25 tsp.)
- Coconut cream (3 oz.)

Method of Prep:
1. Chop the onion, garlic, and carrots.

2. Heat a soup pot using the medium temperature setting. Pour in the oil to heat until hot. Toss in the onion and garlic to sauté for about five minutes.
3. Pour in the tomato sauce, tomato paste, carrots, stock, tomatoes, basil, oregano, and black pepper.
4. Stir the fixings well and continue cooking for another 15 minutes.

Tips for Meal Prep:
1. Cool the soup and pour it into a large container until time to eat.
2. When it is time to eat, pour in the cream, and blend using an immersion blender.
3. Portion the tomato soup into serving bowls and serve.

Dinner: Turkey Sloppy Joes

Yields Provided: 4 -1 cup each Ingredients for Prep:

- Raw ground 93% lean turkey breast (1 lb.)
- Olive oil (1 tsp.)
- Medium onion (1)
- Garlic (2 cloves)
- Medium red bell pepper (1)
- Sea salt (.5 tsp.)
- Ground black pepper (.25 tsp.)
- All-natural tomato sauce, no salt or sugar added (1 cup)
- Worcestershire sauce, gluten-free (1 tbsp.)
- Raw honey/Pure maple syrup (1 tbsp.)
- Hot pepper sauce (1.5 tsp.)

- Optional: Fresh parsley (to taste)

Method of Prep:

1. Warm the oil in a large frying pan using the medium heat temperature setting.
2. Chop and add the garlic, onion, and bell pepper. Sauté for about one minute and add to a medium bowl. Set aside in a mixing bowl.
3. Add the turkey, salt, and pepper to the skillet. Simmer using the medium temperature heat. Stir often until the turkey is no longer pink (8 to 10 minutes).
4. Mix in the onion mixture, tomato sauce, hot sauce, Worcestershire sauce, and maple syrup.
5. Lower the heat to med-low, stirring occasionally until the sauce has thickened (15 to 20 minutes).

Tips for Meal Prep:

1. They are good in the fridge for 3-4 days.
2. Cool the *Sloppy Joes* thoroughly in the fridge before you freeze them in labeled freezer bags. Lay them flat in your freezer, so you can stack the frozen meals for three to six months.
3. Chop and sprinkle each serving with parsley before serving.
4. Place on 1 piece of whole-wheat toast or romaine lettuce leaves.

Snack: Fried Queso Fresco

Yields Provided: 5

Ingredients for Prep:

- Coconut oil (1 tbsp.)
- Queso fresco (1 lb.)
- Olive oil (.5 tbsp.)

Method of Prep:
1. Chop the cheese into cubes.
2. Warm both of the oils to the smoking point, and toss in the cheese.
3. Fry the cheese, flipping once until well browned.
4. Remove and let the cheese rest to cool.

Tips for Meal Prep:
1. Drain on towels to remove the oil.
2. Store in a closed container to enjoy anytime.

Day 6

Breakfast: Omelet Waffles

Yields Provided: 2

Ingredients for Prep:

- Black pepper (1 pinch)
- Eggs (4)
- Low-fat shredded cheddar cheese (.25 cup)
- Chopped ham (2 tbsp.)
- Chopped parsley (2 tbsp.)

Method of Prep:
1. Warm and lightly grease a waffle iron with a spritz of the cooking oil spray.
2. Combine all the fixings in a mixing container.
3. Empty the mixture into the iron and cook for four to five minutes.

Tips for Meal Prep:
1. Cool the waffles entirely before freezing, so they don't collect ice in the freezer.
2. Place them on a cookie tin, so they do not touch and let them fully freeze. If you want to prepare more, stack the trays for a few hours.
3. Place into resealable freezer bags until needed.

Lunch: Chicken – Apple Spinach Salad

Yields Provided: 4

Ingredients for Prep:

- Onion (.5 cup)
- Spinach (4 cups)
- Chopped toasted pecans (.25 cup)
- Acai dressing or your favorite (.75 cup)
- Cooked breast of chicken (2 cups)
- Granny Smith apples (2 cups)

Method of Prep:
1. Prep the Fixings: Dice the chicken. Chop the apples, pecans, and spinach. Slice the onion.
2. Use individual containers or one large salad dish to prep the salad, beginning with a layer of spinach.
3. Arrange the remainder of the fixings.

Tips for Meal Prep:
1. Note: You can wait to slice the apple if desired.
2. Cover the prepared salad with a lid or a layer of plastic wrap until serving time.
3. Sprinkle with the dressing to serve.

Dinner: Apricot BARBECUE Chicken

Yields Provided: 6

Ingredients for Prep:

- Breasts of chicken (1 lb.)
- Sugar-free BARBECUE sauce (.5 cup)
- Sugar-free Apricot jam (.5 cup)
- Low-sodium soy sauce (2 tbsp.)
- Ground ginger (1 tsp.)
- Onion powder (1 tsp.)
- Garlic powder (1 tsp.)

Method of Prep:
1. Warm the oven temperature at 350° Fahrenheit.
2. Trim away the skin and bones from the chicken. Prepare a baking sheet with foil and add the chicken.
3. Whisk the barbecue sauce, jam, seasonings, and soy sauce together in a mixing container. Pour over the chicken and bake for about 30 minutes.

Tips for Meal Prep:
1. This is a great choice for meal prep. Make this entire recipe and let it cool.
2. Store in the refrigerator for up to two days or freeze for later use.

3. Enjoy with your favorite side dishes.

Snack: Veggie Egg Cups

Yields Provided: 6 (2 each)

Ingredients for Prep:

- Homemade salsa (12 tbsp.)
- Green onions (2)
- Medium red bell pepper (1)
- Mushroom (1 cup)
- Large eggs (12)
- Nonstick cooking spray
- Sea salt and black pepper (as desired)

Homemade Salsa:
- Fresh cilantro (1 bunch)
- Small sweet onion (1)
- Garlic (3 cloves)
- Sea salt (.5 tsp.)
- Medium tomatoes (3)
- Medium jalapeno (1)

Method of Prep:

1. Prepare the salsa. Roast the jalapeno with the veins and seeds removed. Chop the cilantro with the stems removed. Finely chop and combine the jalapeno, tomatoes, garlic, onion, cilantro, and salt in a medium mixing container.
2. Prepare oven to 375° Fahrenheit. Spray a muffin tin with cooking spray.

3. Add the eggs, salt, and pepper in a large mixing bowl and whisk until blended. Finely chop and mix in the mushrooms, green onions, and bell peppers.
4. Fill each muffin cup evenly with the egg mixture.
5. Bake in the oven until a toothpick inserted into the center of the cups comes out clean (15-20 min.).

Tips for Meal Prep:
1. Freeze for Later: When completely cooled, put them in a gallon-sized freezer bag or container, squeeze out any air, seal, and freeze for up to 3 months.
2. Prepare from Frozen: Thaw overnight in refrigerator or pop into the microwave for a quick defrost.
3. To Serve: Top each egg cup with 1 teaspoon of homemade salsa.

Day 7

Breakfast: Banana Oat Pancakes

Yields Provided: 8 (2 pancakes each serving)

Ingredients for Prep:

- Extra-virgin coconut oil (.5 tsp.)
- Old-fashioned rolled oats - dry (2 cups)
- Sea salt (1 dash)
- Ground cinnamon (.5 tsp.)
- Baking powder (1 tsp.)
- Large ripe banana (1)
- Large eggs (2)
- Unsweetened almond milk (1 cup)
- Pure vanilla extract (1 tsp.)
- Fresh mixed berries (3 cups)

Method of Prep:
1. Combine the almond milk, salt, baking powder, cinnamon, eggs, banana extract, and oats in a blender. Blend until it's creamy.
2. Pour the oil in a frying pan using the med-low heat setting.
3. Pour ¼ cup of batter into the skillet and cook for two to three minutes. The edges of the pancake will

bubble when they're ready to flip. Cook for another 1.5 minutes.
4. Repeat the process until all of the batters are gone.

Tips for Meal Prep:
1. The pancakes that are not eaten can be frozen and reheated in a toaster.
2. Cool thoroughly, and place in freezer bags for longer storage.
3. When ready to eat, top with fresh mixed berries.

Lunch: Ham Salad

Yields Provided: 4

Ingredients for Prep:

- Mango chutney (1 tbsp.)
- Onion powder (2 tsp.)
- Light mayonnaise (2 tbsp.)
- Dried mustard (2 tsp.)
- Plain Greek yogurt - Nonfat (2 tbsp.)
- Cooked - chopped ham (1 cup)

Method of Prep:
1. Pulse the fixings (omit the ham or not) in a processor until creamy smooth.
2. Put the container in the fridge for 30-45 minutes or until needed.

Tips for Meal Prep:
1. For meal prep, place the salad into four individual bowls.
2. Leave in the refrigerator and enjoy on-the-run.

Dinner: Baked Chicken Fajita

Yields Provided: 4

Ingredients for Prep:

- Chicken breasts (1 lb.)
- Bell pepper (1)
- Onion (1 medium)
- Tomato (1 ripe)
- Cumin (1 tbsp.)
- Garlic powder (2 tsp.)
- Salt (1 tsp.)
- Black pepper (1 tsp.)
- Onion powder (1 tsp.)
- Chili powder (.5 tsp.)

Method of Prep:
1. Slice or chop the veggies. Slice the chicken into strips making sure to remove all of the skin and bone fragments.
2. Combine all of the seasonings in a mixing container and add the chicken. Toss.
3. Set the oven temperature at 375° Fahrenheit.

4. Use a misting of cooking spray on the casserole dish and add the prepared chicken in a single layer. Top with the veggies.
5. Bake 35-40 minutes.

Tips for Meal Prep:
1. This is yet another great option for meal prep.
2. Prepare as above and let it cool thoroughly.
3. You can put it into four separate containers for storage or freezing.
4. Enjoy with some salsa, cheese, on a tortilla, or any way you like it.

Snack: Mini Crustless Quiche

Yields Provided: 12

Ingredients for Prep:

- Large eggs (15)
- Plum tomatoes (3)
- Pepper jack cheese (.5 cup)
- Mozzarella cheese (1 cup)
- Sweet onion (.33 cup)
- Pickled jalapenos (.33 cup)
- Salami (1 cup)
- Heavy cream (.5 cup)
- Also Needed: Muffin tins - 11x15-inch

Method of Prep:
1. Warm up the temperature in the oven to 325° Fahrenheit.
2. Prep the veggies. Dice the tomatoes, onions, jalapenos, and salami. Shred the cheese.
3. Spritz the muffin tins lightly with a misting of cooking oil.
4. Whisk all of the fixings together and split the batter in the muffin tins.
5. Bake for 25 minutes.

Tips for Meal Prep:
1. Cool thoroughly and slice the quiche into 12 portions.
2. Wrap it in plastic wrap.
3. When ready to eat, microwave from frozen, using the high setting at 30-second intervals - probably no more than one minute.
4. If you don't slice it, cover it in foil. Place the prepared dish into an oven-proof container, and heat for 20 minutes using a 350° Fahrenheit oven.

Week 2

Day 8

Breakfast: Veggie Egg Scramble

Yields Provided: 6

Ingredients for Prep:

- Diced tomato (1)
- Large eggs (6)
- Baby spinach (3 cups)
- Minced garlic clove (1)
- Red or purple diced onion (half of 1)
- Freshly cracked black pepper and kosher salt (1 tsp. each)
- Olive oil (1.5 tbsp.)
- 2% sharp cheddar cheese - ex. Cabot (.5 cup)

Method of Prep:
1. Whisk the eggs, pepper, and salt.
2. Warm up the oil in a skillet. Toss in the spinach, onions, tomato, and garlic. Simmer until done or 5 to 7 minutes.
3. Pour in the eggs and simmer 3 to 4 minutes – stirring occasionally.

4. When set, let the container become room temperature and take it away from the burner.
5. Sprinkle the cheese. Serve and enjoy.

Tips for Meal Prep:
1. Prepare the eggs and set aside to cool.
2. Place in the fridge and take the fixings with you to work tomorrow for a healthy breakfast.

Lunch: Asparagus Soup

Yields Provided: 6

Ingredients for Prep:

- Cooked chicken breasts (2)
- Salt & black pepper (1 pinch each)
- Carrots (2)
- Chopped asparagus spears (12)
- Yellow onion (1)
- Spinach (4 cups)
- Minced garlic cloves (3)
- Low-sodium veggie stock (6 cups)
- Lime (half of 1)
- Olive oil (1 tbsp.)
- Chopped cilantro (1 handful)

Method of Prep:
1. Cook the chicken and remove the skin and bones. Finely chop the asparagus, yellow onion, and carrots. Mince the garlic cloves.
2. Use the medium heat setting on the stovetop, and add the oil to a soup pot.
3. When hot, toss in the onions and sauté for five minutes.
4. Next, toss in the garlic, asparagus, and carrots. Continue cooking for an additional five minutes.
5. Toss in the spinach with a dusting of the pepper and salt. Add the chicken and stock. Continue cooking for about 20 minutes.

Tips for Meal Prep:
1. Chill thoroughly before placing it in the fridge.
2. When it is time to eat, toss in the lime zest and cilantro.
3. Stir well and ladle the soup into serving dishes.

Dinner: Asian Glazed Chicken

Yields Provided: 4

Ingredients for Prep:

- Coconut aminos (.33 cup)
- Chicken thighs (8)
- Garlic (3 tbsp.)
- Balsamic vinegar (.5 cup)
- Olive oil (.25 cup)

- Black pepper (1 pinch)
- Garlic chili sauce (3 tbsp.)
- Green onion (1 tbsp.)

Method of Prep:
1. Set the oven temperature at 425° Fahrenheit.
2. Discard the bones and skin from the chicken. Mince the garlic and chop the green onion.
3. Prepare a baking sheet with a spritz of cooking oil spray.
4. Add oil to the pan along with the chicken, vinegar, aminos, chili sauce, onion, black pepper, and garlic.
5. Toss well and bake for 30 minutes.
6. When done, serve with the sauce.

Tips for Meal Prep:
1. This is super for meal prep since all you do is let it thoroughly cool.
2. Arrange the chicken into individual freezer bags or another type of storage container.
3. Be sure to label its contents and freeze.

Snack: Veggie Snack Pack

Ingredients for Prep:
- Foster Farms Bold Bites Pouch
- Cherry tomatoes (5)
- Red bell pepper (.25 of 1)

- Sugar snap peas (.33 cup)
- Baby carrots (.5 cup)
- English cucumber (.33 cup)
- Hummus (2 tbsp.)

Method of Prep:
1. Rinse all of the veggies.
2. Discard the seeds from the pepper and slice.
3. Slice the cucumber.
4. Measure out the rest of the fixings.

Tips for Meal Prep:
1. Fill a small reusable dipping sauce container with two tablespoons of hummus. Secure the lid and place it into the container.
2. Arrange the prepared vegetables into portions (bell peppers, cucumbers, tomatoes, carrots, and peas) and close the container.
3. Place in the fridge until you need a quick on-the-go snack. Serve with one package of *Bold Bites*.

Day 9

Breakfast: Spinach – Feta & Egg Breakfast Quesadillas

Yields Provided: 5

Ingredients for Prep:

- Olive oil (2 tsp.)
- Red bell pepper (1)
- Red onion (half of 1)
- Eggs (8)
- Milk (.25 cup)
- Black pepper and salt (.25 tsp. each)
- Spinach leaves (4 handfuls)
- Feta (.5 cup.)
- Mozzarella cheese (1.5 cups)
- Tortillas (5)

Method of Prep:

1. Warm the olive oil in a skillet using the medium temperature setting.
2. Dice the onion and peppers. Toss into the pan to sauté for 4-5 minutes.
3. Whisk the eggs, salt, pepper, and milk. Stir often and toss in with the onions and peppers until the eggs are done.

4. Fold the feta and spinach into the eggs, stirring until the spinach is wilted. Take the pan from the burner.
5. Spray another frying pan with a spritz of cooking oil and warm using the medium temperature setting. Add the tortilla and spread ½ cup of egg mixture on one side of the tortilla. Garnish with ⅓ cup of the mozzarella and fold over the tortilla. Cook until browned (2 min.).
6. Flip it and cook another minute. Continue until all are done. It should take no more than 25 minutes from start to finish.

Tips for Meal Prep:
1. Cool thoroughly on a rack and wrap in plastic or store in a resealable container.
2. Reheat on top of a paper towel in the microwave for 30 to 60 seconds.
3. Crisp on a grill or in a frying pan for two to three minutes.

Lunch: Salmon Vegetable Frittata

Yields Provided: 6

Ingredients for Prep:

- Eggs (6)
- Mushrooms (2 cups)
- Green onion (.25 cup)

- Butter or margarine (1 tbsp.)
- Smoked salmon (4 oz.)
- Skim milk (1 cup)
- Paprika (.25 tsp.)
- Pepper (.25 tsp.)
- *Also Needed*: Ovenproof skillet

Method of Prep:
1. Warm up the oven to reach 350° Fahrenheit.
2. Chop the onions and mushrooms. Sauté in melted butter in the pan for about three to five minutes.
3. Whisk the eggs with the milk, pepper, and paprika with a wire whisk until mixed.
4. Dice the salmon into small chunks. Fold into the egg mixture with the cooked onions and mushrooms. Toss well.
5. Bake for 30 minutes.

Tips for Meal Prep:
1. Carefully transfer the pan to the stovetop to cool.
2. Slice into six wedges and store in the fridge.
3. *Option #1*: You can individually wrap the frittatas or leave them in the pan to enjoy for a full meal.
4. Option #2: Portion the frittata into sealed containers with your favorite veggies for another meal.
5. Freeze after the first or second day.

Dinner: Thai Peanut Chicken

Yields Provided: 6-8

Ingredients for Prep:

- Chicken thighs (2 lb.)
- Minced garlic (2 tsp.)
- Coconut milk (14 oz. can)
- Creamy peanut butter (.5 cup)
- Lime juice (3 tbsp.)
- Ginger (1 tbsp. - grated)
- Tamari or soy sauce (2 tbsp.)
- Honey (3 tbsp.)
- Toasted sesame oil (1 tbsp.)
- Garam masala (1 tsp.)
- Curry powder yellow (2 tsp.)
- Cumin (1 tsp.)
- Red pepper flakes (.5 tsp.)

Method of Prep:
1. Trim and discard the bones from the chicken.
2. This is a great prep recipe since you put it together and freeze it to pop into a slow cooker at a later date.
3. In a medium container, mix the coconut milk, lime juice, ginger, tamari, honey, sesame oil, garlic, curry powder, cumin, garam masala, peanut butter, and red pepper flakes.

4. Whisk it all together until smooth. Add the chicken.
5. To Eat Now: Add the chicken and sauce to a crockpot and cook.

Tips for Meal Prep:
1. Transfer chicken and sauce to a labeled container or freezer bag and freeze.
2. From thawed or freshly made, transfer the chicken and sauce into a slow cooker. Cook using the low setting for six hours or the high setting for four hours.

Snack: Beef & Cheddar Roll-Ups

Yields Provided: 1

Ingredients for Prep:

- Cheddar cheese (half of 1 slice)
- Thousand Island yogurt/Regular dressing (1 tbsp.)
- Tomatoes & onions (as desired)

Method of Prep:
1. Thinly slice and lay the roast beef onto a preparation surface.
2. Place the cheese, dressing, and veggies on top.
3. Roll it up and secure with toothpicks.

Tips for Meal Prep:
1. When you are ready to eat, cut them into halves.

Day 10

Breakfast: Breakfast Bowls

Yields Provided: 6

Ingredients for Prep:

- Yukon gold potatoes (2 lb.)
- Green pepper (1)
- Onion (1)
- Olive oil
- Seasoned salt
- Eggs (12)
- Freshly shredded cheddar cheese (4 oz.)
- Green onions (3)
- Optional Toppings: Salsa - tortilla & avocado
- Individual-sized glass containers with lids or Tupperware type (6)

Method of Prep:
1. Dice the cucumber, onions, and potatoes into 1-inch cubes. Deseed and chop the green peppers.
2. Warm the oven at 425° Fahrenheit.
3. Prepare a baking tray with a drizzle of oil and add the onions, potatoes, and peppers. Dust with the pepper and seasoned salt.
4. Split the veggies onto two baking trays and roast for 30-40 minutes. Rotate and toss the potatoes about halfway through the baking cycle.

5. Whisk the eggs pepper and salt until smooth.
6. Prepare a skillet using the medium temperature setting with a spritz of cooking oil. Lower the heat to the low-temperature setting, cooking until the eggs until barely incorporated.

Tips for Meal Prep:
1. Divide the fixings evenly into two containers. Cool thoroughly and sprinkle with green onions and cheese. Place a lid on each container.
2. Eat the meal within three days or freeze.
3. When ready to reheat from frozen, set the microwave at 50% power, and set the timer for 1.5 minutes. Stir until fully heated. Top to your liking.

Lunch: Chili Con Carne

Yields Provided: 12 Ingredients for Prep:

- Ground chuck (5 lb.)
- Large onion (1)
- Green and red bell pepper (1 each)
- Garlic cloves (2)
- Chili powder (.5 cup)
- Cumin (2 tbsp.)
- Chipotle (1 tsp.)
- Pinto/kidney beans (2 - 15 oz. cans)
- Tomato paste (10 oz. can)
- Tomato sauce (2 - 10 oz. cans)
- Black pepper (1 tbsp.)
- Salt (2 tsp.)
- Water (2 cups or as needed)

- Cayenne (as desired)

Method of Prep:
1. Gather the fixings. Drain the beans in a colander. Seed and dice the peppers. Mince the onion and garlic.
2. Add the ground beef to a large pot using med-high heat. Cook it until browned. Drain the grease and mix in the onions, bell peppers, and garlic. Simmer for about three minutes.
3. Toss the remainder of the fixings into the pan. Simmer using the low-heat temperature setting (lid off) until the meat is tender or about one hour. Add more water as needed. Adjust the spices and serve hot.

Tips for Meal Prep:
1. Scoop the chili (1 cup) into a container or a plastic freezer bag. Seal, leaving ½ inch of empty space at the top.
2. Label it with the date you made it and also the time you placed it in the freezer. Usually, chilies that are frozen are good for one week.
3. Place each bag of chili at the end of the freezer, as this is the coldest part of the freezer.
4. To Eat: Thaw the chili in the refrigerator for 1 hour. Place it in a pot over medium heat (rolling boil). Keep the pot covered to retain moisture.
5. Upon boiling, lower the temperature. At this point, it's necessary to season it because the flavor has diminished a little during the freezing process.
6. Serve it piping hot.

Dinner: Cajun Chicken

Yields Provided: 4-5

Ingredients for Prep:

- Chicken breast (1 lb.)
- Black pepper (1 pinch)
- Olive oil (1 tbsp.)
- Dried oregano (.5 tsp.)
- Low-sodium vegetable stock (.25 cup)
- Cajun seasoning (1 tbsp.)
- Chopped green onions (4)
- Cherry tomatoes - cut in half (2 cups)
- Minced cloves of garlic (3)
- Coconut cream (.66 cup)
- Sweet paprika (.5 tsp.)
- Lemon juice (2 tbsp.)

Method of Prep:
1. Heat a skillet using the med-high temperature setting.
2. Once the oil is hot, toss in the chicken and portion of pepper. Cook on each side for five minutes.
3. Pour in the stock, oregano, lemon juice, cream, paprika, garlic, green onions, and the Cajun seasoning.
4. Simmer for about ten minutes. Divide into serving bowls and enjoy.

Tips for Meal Prep:
1. Let everything cool.
2. Portion the fixings into storage containers to freeze.

Snack: Fruit Snack Pack

Yields Provided: 3 packs

Ingredients for Prep:

- Raspberries (.5 cup)
- Sliced oranges (¼ of 1)
- Strawberries (4)
- Grapes (1 cup)
- Trail mix (2 tbsp.)
- Foster Farms <u>Bold Bites</u> Pouch (1)

Method of Prep:
1. Slice the orange before you begin.

Tips for Meal Prep:
1. Add the trail mix to a reusable dipping container.
2. Fill a small reusable dipping sauce container with 2 tablespoons of the trail mix. Close the top tightly and transfer to a single- compartment container.
3. Arrange the prepared fruit (orange, strawberries, grapes, raspberries) within the container and cover.
4. Serve with 1 pouch of your favorite Bold Bites and store in the fridge until ready to enjoy.

Day 11

Breakfast: Carrot Muffins

Yields Provided: 5

Ingredients for Prep:

- Whole wheat flour (1.5 cups)
- Stevia/your preferred sweetener (.5 cup)
- Baking soda (.5 tsp.)
- Cinnamon (.5 tsp.)
- Baking powder (1 tsp.)
- Natural apple juice (.25 cup)
- Egg (1)
- Olive oil (.25 cup)
- Freshly picked cranberries (1 cup)
- Grated carrots (2)
- Chopped pecans (.25 cup)
- Grated ginger (2 tsp.)
- Cooking oil spray (as needed)

Method of Prep:
1. Warm the oven to reach 375° Fahrenheit.
2. Drain the cranberries.

3. Sift or whisk the stevia, flour, cinnamon, baking soda, and baking powder in a mixing container.
4. Pour in the apple juice, whisked egg, oil, cranberries, carrots, pecans, and ginger. Stir thoroughly.
5. Lightly grease a muffin tray with a spritz of cooking oil spray. Divide the mix and to each of the containers.
6. Bake for 30 minutes. When ready, take out of the oven.

Tips for Meal Prep:
1. Leave in the muffin pan for 5 to 10 minutes to cool.
2. Remove each muffin from the pan and thoroughly cool before storing it in the refrigerator. Freeze for longer storage.
3. If frozen, leave them on the countertop to defrost for about 30 minutes.
4. You can also add them in a lunchbox for a quick pick-up at work.

Lunch: Classic Stuffed Peppers

Yields Provided: 6

Ingredients for Prep:

- Green peppers (6 large)
- Lean ground beef (1 lb.)
- Onion (.25 cup)
- Diced tomatoes (16 oz. can)

- Tomato sauce (16 oz. can)
- Basil (1 tsp.)
- Oregano (1 tsp.)
- Black pepper & salt (as desired)
- Instant white rice (1 bag)
- Shredded cheddar cheese (1 cup)

Method of Prep:
1. Warm the oven in advance to reach 350° Fahrenheit.
2. Brown the beef and finely chopped onion in a large skillet using the low-temperature setting.
3. Slice the tops off of each pepper, discard the seeds, and arrange in a lightly greased baking dish.
4. Prepare the rice according to package instructions and drain.
5. In a large mixing container, combine the tomato sauce, basil, oregano, salt, black pepper, rice, and diced tomatoes. Stir in the cooked beef and onions with a few chopped peppers if desired.
6. Spoon the mixture into each shell. Bake for 35 minutes.
7. Remove and add a portion of cheddar cheese on top. Place back into the oven. Bake until the cheese has melted (5 min.).

Tips for Meal Prep:
1. Cool thoroughly and wrap each pepper in plastic wrap. Place into freezer zipper bags or individual containers to keep for up to six months.
2. Defrost them in the microwave when desired. Reheat them for five minutes. Remove the dish

from the microwave and sprinkle with a portion of fresh cheese. Serve when ready.

Dinner: Cilantro Lime Chicken

Yields Provided: 6

Ingredients for Prep:

- Chicken breast (1 lb.)
- Orange juice (1 cup)
- Chicken broth (1 cup)
- Juice (2 fresh limes)
- Garlic (2 tsp.)
- Cilantro leaves (.5 cup)
- Black beans (1 can)
- Frozen corn (2 cups)
- Ground cumin (1 tbsp.)

Method of Prep:
1. Rinse and drain the beans, mince the garlic, and chop the cilantro leaves. Remove the skin and bones from the chicken.
2. This is great to prepare and set aside for those days when you are pressed for time. Add all ingredients to a gallon-sized freezer bag or container.

Tips for Meal Prep:

1. From thawed or freshly made, transfer into a slow cooker. Cook on high for three to four hours or low for six hours.
2. Serve as a homemade burrito bowl. Just add rice, sour cream, guacamole, and cilantro for a super delicious meal. Tacos and nachos are great ways to serve this as well.

Snack: Avocado Hummus Snack Jars

Yields Provided: 4 jars

Ingredients for Prep:

- Chickpeas (1 can)
- Tahini (.5 cup)
- Avocado (1)
- Garlic (2 cloves)
- Lemon juice (1 tbsp.)
- Salt (.5 tsp.)
- Water (.25 cup)
- Optional Toppings: Sliced sun-dried tomatoes/antipasto
- Celery, cucumber & carrot sticks
- Assorted chips & crackers

Method of Prep:
1. Rinse and drain the chickpeas. Dice the avocado and garlic. Cut the carrots, celery, and cucumber into wedges/sticks.
2. Toss all of the fixings (omit the optional/final toppings) into a Vitamix.
3. Blend using the lowest speed setting for about 30 seconds. Stir as needed until full mixed (5 min.).

Tips for Meal Prep:
1. Scoop into jam jars, and top with antipasto or sundried tomatoes.
2. Serve alongside cut-up veggies, crackers, chips, or whatever other snacks you're craving.
3. Enjoy within the first two to three days after preparation.

Day 12

Breakfast: Buckwheat Pancakes

Yields Provided: 6

Ingredients for Prep:

- All-purpose flour (.5 cup)
- Buckwheat flour (.5 cup)
- Baking powder (1 tbsp.)
- Sugar (1 tbsp.)
- Egg whites (2)
- Fat-free milk (.5 cup)
- Sparkling water (.5 cup)
- Fresh strawberries (3 cups)
- Canola oil (1 tbsp.)

Method of Prep:
1. Slice the berries. Whisk the oil, eggs, and milk in a small mixing container.
2. Use another dish to blend the sugar, baking powder, and each of the flours. Blend in the egg white mixture along with the water until barely moist.
3. Using the medium heat setting to prepare a nonstick griddle or skillet, and spoon the batter in ½ cup increments.
4. Continue cooking for about two minutes (bubbles will appear on the top).

5. Flip and continue to cook for about one to two more minutes.

Tips for Meal Prep:
1. Either serve now or cool for storage.
2. Store in freezer bags until ready to serve.
3. Place the frozen pancakes in a heated 375° Fahrenheit oven for 8-10 minutes.
4. Garnish each one with 1/2 of a cup of sliced berries and serve.

Lunch: One-Tray Caprese Pasta

Yields Provided: 2

Ingredients for Prep:

- Pasta (2 cups - cooked al dente)
- Onion (.75 cup)
- Marinara sauce (1 cup)
- Fresh basil (.33 cup)
- Black pepper and salt (1 tsp. each)
- Optional: Mozzarella cheese
- Also Needed: Aluminum foil (2 sheets @ 12 by 12)

Method of Prep:
1. Set oven to 400° Fahrenheit.
2. Chop the veggies and shred the cheese.
3. Stack the sheets of foil on top of each other.

4. Fold one side of the foil about ⅓ of the way across the sheet, repeat for the opposite side.
5. Pinch the corner to form a point and then flatten it to the short side of the foil, forming a raised corner. Repeat for all four sides (make 4).
6. Add all of the ingredients to the foil boats and stir.
7. Bake for 12 minutes.

Tips for Meal Prep:
1. Cool for 10-15 minutes.
2. Refrigerate for no longer than three to five days.

Dinner: Shrimp Taco Bowls

Yields Provided: 4

Ingredients for Prep:

Spicy Shrimp:
- Medium shrimp (20)
- Garlic clove (1 minced)
- Olive oil (1 tbsp.)
- Ground cumin (.5 tsp.)
- Chili powder (.5 tsp.)
- Optional: Onion powder (.25 tsp.)
- Kosher salt (.25 tsp.)

To Serve:
- Brown rice (2 cups - cooked)
- Corn (1 cup)
- Black beans (1 cup)

- Tomatoes (1 cup - diced)
- Cheddar cheese (.5 cup)
- Cilantro (2 tbsp. - minced)
- Lime (1 cut into 4 slices)
- Meal prep containers (4)

Method of Prep:
1. Drain and rinse the corn and black beans.
2. Peel and devein the shrimp. Toss them into a medium mixing bowl.
3. Whisk the olive oil, salt, cumin, garlic, chili powder, and onion powder. Fold in the shrimp and toss gently.
4. Cover and pop into the fridge to marinate for at least ten minutes or up to 24 hours.
5. Heat a large heavy-duty or cast-iron skillet using the high heat temperature setting for two minutes. Add the olive oil and shrimp.
6. Cook the shrimp in a skillet over med-high heat until pink and cooked thoroughly (5 min.)

Tips for Meal Prep:
1. Divide the brown rice into four containers (.5 cup each). Top with five shrimp, corn, tomatoes, a scoop of black beans, cheese, cilantro, and a lime wedge.
2. Cover and place in the fridge for a maximum of four days.
3. Time to Eat: Warm the bowls in the microwave for two minutes or until heated thoroughly. Top with salsa, sour cream, or guacamole to your liking along with a drizzle of lime juice.

Snack: Vanilla Cashew Butter Cups

Yields Provided: 12 large or 24 small cups

Ingredients for Prep:

- Dark chocolate or chocolate chips (7 oz. - chopped)
- Cashew butter (1 cup)
- Honey/maple syrup for vegan (2 tbsp.)
- Vanilla (1 tbsp.)
- Sea salt (1 pinch)
- Flaky sea salt - for the tops
- Also Needed: 12-count or 24-count muffin tin with liners

Method of Prep:
1. Line the muffin tin with liners.
2. Place about two-thirds of the chocolate in a pan using the low- temperature heat setting. After it's mostly melted, remove it from the heat and add the remaining chocolate. Stir a few times while the residual heat melts the chocolate.
3. Working one at a time, add slightly less than a tablespoon of the melted chocolate to one of the cupcake liners. Tip it on its side and rotate it so that the chocolate comes one-third of the way up the side of the liner. Repeat until all the liners have a chocolate coating then place them in the fridge to harden.
4. Add the cashew butter, honey, vanilla, and salt to a medium- sized bowl. Gently fold them together. Once the chocolate cups have hardened, divide the

5. cashew butter between the cups. Use your finger to press it down into the cups.
6. Pour the remaining chocolate over the tops of the cashew butter cups, then pop them back into the fridge to harden.
7. Sprinkle a little flaky sea salt on top to make them irresistible.

Tips for Meal Prep:
1. In a microwave, melt the chocolate for 20 to 30 seconds. Drizzle and serve.
2. Cashew butter can be pricey. You can make your own with a food processor or high-powered blender and about ten minutes. You'll need two cups of raw cashews plus one tablespoon of coconut oil to make 1 cup of cashew butter.

Day 13

Breakfast: Corn & Apple Muffins

Yields Provided: 12

Ingredients for Prep:

- All-purpose flour (2 cups)
- Packed brown sugar (.25 cup)
- Yellow cornmeal (.5 cup)
- Baking powder (1 tbsp.)
- Salt (.25 tsp.)
- Egg whites (2)
- Apple (1)
- Corn kernels (.5 cup)

Method of Prep:
1. Peel and coarsely chop the apple.
2. Use a 12-cup muffin pan and line the containers with foil or paper liners.
3. Set the oven temperature to reach 425° Fahrenheit.
4. Mix the brown sugar, cornmeal, salt, flour, and baking powder completely in a big container.
5. Use a separate mixing container to beat the egg whites and milk. Blend in the corn kernels and apple bits.

6. Whisk again and pour the batter into the flour mixture. Continue to gently stir the fixings until slightly moistened.
7. Fill the cups 2/3 of the way full. Bake for about 30 minutes.
8. Test the muffins for doneness by gently pressing the center. They should spring back.

Tips for Meal Prep:
1. Cool thoroughly before placing the muffins into a storage container.
2. Store in the fridge for longer storage times.

Lunch: Smoked Sausage & Orzo

Yields Provided: 6-8

Ingredients for Prep:

- Jennie-O Hardwood Smoked Turkey Sausage (16 oz.)
- Olive oil (1 tbsp.)
- Yellow onion (1 small)
- Red bell pepper (1 small)
- Garlic (3 cloves)
- Cajun seasoning (1 tbsp.)
- Crushed red pepper flakes (.5 tbsp.)
- Chicken broth - Low-sodium (14.5 oz. can)
- Crushed tomatoes (15 oz. can)
- Uncooked orzo pasta (8 oz.)
- Medium zucchini (1 shredded)

- Kosher salt (.5 tsp.)
- Freshly cracked black pepper (as desired)
- For the Garnish: Flat-leaf parsley

Method of Prep:
1. Slice the sausage diagonally and add to a large skillet with olive oil. Dice and toss in the onions, bell peppers, garlic, kosher salt, black pepper, Cajun seasoning, and pepper flakes.
2. Pour in the chicken broth, orzo, and tomatoes. Wait for it to boil.
3. Reduce the heat setting to med-low and cover. Set a timer for 8 minutes, or until the orzo is tender.

Tips for Meal Prep:
1. Pour the fixings into resealable plastic bags or shallow airtight containers for up to three to five days.
2. Time to Eat: Stir in shredded zucchini, freshly chop flat-leaf Italian parsley and a sprinkle of Cajun seasoning.

Dinner: Chicken & Broccoli

Yields Provided: 4

Ingredients for Prep:

- Breasts of chicken (4)
- Olive oil (1 tbsp.)
- Red onions (1 cup)
- Garlic cloves (2)

- Oregano (1 tbsp.)
- Coconut cream (.5 cup)
- Broccoli florets (2 cups)

Method of Prep:
1. Cut the skin and bones from the chicken breasts.
2. Mince the garlic cloves. Chop the red onions and oregano.
3. Heat a skillet to warm the oil using the med- high heat setting.
4. Arrange the chicken breasts in the pan and simmer for about 5 minutes per side.
5. Toss in the onions and garlic. Stir and cook for approximately 5 more minutes.
6. Add in the broccoli, cream, and oregano. Continue cooking for 10 more minutes.
7. When ready, portion into the plates and serve.

Tips for Meal Prep:
1. It will keep for 3-5 days in the fridge.
2. For further prep time, cover with foil and place in a freezer bag or container.

Snack: Protein Snack Pack

Yields Provided: 3

Ingredients for Prep:

- Foster Farms Bold Bites Pouch
- Hard-Boiled egg (1)
- Chopped cheese (.25 cup)
- Avocado (half of 1)
- Chickpeas (.5 cup)

- Hazelnuts/your preference (2 tbsp.)

Method of Prep:
1. Chop the cheese into cubes.
2. Fill a dipping sauce <u>container</u> with two tablespoons of hazelnuts.
3. Close the top and place it into a storage container alongside the rest of the fixings.

Tips for Meal Prep:
1. Arrange the egg, chickpeas, cheese, and avocado within the storage container and securely close the lid or use plastic wrap.
2. Place in the fridge until needed. It's best used within 24 to 48 hours.
3. When it is time to eat, serve with a pouch of the bold bites.

Day 14

Breakfast: Veggies & Eggs

Yields Provided: 4

Ingredients for Prep:

- Large eggs (8)
- Broccoli crowns (2)
- Small head cauliflower (half of 1)
- Bell peppers (2)
- Garlic powder (1 tsp.)
- Black pepper (as desired)
- Salt (.5 tsp.)
- Avocado/coconut oil (3 tbsp.)
- Water (.25 cup)
- Optional: Cheese of choice
- Sprouted bread slices (2 toasted)
- For Serving: Salsa

Method of Prep:
1. Coarsely chop the broccoli and cauliflower. Dice the peppers.

2. Warm a large ceramic skillet using the medium temperature heat setting and swirl two tablespoons of oil to coat. Toss in the broccoli and cauliflower. Cover and cook for two to three minutes. Stir, cover, and cook for another two to three minutes.
3. Meanwhile, in a small dish, whisk the eggs, water, pepper, and ¼ teaspoon of salt. Whisk well and set aside.
4. Add the bell pepper, rest of the salt, garlic powder, and black pepper to the skillet with the vegetables. Stir and cook for two to three more minutes.

Tips for Meal Prep:
1. Divide between four plastic or glass meal prep containers, add a small container of salsa, 1/2 slice of toast, and sprinkle of cheese if desired.
2. Refrigerate for up to 5 days. Heat in a skillet on the stovetop.
3. Swirl one tablespoon of oil into the pan and pour in the egg mixture. Cook until it's scrambled, stirring (folding) constantly.

Lunch: Starbucks™ Protein Bistro Box

Yields Provided: 8

Ingredients for Prep:

- Hard-boiled eggs (8)
- Grapes (2 cups)
- Large apples (2)
- Mini Babybel cheese - Reduced-fat (4)

- Multi-grain flatbread sandwich thins (2 cuts in quarters)
- Honey-Roasted Peanut Butter (portioned into 2 oz. containers)
- Optional: Freshly squeezed lemon juice
- Freshly cracked pepper and kosher salt (as desired)

Method of Prep:
1. Rinse the apples and grapes. Brush the apple slices lightly using the juice to prevent browning.
2. Boil and peel the eggs. Cool and dust eggs using salt and pepper to taste.

Tips for Meal Prep:
1. Assemble the protein bistro boxes and store refrigerated.
2. It is recommended to store the eggs whole.

Dinner: Sweet & Sour Meatballs

Yields Provided: 8-12

Ingredients for Prep:

- *The Meatballs*:
- Ground chuck (1.5 lb.)
- Water chestnuts (3-4 tbsp. - chopped)
- Quick oats (.75 cup)

- Garlic powder (.5 tsp.)
- Onion powder (.5 tsp.)
- Salt (.5 tsp.)
- Egg (1 beaten)
- Milk (.5 cup)
- Soy sauce - reduced-sodium (.5 tsp.)
- *The Sauce:*
- Brown sugar (1 cup)
- Beef bouillon (.5 cup)
- Vinegar (.5 cup)
- Cornstarch (2 tbsp.)
- Reduced-sodium soy sauce (2 tsp.)
- Pineapple tidbits - drained (8-9 oz. can)
- Chopped bell pepper - green (.5 cup)

Method of Prep:
1. Combine the meatball fixings preparing them into one-inch balls.
2. Brown, drain the grease and set aside.
3. Whisk the sugar, vinegar, bouillon, cornstarch, and soy sauce in a Dutch oven or large deep skillet, bringing it to a boil.
4. Simmer the sauce mixture until thickened. Drain and stir in the pineapple, peppers, and meatballs.
5. Continue cooking for about half an hour.

Tips for Meal Prep:
1. Cool the meatballs until thoroughly chilled.

2. Measure your required number of meatballs per serving into a freezer bag.
3. Pop the package into the freezer for a quick meal.
4. Be sure to label it with its contents and date to ensure you don't overlook it.

Snack: Ham – Swiss & Spinach Roll-Ups

Yields Provided: 1

Ingredients for Prep:

- Uncured organic deli ham/your preference (1 slice)
- Hummus (1 tbsp.)
- Swiss cheese (half of 1 slice)
- Baby spinach leaves (4-5)

Method of Prep:
1. Spread hummus onto the slice of ham.
2. Top that with swiss cheese and spinach leaves.
3. Roll them up.

Tips for Meal Prep:
1. Prepare as many snacks as you want to prep.
2. The roll-ups can be made 1-2 days ahead of time.

Chapter 4: Keto Diet

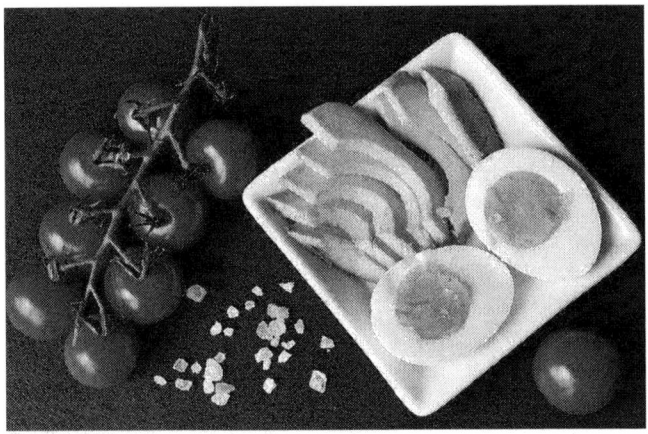

What Is the Keto Diet?

The term keto in ketogenic comes from ketones. Ketones are small fuel molecules produced in the body. These molecules provide an alternative source of fuel for the body when there's a short supply of glucose in the blood.

When you consume very few carbs, your body will not have sufficient glucose or blood sugar needed to power the cells. Since glucose is unavailable, the body will reach into its fat reserves to produce blood sugar.

The ketogenic process takes place in the liver. It is the liver that produces ketones from fat stores in the body. These ketones then

> provide the necessary fuel needed throughout the body and mostly for the brain. The brain is an organ that is continuously working and has a high demand for energy. However, it cannot run on fat. It only functions on glucose or ketones.

When you consume no carbs, the body will lack glucose to produce energy, and the body will convert the fat that you consume into ketones. This happens when your insulin levels fall drastically. When this happens, fat burning occurs quite fast. Your body can easily access stored fat, including the stubborn fat around the belly and waistline.

The ketogenic process is excellent for weight loss and fat burning. If you are looking to lose weight and shed off the pounds, then the ketogenic diet is highly recommended. However, apart from the benefit of weight loss occasioned by the keto diet, you will also enjoy a host of other benefits as well. For instance, you will lose weight but without the need to fast.

Variations of the Ketogenic Diet Plan

- ***Standard Ketogenic Diet:*** It's also known as SKD, which is a high-fat, very low-carb, and moderate-protein diet. This diet consists of 20% protein, 75% carbs, and only 5% carbs.

- ***Targeted Ketogenic Diet:*** The technique used in this dieting phase is similar to the standard keto diet except that it allows variations in carbs intake based on workout demands.

- ***Cyclic Ketogenic Diet:*** This variation of the keto diet involves varying periods where you enjoy five days of ketogenic diet followed by two days where you have a diet high in carbs; hence, the 5:2 diet.

- ***High-Protein Ketogenic Diet:*** You can also enjoy a high-protein keto diet, which is somewhat similar to the standard keto diet. However, it consists of higher protein levels compared to the SKD diet. The ratios here are 35% protein, 60% fat, and 5% carbs.

Most people follow the standard ketogenic diet and sometimes the high-protein keto diet. For purposes of learning more about the ketogenic diet, we will focus more on the standard version.

Benefits of the Keto Diet

Ketosis has numerous benefits. At the onset, it provides the brain and body an endless supply of energy. This energy is crucial for the brain and helps you to be sharp and focused. This also enhances your physical and mental endurance.

Other benefits of ketosis include the facilitation of effortless weight loss. Ketosis is one of the most efficient weight loss processes known. People who have type 2 diabetes can get relief from the condition. Type II diabetes is aggravated by excessive blood sugar, which is controlled via ketosis. Other conditions, such as epilepsy, can easily be controlled using ketosis even without the use of medication.

Let's see how tasty the foods are in this segment! You'll be surprised!

Week 1

Day 1

Breakfast: Almost McGriddle Casserole

Yields Provided: 8

Total Net Carbs: 3 grams

Ingredients for Prep:

- Breakfast sausage (1 lb.)
- Flaxseed meal (.25 cup)
- Almond flour (1 cup)
- Large eggs (10)
- Maple syrup (6 tbsp.)
- Cheese (4 oz.)
- Butter (4 tbsp.)
- Onion (.5 tsp.)
- Sage (.25 tsp.)
- Garlic powder (.5 tsp.)
- *Also Needed*: 9 by 9-inch casserole dish & parchment baking paper

Method of Prep:
1. Warm the oven temperature to reach 350° Fahrenheit.
2. Use the medium heat setting on the stovetop to prepare the sausage in a skillet.
3. Add all of the dry fixings (the cheese also), and stir in the wet ones. Add four tablespoons of syrup. Stir and blend well.
4. After the sausage is browned, combine everything (the grease too).
5. Prepare the casserole dish using a sheet of baking paper. Dump the mixture into the casserole dish. Drizzle using the rest of the syrup and bake for 45 to 55 minutes.
6. Transfer to the countertop to cool.

Tips for Meal Prep:
1. The casserole should be easily removed by using the edge of the parchment paper.
2. After the casserole has cooled, slice it into eight portions to enjoy for a couple of days.
3. Place the muffins in a storage container or freezer baggie. Store in the fridge for about five days or freeze for later.

Lunch: Caesar Salmon Salad

Yields Provided: 2

Total Carbohydrates: 2 grams

Ingredients for Prep:

- Salmon fillets (2 - 6 oz. portions)
- Bacon slices (4)

- Ghee (1 tbsp. or as needed)
- Pink salt (1 pinch)
- Freshly ground black pepper (1 pinch)
- Avocado (.5 of 1)
- Romaine hearts (2 cups)
- Caesar dressing (2 tbsp.)

Method of Prep:
1. Cook the bacon until crispy for 8 minutes using the med-high heat setting on the stovetop. Drain on a platter using paper towels.
2. Remove the excess water from the fillets. Give them a shake of pepper and salt.
3. Use the same pan to prepare the salmon. Add butter if needed.
4. Cook the salmon for five minutes per side for medium-rare.

Tips for Meal Prep:
1. Break the bacon into bits.
2. Chop the romaine hearts and slice the avocado.
3. Prepare two salad dishes or a closed container for the meal prep with equal parts of romaine, avocado, and the bacon.
4. Place the bacon into separate containers to keep them crunchy.
5. When ready to serve, enjoy with a drizzle of the dressing.

Dinner: Chipotle Roast

Yields Provided: 4

Total Carbohydrates: 1 gram

Ingredients for Prep:

- Diced tomatoes (7.25 oz.)
- Bone broth (6 oz.)
- Diced green chilis (2 oz.)
- Pork roast (2 lb.)
- Chipotle powder (1 tsp.)
- Cumin (.5 tsp.)
- Onion powder (.5 tsp.)

Method of Prep:
1. Combine each of the fixings in the Instant Pot and close the lid.
2. Manually set the timer for 1 hour. Natural-release the pressure.

Tips for Meal Prep:
1. Cool the roast and slice into four portions.
2. Freeze in individual compartment storage containers. Add your favorite vegetable and freeze for later.
3. When it's dinner time, defrost the meat, and heat as desired.

Snack: Peanut Butter Protein Bars

Yields Provided: 12 bars **Total Carbohydrates:** 3 grams

Ingredients for Prep:

- Keto-friendly chunky peanut butter (1 cup)
- Egg whites (2)
- Almonds (.5 cup)
- Cashews (.5 cup)
- Almond meal (1.5 cups)

Method of Prep:
1. Warm up the oven ahead of time to 350° Fahrenheit.
2. Combine all of the fixings and add them to the prepared dish.
3. Bake for 15 minutes, and cut into 12 pieces once they're cooled.

Tips for Meal Prep:
1. Store in the fridge to keep them fresh using a closed, airtight container.

Day 2

Breakfast: Jalapeno Cheddar Waffles

Yields Provided: 1

Total Carbohydrates: 6 grams

Ingredients for Prep:

- Large eggs (3)
- Jalapeno (1 small)
- Cream cheese (3 oz.)
- Psyllium husk powder (1 tsp.)
- Coconut flour (1 tbsp.)
- Cheddar cheese (1 oz.)
- Baking powder (1 tsp.)
- *Also Needed:* Immersion blender

Method of Prep:
1. Mix all of the fixings using the blender, except for the jalapeno and cheese.
2. After you have a smooth texture, add the cheese and jalapeno. Blend and pour the batter into the waffle iron.
3. Cook for 5 to 6 minutes. Set aside when done.

Tips for Meal Prep:
1. Let the waffles cool off for prep.

2. Put them into a plastic freezer bag and pop them in the freezer until you have the desire for a delicious waffle.
3. To reheat, preheat the oven temperature to 400° Fahrenheit. When it's hot, place the waffles on a baking tin. Warm them up for 5 minutes. Serve and enjoy!
4. *Tip*: It isn't recommended to warm them in a regular toaster.

Lunch: Chicken 'Zoodle' Soup

Yields Provided: 2

Total Carbohydrates: 4 grams

Ingredients for Prep:

- Chicken broth (3 cups)
- Chicken breast (1)
- Avocado oil (2 tbsp.)
- Green onion (1)
- Celery stalk (1)
- Cilantro (.25 cup)
- Salt (to taste)
- Peeled zucchini (1)

Method of Prep:
1. Chop or dice the breast of the chicken. Pour the oil into a saucepan and cook the chicken until done. Pour in the broth and simmer.
2. Chop the celery and green onions and toss into the pan. Simmer for 3 to 4 more minutes.

3. Chop the cilantro and prepare the zucchini noodles. Use a spiralizer or potato peeler to make the 'noodles.' Add to the pot.
4. Simmer for a few more minutes and season to your liking.

Tips for Meal Prep:
1. Store in a glass container in the fridge. It will remain tasty for 2 to 3 days.

Dinner: Chicken Nuggets

Yields Provided: 6

Total Carbohydrates: 2 grams

Ingredients for Prep:

- Cooked chicken (2 cups)
- Cream cheese (8 oz.)
- Egg (1)
- Garlic salt (1 tsp.)
- Almond flour (.25 cup)

Method of Prep:
1. Set the oven temperature to 350° Fahrenheit.
2. Lightly spritz a baking tray using a misting of cooking oil spray. You can also use a layer of parchment paper.

3. Shred the chicken using a food processor or by hand. (Try using a combination of dark and light meat.)
4. Combine the rest of the fixings and mix well.
5. Scoop the nugget mixture onto the baking tin.
6. Bake until firm and slightly browned (12 to 14 min.).

Tips for Meal Prep:
1. You will love this one. Just prepare the mixture and bake.
2. Store in the fridge for one or two days.
3. Freeze and enjoy at another time for lunch, dinner, or just a snack

Snack: Blueberry Cream Cheese Fat Bombs

Yields Provided: 12

Total Carbohydrates: 1 gram

Ingredients for Prep:

- Unchilled cream cheese (1.5 cups)
- Fresh/frozen berries (1 cup)
- Swerve (2-3 tbsp.)
- Vanilla extract (1 tbsp.)
- Coconut oil (.5 cup)

Method of Prep:
1. About 30 to 60 minutes before preparation time, place the cream cheese on the countertop to become room temperature.
2. Take the stems off the berries and rinse. Pour into a blender. Mix well until smooth.
3. Pour in the Swerve and extract. Blend in the oil and cream cheese.
4. Add the mixture to candy molds and freeze for approximately two hours.

Tips for Meal Prep:
1. Once the bombs are solid, just pop them out.
2. Store in freezer bags or another safe freezer container.

Day 3

Breakfast: Baked Green Eggs

Yields Provided: 6

Total Carbohydrates: 5 grams

Ingredients for Prep:

1. Sun-dried tomatoes (.25 cup)
2. Feta cheese (.5 cup)
3. Oregano (.5 tsp.)
4. Chopped kale (1 cup)
5. Eggs (12)

Method of Prep:
1. Warm up the oven to reach 350° Fahrenheit.
2. Cover a baking tin with a layer of foil and a spritz of nonstick cooking spray.
3. Whisk the eggs and combine with the rest of the fixings. Stir well and pour into the pan to bake for approximately 25 minutes.
4. Transfer to the countertop to entirely cool and slice.
5. Warm up the oven to reach 350° Fahrenheit.
6. Cover a baking tin with a layer of foil and a spritz of nonstick cooking spray.
7. Whisk the eggs and combine with the rest of the fixings. Stir well and pour into the pan to bake for approximately 25 minutes.
8. Transfer to the countertop to entirely cool and slice.

Tips for Meal Prep:

1. Place the package in the refrigerator to use within four to five days in an airtight container.
2. You can also place them into individual containers for convenience.

Lunch: Mushroom & Cauliflower Risotto

Yields Provided: 4

Total Carbohydrates: 4 grams

Ingredients for Prep:

- Cauliflower (1)
- Vegetable stock (1 cup)
- Chopped mushrooms (9 oz.)
- Butter (2 tbsp.)
- Coconut cream (1 cup)
- Pepper and Salt (to taste)

Method of Prep:
1. Pour the stock in a saucepan. Boil and set aside.
2. Prepare a skillet with butter and sauté the mushrooms until golden.
3. Grate and stir in the cauliflower and stock.

Tips for Meal Prep:
1. Simmer and add the cream, cooking until the cauliflower is al dente. Serve.
2. Let it cool before placing it in the fridge for storage.

Dinner: Chili Lime Cod

Yields Provided: 2

Total Carbohydrates: 3 grams

Ingredients for Prep:

- Wild-caught cod (10-12 oz.)
- Coconut flour (.33 cup)
- Egg (3)
- Lime (1)
- Garlic powder (1 tsp.)
- Cayenne pepper (.5 tsp.
- Salt (1 tsp.)
- Crushed red pepper (1 tsp.)

Method of Prep:
1. Heat the oven temperature to reach 400° Fahrenheit.
2. In separate dishes, whip the egg, and remove any lumps from the flour.
3. Let the fillet soak in the egg dish for one minute per side. Dip it into the flour dish, and then add it to a baking sheet.
4. Sprinkle the spices and drizzle the lime juice over the cod, and bake it for 10 to 12 minutes or when it easily flakes apart.

Tips for Meal Prep:
1. Cool the fish entirely once it is like you like it.

2. Use foil to keep the fish safe for a day. Freeze and enjoy later.
3. Once it is time to eat, just drizzle with some Sriracha if you wish, and enjoy.

Snack: *Coffee Fat Bombs*

Yields Provided: 15

Total Carbohydrates: 0 grams

Ingredients for Prep:

- Unchilled cream cheese (4.4 oz.)
- Powdered xylitol (2 tbsp.)
- Instant coffee (1 tbsp.)
- Unsweetened cocoa powder (1 tbsp.)
- Coconut oil (1 tbsp.)
- Unchilled butter (1 tbsp.)

Method of Prep:
1. Put the butter and creamcheese on the countertop for about an hour before it's time to begin.
2. Use a blender/food processor to blitz the xylitol and coffee into a fine powder. Add the hot water to form a pasty mix.
3. Blend in the cream cheese, cocoa powder, butter, and coconut oil.
4. Add to ice cube trays and freeze for a minimum of one to two hours.

Tips for Meal Prep:
1. Use zipper-type bags to keep them fresh in the freezer.

Day 4

Breakfast: Vegan Gingerbread Muffins

Yields Provided: 5

Total Carbohydrates: 2 grams

Ingredients for Prep:

- Non-dairy milk or water (.75 cup)
- Granulated sweetener - your preference (.25 cup)
- Ground flax seeds (.5 cup)
- Melted coconut oil or MCT oil (2 tbsp.)
- Vanilla extract (1 tsp.)
- Coconut flour (.5 cup)
- Freshly grated ginger (1.5 tsp.)
- Allspice (.25 tsp.)
- Cinnamon (1.5 tsp.)
- Ground cloves (.25 tsp.)
- Nutmeg (.25 tsp.)
- *Also Needed*: Standard-size muffin pan with paper liners

Method of Prep:
1. Heat the oven to 375° Fahrenheit.

2. Line five of the wells of the pan with a layer of parchment baking paper.
3. Combine the sweetener, flax seeds, oil, milk, and vanilla. Whisk well and set aside for approximately five minutes for the seeds to rest.
4. In another mixing container, whisk the remainder of the fixings until the mixture has thickened.
5. Empty the batter mixture into the muffin pan.
6. Bake until the tops are firm to the touch (30-35 min.).

Tips for Meal Prep:
1. Remove and transfer to the countertop to cool in the pan for at least 15 minutes.
2. Once cool, the muffins should easily pop out of the pan.
3. Place the container in the refrigerator for the best storage results.

Lunch: Spicy Beef Wraps

Yields Provided: 2

Total Carbohydrates: 4 grams

Ingredients for Prep:

- Coconut oil (1-2 tbsp.)
- Onion (¼ of 1)

- Ground beef (.66 lb.)
- Chopped cilantro (2 tbsp.)
- Red bell pepper (1)
- Fresh ginger (1 tsp.)
- Cumin (2 tsp.)
- Garlic cloves (4)
- Pepper and salt (as preferred)
- Large cabbage leaves (8)

Method of Prep:
1. Dice the bell pepper, onion, ginger, and garlic.
2. Heat a frying pan and pour in the oil.
3. Sauté the peppers, onions, and ground beef using medium heat.
4. When done, add the pepper, salt, cumin, ginger, cilantro, and garlic.

Tips for Meal Prep:
1. Cool the burger entirely and add to storage containers.
2. *Time to Eat:* Prepare a large pot of boiling water (3/4 full).
3. Cook each leaf for 20 seconds, plunge it in cold water and drain before placing it on your serving dish.
4. Reheat the beef mixture.
5. Scoop the mixture onto each leaf, fold, and enjoy.

Dinner: Asparagus & Chicken

Yields Provided: 8

Total Carbohydrates: 4 grams

Ingredients for Prep:

- Chicken breasts (4 lbs.)
- Avocado oil (1 tbsp.)
- Trimmed asparagus (1 lb.)
- Sun-dried tomatoes (4)
- Thick-cut bacon slices (4)
- Salt (1 tsp.)
- Pepper (.25 tsp.)
- Provolone cheese slices (8)
- *Also Needed*: 1 baking pan

Method of Prep:

1. Slice the chicken into eight thin pieces. Chop the bacon and tomatoes into one-inch pieces.
2. Warm up the oven temperature to 400° Fahrenheit.
3. Add the oil to the baking pan along with the chicken and asparagus. Top it off with the tomatoes and bacon. Sprinkle some pepper and salt for seasoning.
4. Bake until the chicken reaches 160° Fahrenheit internally - or about 25 minutes.
5. Toss in the asparagus and cheese.

6. Garnish with some bacon and tomatoes. Bake another three to four minutes until the cheese has melted.

Tips for Meal Prep:

1. Prepare the chicken and store it in the fridge for several days.
2. Place into plastic bins or freezer bags until ready to use.
3. Prepare the asparagus when ready to eat and combine with the cheese. Garnish and serve.

Snack: Mocha Cheesecake Bars

Yields Provided: 16

Total Carbohydrates: 3 grams

Ingredients for Prep:

- Vanilla extract (2 tsp.)
- Unsalted butter (6 tbsp.)
- Large eggs (3)
- Almond flour (1.5 cups)
- Hershey's Baking Cocoa (.5 cup)
- Erythritol (1 cup)
- Salt (.5 tsp.)
- Instant coffee (.5 tbsp.)
- Baking powder (1 tsp.)

The Cream Cheese Layer

- Erythritol (.5 cup)
- Softened cream cheese (1 lb.)

- Large egg (1)
- Vanilla extract (1 tsp.)
- Also Needed: 8 by 8-inch baking pan

Method of Prep:
1. Heat the oven to 350° Fahrenheit. Lightly grease or spray the pan with a spritz of oil cooking spray.
2. Combine the wet fixings, starting with the vanilla, butter, and eggs.
3. In another container, combine the dry fixings and whisk with the wet ones. Reserve .25 cup of the batter for later. Pour the mixture into the pan.
4. Mix the cream cheese (room temperature) with the rest of the ingredients for the second layer. Spread it on the layer of brownies.
5. Use the reserved batter as the last layer (will be thin). Bake it for 30 to 35 minutes.

Tips for Meal Prep:
1. When cooled, slice the cheesecake bars.
2. They will store in the refrigerator for several days or freeze in containers or freezer bags for extended use. Be sure to date and add the name of the contents.

Day 5

Breakfast: Egg Loaf

Yields Provided: 6

Total Carbohydrates: 0 grams

Ingredients for Prep:

- Eggs (6)
- Water for steaming (2 cups)
- Unsalted butter (for the bowl)

Method of Prep:
1. Prepare a heat-proof container with the butter.
2. Break the eggs into the dish (yolks intact) and cover with a sheet of aluminum foil. Set aside.
3. Add the trivet and two cups of water into the Instant Pot cooker. Arrange the bowl in the cooker.
4. Secure the lid and choose the manual pressure cooker function for 4 minutes using the high-temperature setting.
5. When the egg loaf is done, quick-release the pressure, and remove the pot.

Tips for Meal Prep:
1. Let it cool slightly and place in the refrigerator for up to four days.
2. Chop to your liking and mix with a little egg for salad or a little butter, pepper, and salt.

Lunch: BARBECUE Pork Loin

Yields Provided: 4

Total Carbohydrates: 3 grams

Ingredients for Prep:

- Pork loin (1 lb.)
- Tomato paste (4 tbsp.)
- Worcestershire sauce (1 tsp.)
- Avocado oil (2 tbsp.)
- Smoked paprika (.5 tsp.)
- Minced garlic (.5 tsp.
- Chopped onion (1 tbsp.)

Method of Prep:
1. Whisk the minced garlic, chopped onion, paprika, tomato paste, and Worcestershire sauce. Use the rub to prepare the pork and wrap it in foil.
2. Marinate the pork loin in the fridge for at least 1/2 hour for the spices to be absorbed.
3. Add the trivet to the Instant Pot and pour the water into the cooker. Secure the lid.
4. Set the timer for 60 minutes. Natural-release the pressure, when it's done.

Tips for Meal Prep:
1. Open the lid and let it cool slightly.

2. Let the pork completely cool.
3. Place into individual containers along with your favorite prepped veggie.
4. When it's time to eat, just thaw the container.
5. Warm it up and serve as desired.

Dinner: Short Ribs

Yields Provided: 4

Total Carbohydrates: 2.5 grams

Ingredients for Prep:

- Keto-friendly soy sauce (.25 cup)
- Beef short ribs (6 - 4 oz. each)
- Fish sauce (2 tbsp.)
- Rice vinegar (2 tbsp.)
- Red pepper flakes (.5 tsp.)
- Sesame seeds (.5 tsp.)
- Onion powder (.5 tsp.)
- Salt (1 tbsp.)
- Minced garlic (.5 tsp.)
- Ground ginger (1 tsp.)
- Cardamom (.25 tsp.)

Method of Prep:
1. Mix the fish sauce, vinegar, and alternative soy sauce.
2. Arrange the ribs in a dish with high sides. Add the sauce and marinate for up to 1 hour.
3. Combine all of the spices together. Take the ribs from the dish and sprinkle with the rub.
4. Warm up the grill (med-high) and cook for three to five minutes per side.

Tips for Meal Prep:
1. Put the ribs in a platter to cool.
2. Place in freezer bags or into plastic containers (4 portions) until it's time to serve and enjoy.

Snack: Delicious No-Bake Coconut Cookies

Yields Provided: 20

Total Carbohydrates: 0 grams

Ingredients for Prep:

- Melted coconut oil (1 cup)
- Monk fruit sweetened maple syrup or sweetener of choice (.5 cup)
- Shredded unsweetened coconut flakes (3 cups)

Method of Prep:

1. Prepare a cookie tray with a layer of parchment baking paper.
2. Combine all of the fixings. Run your hands through some water from the tap and shape the mixture into small balls. Arrange them in the pan around one to two inches apart.
3. Press them down to form a cookie and refrigerate until firm.

Tips for Meal Prep:

1. Prepare these into individual bags if you're an on-the-go kind of person.
2. The cookies will remain fresh covered for up to 7 days at room temperature.
3. Store in the fridge for up to a month.
4. If you choose, you can freeze the cookies for up to two months.

Day 6

Breakfast: Spinach Quiche

Yields Provided: 6

Total Carbohydrates: 0 grams

Ingredients for Prep:

- Chopped onion (1)
- Olive oil (1 tbsp.)
- Frozen & thawed spinach (10 oz. pkg.)
- Shredded muenster cheese (3 cups)
- Organic eggs – whisked (5)
- To Taste: Black pepper and salt
- Also Needed: 9-inch pie plate

Method of Prep:

1. Heat the oven at 350° Fahrenheit. Lightly grease the dish.
2. Use the medium temperature setting to warm a skillet with the oil.
3. Toss in the onion and sauté for 4-5 minutes. Raise the heat setting to med-high.
4. Fold in the spinach. Sauté for about two to three minutes or until the liquid is absorbed. Cool slightly.
5. Combine the rest of the fixings in a large mixing container, and toss with the cooled spinach. Dump

into the prepared dish. Set a timer to bake for 30 minutes.
6. Take the quiche out of the oven to cool for at least ten minutes.
7. Slice into six wedges.

Tips for Meal Prep:
1. Add the cooled pieces into plastic baggies.
2. It will store in the fridge for two to four days.
3. To warm up, prepare in the microwave for one minute on the high setting before serving.

Lunch: BLT Salad in a Jar

Yields Provided: 8

Total Carbohydrates: 7 grams

Ingredients for Prep:

Method of Prep:
1. Combine all of the dressing components.
2. Slowly pour into the jars.
3. Layer the veggies, croutons, and garnish of bacon.
4. Heat a skillet using the high heat setting. Add the fat and patties. Prepare the burgers for 2 to 3 minutes per side.
5. Serve when crispy brown.

Tips for Meal Prep:
1. Tightly close each of the jars.
2. Place in the refrigerator and enjoy it within three days.

- Romaine lettuce (2 cups)
- Iceberg lettuce (2 cups)
- Chopped scallions (2)
- Diced tomatoes (2)
- Bacon slices (4 crumbled)

Dinner: Buffalo Chicken Burgers

Yields Provided: 2 burgers Total Carbohydrates: 1 gram

Ingredients for Prep:

- Cooked chicken breasts (8 oz.)
- Room-temperature cream cheese (2 oz.)
- Shredded mozzarella cheese (.5 cup)
- Frank's Red-Hot Sauce or your choice (2 tbsp.)
- For Frying: Ghee or Coconut oil

Method of Prep:
1. Either chop or shred the prepared chicken and combine it with the rest of the fixings.
2. Place the fixings in the microwave for 15 to 20 seconds to help compact the ingredients. Form two medium patties and place them on a plate. Store in the freezer for about 15 minutes.
3. Heat a skillet using the high heat setting. Add the fat and patties. Prepare the burgers for 2 to 3 minutes per side.

4. Serve when crispy brown.

Tips for Meal Prep:
1. Prepare the chicken and shape the mixture into patties.
2. Freeze, or cook and freeze the patties.

Snack: Spice Cakes

Yields Provided: 12

Total Carbohydrates: 3 grams

Ingredients for Prep:

- Eggs (4)
- Baking powder (2 tsp.)
- Almond flour (2 cups)
- Salted butter (.5 cup)
- Nutmeg (.5 tsp.)
- Allspice (.5 tsp.)
- Ginger (.5 tsp.)
- Cinnamon (.5 tsp.)
- Erythritol (.75 cup)
- Ground cloves (.25 tsp.)
- Vanilla extract (1 tsp.)
- Water (5 tbsp.)

Method of Prep:
1. Set the temperature in the oven to 350° Fahrenheit. Prepare a cupcake tray with liners (12).
2. Mix the butter and erythritol with a hand mixer. Once it's smooth, combine with two eggs and the vanilla. Mix and stir in the remainder of the eggs, stirring until creamy.
3. Grind the clove to a fine powder and add with the rest of the spices. Whisk into the mixture. Stir in the baking powder and almond flour. Blend in the water. When the batter is smooth, add to the prepared tin.
4. Bake for 15 minutes. Enjoy any time.

Tips for Meal Prep:
1. Cool thoroughly for the prep.
2. It's recommended to place them in the refrigerator for a few days or in the freezer to enjoy later.

Day 7

Breakfast: Morning Hot Pockets

Yields Provided: 2

Total Carbohydrates: 4 grams

Ingredients for Prep:
- Shredded mozzarella - not fresh (.75 cup)
- Almond flour (.33 cup)
- Scrambled eggs (2 large)
- Ghee or unsalted butter (2 tbsp.)
- Slices of bacon (3 cooked)

Method of Prep:
1. Cook the bacon and eggs. Prepare the dough by melting the shredded mozzarella (stovetop @ low heat or in a microwave). Fold in the almond flour. Stir until the dough is well-combined.
2. Arrange the bacon strips in a large pan. Add two to three tablespoons of water. Steam-fry using the med-high heat setting until the water starts to boil.
3. Lower the temperature setting to medium. Simmer until the water evaporates and bacon fat is rendered. Reduce the temperature setting to low. Continue cooking until the bacon is crispy.
4. Grease the same skillet with half of the butter/ghee and add both eggs. Simmer using the med-low temperature until done, stirring continuously.

Transfer to the countertop and add the rest of the butter.

5. Roll the dough out between two sheets of parchment paper (A silicone mat and silicone rolling pin are useful).
6. Place the bacon slices and scrambled eggs along the center.
7. Fold over and seal the dough. Make several holes for releasing the steam while baking.
8. Set the oven temperature to 400° Fahrenheit. Bake for about 20 minutes, or it is firm to the touch.

Tips for Meal Prep:
1. Transfer the hot pockets from the oven and let them cool.
2. Wrap in foil and toss into a freezer bag. Place on a baking tin to freeze solid.
3. *Note*: It is advisable to not leave in the refrigerator for storage.

Lunch: Greek Salad

Yields Provided: 1

Total Carbohydrates: 8 grams

Ingredients for Prep:

- Red onion (.25 cup)
- Tomato (.25 cup)

- Cucumber (.25 cup)
- Bell pepper (.25 cup)
- Feta cheese (.5 cup)
- Olive oil (3 tbsp.)
- Olives (1 tbsp.)
- Red wine vinegar (.5 tbsp.)

Method of Prep:
1. Dice the tomato, chop the olives, and slice the onion, cucumber, and pepper.
2. Combine the bell pepper, tomato, cucumber, crumbled feta cheese, and onion.

Tips for Meal Prep:
1. You can prepare the salad and pop into the fridge until time to eat.
2. Spritz using the oil and vinegar with a shake of salt and black pepper to your liking.
3. Toss until all of the ingredients are well mixed before serving.

Dinner: Buffalo Sloppy Joes

Yields Provided: 8

Total Carbohydrates: 2 grams

Ingredients for Prep:

- Coconut oil (1 tbsp.)

- Celery stalk (1 medium)
- Baby carrots (.25 cup)
- White onion (1 small)
- Garlic powder (1 tsp.)
- Red hot sauce (.5 cup)
- Mayonnaise (.25 cup)
- Ground chicken or turkey (1 lb.)

Method of Prep:
1. Pulse the baby carrots, celery stalk, and onion using a food processor. (You can also finely chop the veggies.)
2. Heat a skillet using the med-high temperature setting.
3. Pour in the coconut oil to heat. Toss in the minced veggies. Sauté for five to eight minutes. When it's ready, the carrots and onions will be fork tender.
4. Fold in the ground chicken. Continue to sauté until the chicken is thoroughly cooked.
5. Adjust the heat setting to low. Stir in the hot sauce and garlic powder.
6. Simmer for another five minutes. Remove from the burner.

Tips for Meal Prep:
1. Cool the chicken completely. Add to eight containers or freezer bags.
2. Store in the freezer until needed.
3. Defrost the portions needed to thaw.
4. Once it's dinner time, stir in the mayonnaise.
5. Note: Be sure the mixture is cool, or mayonnaise could curdle.
6. Spoon into your wrap or bun to serve.

Snack: Brownie Muffins

Yields Provided: 6

Total Carbohydrates: 4.4 grams

Ingredients for Prep:

- Salt (.5 tsp.)
- Flaxseed meal (1 cup)
- Cocoa powder (.25 cup)
- Cinnamon (1 tbsp.)
- Baking powder (.5 tbsp.)
- Coconut oil (2 tbsp.)
- Large egg (1)
- Vanilla extract (1 tsp.)
- Pumpkin puree (.5 cup)
- Sugar-free caramel syrup (.25 cup)
- Slivered almonds (.5 cup)
- Apple cider vinegar (1 tsp.)

Method of Prep:
1. Set the oven temperature to 350° Fahrenheit.
2. Use a deep mixing container—mix all of the fixings and stir well.
3. Use six paper liners in the muffin tin, and add ¼ cup of batter to each one.

4. Sprinkle several almonds on the tops, pressing gently.
5. Bake approximately 15 minutes or when the top is set.

Tips for Meal Prep:
1. Cut the brownies into six portions.
2. Store in plastic baggies for the fridge or freezer bags if you want to have them last longer than three to four days.

Week 2

Day 8

Breakfast: Avocado Eggs

Yields Provided: 2

Total Carbohydrates: 9 grams

Ingredients for Prep:

- Eggs (2)
- Avocado (1 ripened)
- Black pepper and salt (to your liking)
- Optional: Hot sauce

Method of Prep:

1. Warm up the oven until it reaches 425° Fahrenheit.
2. Slice the avocado in half and discard the pit. Use a metal scoop to remove about one to two tablespoons of the fleshy insides.
3. Arrange the halves in a small baking pan. Crack an egg into both halves and season with some pepper and salt.
4. Bake for 15-20 minutes.

Tips for Meal Prep:
1. Let the fixings cool and store for a day or so in the refrigerator to enjoy the next morning or for a snack.

2. If you want to spice it up a little, sprinkle in a portion of keto-friendly hot sauce on the second day.

Lunch: Tuna Salad

Yields Provided: 2

Total Carbohydrates: 6 grams

Ingredients for Prep:

- Fresh lemon juice (half of 1)
- Olive oil (1 tbsp.)
- Large chopped boiled eggs (2)
- Tuna packed in oil (2 cans - 15 oz. each)
- Cucumber (half of 1)
- Medium red onions (2)
- Cilantro (half of 1)
- Salt (1 tsp.)
- Mayonnaise (2 tbsp.)
- Dijon mustard (2 tsp.)

Method of Prep:
1. Whisk the oil, lemon juice, mayo, and mustard in a container.
2. Thinly slice the cucumber and onions.
3. Drain the tuna and combine it with the remainder of the ingredients in another bowl.
4. Place each container in the fridge.

Tips for Meal Prep:
1. Add the dressing to the salad and toss to serve.

Dinner: Bacon & Shrimp Risotto

Yields Provided: 2

Total Carbohydrates: 5 grams

Ingredients for Prep:

- Bacon (4 slices)
- Daikon winter radish (2 cups)
- Dry white wine (2 tbsp.)
- Chicken stock (.25 cup)
- Garlic (1 clove)
- Ground pepper (as desired)
- Chopped parsley (2 tbsp.)
- Cooked shrimp (4 oz.)

Method of Prep:

1. Peel and slice the radish, mince the garlic, and chop the bacon. Remove as much water as possible from the daikon once it's shredded.
2. On the stovetop, heat up a saucepan using the medium heat temperature setting. Toss in the bacon and fry until it's crispy. Leave the drippings in the pan and remove the bacon with a slotted spoon to drain.
3. Add the stock, wine, daikon, salt, pepper, and garlic into the pan. Simmer for 6-8 minutes until most of the liquid is absorbed.
4. Fold in the bacon (saving a few bits for the topping), and shrimp along with the parsley. Serve.
5. *Tip*: If you cannot find the daikon, just substitute it using shredded cauliflower.

Tips for Meal Prep:

1. This delicious treat can be cooled and stored in the fridge for a day or two.
2. Save the bacon and shrimp in separate containers until ready to serve.

Snack: Pumpkin Pie Cupcakes

Yields Provided: 6

Total Carbohydrates: 2.9 grams

Ingredients for Prep:

- Coconut flour (3 tbsp.)
- Baking powder (.25 tsp.)
- Salt (1 pinch)

- Baking soda (.25 tsp.)
- Pumpkin pie spice (1 tsp.)
- Large egg (1)
- Pumpkin puree (.75 cup)
- Swerve Granular/Swerve Brown (.33 cup)
- Heavy whipping cream (.25 cup)
- Vanilla (.5 tsp.)

Method of Prep:
1. Warm up the oven to 350° Fahrenheit. Prepare the baking pan.
2. Whisk the coconut flour with the baking powder, pumpkin pie spice, baking soda, and salt.
3. In another container, whisk the pumpkin puree with the cream, sweetener, vanilla, and egg until well combined.
4. Whisk in the dry fixings. If the batter is too thin, whisk in an additional tablespoon of the coconut flour.
5. Portion into the muffin tins. Bake until puffed and barely set (25 to 30 min.).
6. Transfer the pan to the countertop (in the pan) to cool. Store in the fridge for a minimum of one hour before it's time to serve.
7. Top it off using a generous helping of whipped cream.
8. Note: They will sink when you let them cook. It will be that much tastier with the serving of whipped cream!

Tips for Meal Prep:
1. After they are cooled, store in the fridge until you want one to eat.
2. Top it off using the whipped cream.

Day 9

Breakfast: Tomato & Cheese Frittata

Yields Provided: 2

Total Carbohydrates: 6 grams

Ingredients for Prep:

- Eggs (6)
- Soft cheese (3.5 oz./.66 cup)
- White onion (half of 1 medium)
- Halved cherry tomatoes (.66 cup)
- Chopped herbs - ex. Chives or basil (2 tbsp.)
- Ghee/butter (1 tbsp.)

Method of Prep:
1. Set the oven broiler temperature to 400° Fahrenheit.
2. Arrange the onions on a greased - hot iron skillet. Cook with either ghee or butter until lightly browned.
3. In another dish, crack the eggs and flavor with salt, pepper, or add some herbs of your choice. Whisk and add to the pan of onions, cooking until the edges begin to get crispy.
4. Top with cheese (such as feta), and a few diced tomatoes. Put the pan in the broiler for five to seven minutes or until done.
5. Enjoy piping hot or let cool down.

6. Note: You can purge all of the leftover veggies into the recipe (if you wish).

Tips for Meal Prep:
1. Divide into two equal portions. Place in separate containers until you're ready to enjoy a healthy breakfast.
2. Enjoy this readily prepared frittata that you can serve either hot or cold.
3. The deliciously prepared frittata will remain good to serve for up to five days. So, prep enough for several days.

Lunch: Beef & Pepperoni Pizza

Yields Provided: 4

Total Carbohydrates: 2 grams

Ingredients for Prep:

- Large eggs (2)
- Ground beef (20 oz.)
- Pepperoni slices (28)
- Pizza sauce (.5 cup)
- Shredded cheddar cheese (.5 cup)
- Mozzarella cheese (4 oz.)
- Also Needed: 1 Cast iron skillet

Method of Prep:
1. Combine the eggs, beef, and seasonings and place in the skillet to form the crust. Bake until the meat is done or about 15 minutes.
2. Take it out of the oven and add the sauce, cheese, and toppings. Place the pizza back in the oven for a few more minutes until the cheese has melted.

Tips for Meal Prep:
1. After it's cooled completely, slice the pizza into four equal portions for freezing.
2. You can also leave it whole and freeze. Add it to a freezer bag until it's time to serve and enjoy.

Dinner: Chicken & Green Beans

Yields Provided: 3

Total Carbohydrates: 4 grams

Ingredients for Prep:

- Olive oil (2 tbsp.)
- Trimmed green beans (1 cup)
- Whole chicken breasts (2)
- Halved cherry tomatoes (8)
- Italian seasoning (1 tbsp.)
- Salt and pepper (1 tsp.)

Method of Prep:
1. Heat a skillet using the medium heat temperature setting. Pour in the oil.
2. Sprinkle the chicken with pepper, salt, and Italian seasoning.
3. Arrange in the skillet and fry for 10 minutes on each side or until well done.

Tips for Meal Prep:
1. Let the chicken cool. Place in a container until it's time to use.
2. Add the tomatoes and beans. Simmer another 5 to 7 minutes and serve.

Snack: Amaretti Cookies

Yields Provided: 16

Total Carbohydrates: 1 gram

Ingredients for Prep:

- Coconut flour (2 tbsp.)
- Cinnamon (.25 tsp.)
- Salt (.5 tsp.)
- Erythritol (.5 cup)
- Baking powder (.5 tsp.)
- Almond flour (1 cup)
- Eggs (2)
- Almond extract (.5 tsp.)
- Vanilla extract (.5 tsp.)
- Coconut oil (4 tbsp.)
- Sugar-free jam (2 tbsp.)
- Shredded coconut (1 tbsp.)

Method of Prep:
1. Cover the tin with a sheet of paper.
2. Warm up the oven to reach 400° Fahrenheit.
3. Sift the flour and combine all of the dry fixings.
4. After combined, work in the wet ones. Shape into 16 cookies.

5. Make a dent in the center of each one. Bake for 15 to 17 minutes.

Tips for Meal Prep:
1. It is important to let them cool for a few minutes.
2. Add a dab of jam to each one and a sprinkle of coconut bits.

Day 10

Breakfast: Blueberry Pancake Bites

Yields Provided: 24 bites

Total Carbohydrates: 7.5 grams

Ingredients for Prep:

- Baking powder (1 tsp.)
- Water (.33 - .5 cup)
- Melted ghee (.25 cup)
- Coconut flour (.5 cup)
- Cinnamon (.5 tsp.)
- Salt (.5 tsp.)
- Eggs (4)
- Vanilla extract (.5 tsp.)
- Frozen blueberries (.5 cup)

Method of Prep:

1. Set the oven to reach 325° Fahrenheit. Use a spritz of coconut oil spray to grease 24 regular-sized muffin cups.
2. Combine the eggs, sweetener, and vanilla, mixing until well incorporated. Fold in the flour, melted ghee, baking powder, salt, and cinnamon. Stir in .33 cup of water to finish the batter.
3. The mixture should be thick. Next, divide the batter into the prepared cups with several berries in each one.

4. Bake until set (20 to 25 min.). Cool.

Tips for Meal Prep:
1. Store in an airtight container; preferable cool also.
2. It will be good for 8 to 10 days.
3. Freeze for 60 to 80 days.

Lunch: Buffalo Chicken Burgers

Yields Provided: 2 burgers Total Carbohydrates: 1 gram

Ingredients for Prep:

- Chicken breasts (8 oz. cooked)
- Unchilled cream cheese (2 oz.)
- Shredded mozzarella cheese (.5 cup)
- Frank's Red-Hot Sauce or your preference (2 tbsp.)
- Coconut oil or ghee - for frying

Method of Prep:
1. Either chop or shred the prepared chicken and combine it with the rest of the fixings.
2. Place the fixings in the microwave for 15 to 20 seconds to help compact the ingredients. Form two medium patties and place them on a plate. Store in the freezer for about 15 minutes.
3. Heat a skillet using the high-temperature setting. Add the fat and patties. Prepare the burgers for 2 to 3 minutes per side.
4. Serve when crispy brown.

Tips for Meal Prep:
1. Prepare the chicken and mix to form patties.
2. Freeze, or cook and freeze the patties.

Dinner: Roasted Leg of Lamb

Yields Provided: 2

Total Carbohydrates: 1 gram

Ingredients for Prep:

- Reduced-sodium beef broth (.5 cup)
- Leg of lamb (2 lb.)
- Chopped garlic cloves (6)
- Fresh rosemary leaves (1 tbsp.)
- Black pepper (1 tsp.)
- Salt (2 tsp.)

Method of Prep:
1. Grease a baking pan and set the oven temperature to 400° Fahrenheit.
2. Arrange the lamb in the pan and add the broth and seasonings.
3. Roast 30 minutes and lower the heat to 350° Fahrenheit. Continue cooking for about one hour or until done.
4. Let the lamb stand about 20 minutes before slicing to serve.
5. Enjoy with some roasted brussels sprouts and extra rosemary for a tasty change of pace.

Tips for Meal Prep:
1. Cool and wrap any leftovers to use later.

2. Wrap well in plastic wrap and store in a freezer bag.

Day 11

Breakfast: Blueberry Essence

Yields Provided: 1

Total Carbohydrates: 3 grams

Ingredients for Prep:

- Blueberries (.25 cup)
- Coconut milk (1 cup)
- Optional: Whey protein powder (1 scoop)
- Vanilla Essence (1 tsp.)
- MCT Oil (1 tsp.)

Method of Prep:

1. For a quick burst of energy, add all of the fixings into a blender.
2. Puree until it reaches the desired consistency.

Tips for Meal Prep:

1. Store in the fridge until ready to enjoy.
2. Add several chunks of ice if you like.

Lunch: Italian Tomato Salad

Yields Provided: 2

Total Carbohydrates: 6 grams

Ingredients for Prep:

- Minced garlic clove (1)
- Freshly chopped basil (.25 cup)
- Balsamic vinegar (1 tbsp.)
- Olive oil (2 tbsp.)
- Pepper and salt (as desired)
- Sliced ripe tomatoes (2 medium)
- Fresh arugula (2 cups)
- Cubed mozzarella cheese (3 oz.)

Method of Prep:
1. Combine the oil, vinegar, basil, garlic, black pepper, and salt into a blender. Mix until it's creamy smooth.
2. Toss the rest of the fixings in a salad container.

Tips for Meal Prep:
1. Combine the salad and add the dressing mixture or add it to individual containers for an on-to-go method.
2. You can store this way for up to one day.

Dinner: Bacon Cheeseburger

Yields Provided: 12

Total Carbohydrates: 0.8 gram

Ingredients for Prep:

- Low-sodium bacon (16 oz. pkg.)
- Ground beef (3 lb.)
- Eggs (2)
- Medium chopped onion (half of 1)
- Shredded cheddar cheese (8 oz.)

Method of Prep:
1. Fry the bacon and chop to bits. Shred the cheese and dice the onion.
2. Combine the mixture with the beef and blend in the whisked eggs.
3. Prepare 24 burgers and grill them the way you like them. You can make a double-decker since they are small. If you like a larger burger, you can just make 12 burgers as a single-decker.

Tips for Meal Prep:
1. Let the cooked burgers cool.
2. Separate them into freezer bags for later use anytime you need a quick meal or snack.

Snack: Strawberry Cream Cheese Bites

Yields Provided: 12

Total Carbohydrates: 2 grams

Ingredients for Prep:

- Diced strawberries (1 cup)
- Vanilla extract (1 tsp.)
- Coconut oil (.25 cup)
- Unchilled cream cheese (.75 cup)
- Also Needed: 12-count muffin cup tin

Method of Prep:
1. Prepare a muffin tray with liners or grease with a spritz of cooking oil spray.
2. Toss the berries into the blender and mix until pureed.
3. Add in the rest of the fixings and mix until it's all smooth.
4. Scoop into the cups and freeze until solid (2 hrs.).

Tips for Meal Prep:
1. After they are frozen, your job is done.
2. Pop them out and store them in a freezer bag and enjoy any time you desire!

Day 12

Breakfast: Pancakes & Nuts

Yields Provided: 2

Total Carbohydrates: 9 grams

Ingredients for Prep:

- Almond flour (10 tbsp.)
- Baking soda (.5 tsp.)
- Ground cinnamon (1 tsp.)
- Large eggs (3)
- Almond milk (.25 cup)

Method of Prep:

1. Whisk all of the fixings in a container. Let the batter sit for 5-10 minutes so the flour will thicken.
2. Warm-up a greased skillet (low-medium).
3. Measure out .25 cup portions of the batter in the frying pan. Cook for two to three minutes per side.

Tips for Meal Prep:

1. Let the pancakes cool.
2. Pour the nuts into a baggie or plastic container. You can add the nuts in the containers together or separately.
3. You can store the pancakes for 5-7 days in the refrigerator.

4. *Time to Eat*: Heat the pancakes and serve with the prepared almond butter drizzle.

Lunch: Pulled Pork for Sandwiches

Yields Provided: 8

Total Carbohydrates: 2.2 grams

Ingredients for Prep:

- Boneless pork shoulder (3 lb.)
- Chopped white onion (1)
- Bay leaves (3)
- Smoked paprika (1 tsp.)
- Garlic powder (2 tsp.)
- Pink Himalayan salt (3 tsp.)

Method of Prep:
1. Warm a slow cooker using the low setting. Combine the paprika, salt, and garlic powder. Slice the pork into chunks and rub into the spices.
2. Chop the onion and toss it into the cooker along with the pork.
3. Add the bay leaves and close the lid. Cook for 10 hours on low.
4. When ready, shred, and let cool.

Tips for Meal Prep:
1. Add the shredded pork to individual bags for the freezer or into compartmentalized dishes to await a veggie.
2. Be sure to date the containers and label with the name of its content.

Dinner: Shrimp Alfredo

Yields Provided: 4

Total Carbohydrates: 6.5 grams

Ingredients for Prep:

- Raw shrimp (1 lb.)
- Salted butter (1 tbsp.)
- Cubed cream cheese (4 oz.)
- Whole milk (.5 cup)
- Salt (1 tsp.)
- Garlic powder (1 tbsp.)
- Dried basil (1 tsp.)
- Shredded parmesan cheese (.5 cup)
- Baby kale or spinach (.25 cup)
- Whole sun-dried tomatoes (5)

Method of Prep:
1. Warm the butter using the medium heat temperature setting in a skillet.
2. Toss in the shrimp and lower the heat to med-low. After 30 seconds, flip the shrimp and cook until slightly pink. Blend in the cream cheese.

3. Increase the heat and pour in the milk. Stir frequently.
4. Sprinkle with the salt, basil, and garlic. Empty the parmesan cheese in and mix well.
5. Simmer until the sauce has thickened. Cut the sun-dried tomatoes into strips.
6. Lastly, fold in the kale/spinach and dried tomatoes. Serve steaming hot.

Tips for Meal Prep:
1. Cool thoroughly and store in the fridge to enjoy in a day or two.

Snack: Coconut Macaroons

Yields Provided: 40 cookies/20 servings Total

Carbohydrates: 1 gram

Ingredients for Prep:

- Water (.33 cup)
- Low carb sweetener (.75 cup or less to taste)
- Sea salt (.25 tsp.)
- Sugar-free vanilla extract (.75 tsp.)
- Large eggs (2)
- Unsweetened shredded coconut (3-4 cups)
- *Optional*: Sugar-free chocolate chips
- Nonstick cooking oil spray

Method of Prep:

1. Set the oven to reach 350° Fahrenheit.
2. Lightly spray the cookie tin with the oil spray.
3. Combine the sweetener, water, vanilla extract, and salt in the pan.
4. Bring to a boil using the med-high temperature setting. Stir well and remove from the burner.
5. Combine the coconut flakes and egg in a food processor. Pour in the syrup and pulse. Scoop the dough onto the prepared cookie tin (one-inch apart).
6. Bake for eight minutes, rotating the cookie tin in the oven.
7. Continue baking until lightly browned or approximately four additional minutes.

8. Cool on the rack. Garnish with the melted chocolate as desired.

Tips for Meal Prep:
1. Note: Start with 3 cups of dried coconut shredded coconut.
2. You can add more as needed for the desired consistency, depending on taste preference.
3. After they are cooled, melt the chocolate, and serve.

Day 13

Breakfast: Cinnamon Smoothie

Yields Provided: 1

Total Carbohydrates: 5 grams

Ingredients for Prep:

- Cinnamon (.5 tsp.)
- Coconut milk (.5 cup)
- Water (.5 cup)
- Extra-virgin coconut oil/MCT oil (1 tbsp.)
- Ground chia seeds (1 tbsp.)
- Plain/vanilla whey protein (.25 cup)
- Optional: Stevia drops

Method of Prep:
1. Pour the milk, cinnamon, protein powder, and chia seeds in a blender.
2. Empty the coconut oil, ice, and water. Add a few drops of stevia to your liking.

Tips for Meal Prep:
1. Store in the fridge until ready to enjoy.
2. Add several chunks of ice if you like.

Lunch: Pita Pizza

Yields Provided: 2

Ingredients for Prep:

- Marinara sauce (.5 cup)
- Low-carb pita (1)
- Cheddar cheese (2 oz.)
- Pepperoni (14 slices)
- Roasted red peppers (1 oz.)

Method of Prep:
1. Set the oven to 450° Fahrenheit.
2. Slice the pita in half and put on a foil-lined baking tray. Rub with a bit of oil and toast for one to two minutes.
3. Pour the sauce over the bread, sprinkle with the cheese, and other toppings. Bake for an additional five minutes or until the cheese melts.

Tips for Meal Prep:
1. Remove the pizza from the oven and cool it thoroughly.
2. Store in the fridge for a couple of days.
3. Freeze to enjoy later using a freezer bag.

Dinner: Roasted Chicken & Tomatoes

Yields Provided: 2

Total Carbohydrates: 5 grams

Ingredients for Prep:

- Olive oil (1 tbsp.)
- Plum tomatoes (2 quartered)
- Chicken legs – bone-in with skin (2)
- Paprika (1 tsp.)
- Ground oregano (1 tsp.)
- Balsamic vinegar (1 tbsp.)

Method of Prep:
1. Set the oven temperature setting at 350° Fahrenheit. Grease a roasting pan with a spritz of oil.
2. Rinse and lightly dab the chicken legs dry with a paper towel. Prepare using the oil and vinegar over the skin. Season with the paprika and oregano.
3. Arrange the legs in the pan along with the tomatoes around the edges.
4. Cover with a layer of foil and bake one hour. Baste to prevent the chicken from drying out.
5. Discard the foil and increase the temperature to 425° Fahrenheit.
6. Bake 15 to 30 minutes more until browned and the juices run clear.
7. Serve with a side salad.

Tips for Meal Prep:
1. If you plan to use this for meal prep only, stop at step 4. Put in a zipper-type freezer bag.
2. Freeze the contents until another time. Proceed by baking.

Snack: Pecan Turtle Truffles

Yields Provided: 15

Total Carbohydrates: 1

Ingredients for Prep:

- Swerve or your preference (.33 cup)
- Melted butter (.5 cup)
- Vanilla extract (.25 tsp.)
- Caramel extract (.5 tsp.)
- Vanilla protein powder -0- carbs (.33 cup)
- Finely ground pecans (1 cup)
- 85% chocolate - Lindt or your choice (4 squares)
- Pecan halves (15)

Method of Prep:
1. Combine the sweetener, butter, vanilla extract, caramel extracts, finely ground pecans and protein powder in a mixing container.
2. Roll into 15 truffles and place them on a sheet of parchment or waxed paper.
3. Melt the chocolate in a baggie in the microwave for one minute. Snip the corner and squeeze the chocolate over the prepared truffles.

4. Garnish each truffle with a pecan half. Chill and enjoy any time.

Tips for Meal Prep:
1. Store in the fridge for the truffles to remain fresh.

Day 14

Breakfast: Bacon Cheese & Egg Cups

Yields Provided: 6

Total Carbohydrates: 1 gram

Ingredients for Prep:

- Large eggs (6)
- Bacon (6 strips)
- Cheese (.25 cup)
- Fresh spinach (1 handful)
- Pepper & Salt (as desired)

Method of Prep:

1. Warm up the oven to 400° Fahrenheit.
2. Prepare the bacon using medium heat on the stovetop. Place on towels to drain.
3. Grease 6 muffin tins with a spritz of oil.
4. Line each tin with a slice of bacon, pressing tightly to make a secure well for the eggs.
5. Drain and dry the spinach with a paper towel. Whisk the eggs and combine with the spinach.
6. Add the mixture to the prepared tins and sprinkle with cheese Sprinkle with salt and pepper until it's like you like it.
7. Bake for 15 minutes. Remove when done and cool.

Tips for Meal Prep:

1. Prepare the cups and store them in airtight containers.
2. Reheat when ready to eat. It keeps in the fridge for 3-4 days.

Lunch: Caprese Salad

Yields Provided: 4

Total Carbohydrates: 5 grams

Ingredients for Prep:

- Grape tomatoes (3 cups)
- Peeled garlic cloves (4)
- Avocado oil (2 tbsp.)
- Mozzarella balls (19 pearl-sized)
- Fresh basil leaves (.25 cup)
- Baby spinach leaves (4 cups)
- Brine reserved from the cheese (1 tbsp.)
- Pesto (1 tbsp.)

Method of Prep:
1. Use a sheet of aluminum foil to cover a baking tray.
2. Set the oven temperature at 400° Fahrenheit.
3. Arrange the cloves and tomatoes on the baking pan. Drizzle with oil. Bake for 20 to 30 minutes until the tops are lightly browned.
4. Drain the liquid (saving one tablespoon) from the mozzarella. Mix the pesto with the brine.
5. Arrange the spinach in a large serving bowl. Transfer the tomatoes to the dish along with the roasted garlic.

Tips for Meal Prep:
1. Cool the ingredients thoroughly. Place in closed containers until time to use.
2. Drizzle with the pesto sauce. Garnish with the mozzarella balls and freshly torn basil leaves.

Dinner: Enchilada Skillet Dinner

Yields Provided: 4

Total Carbohydrates: 7 grams

Ingredients for Prep:

- Small yellow onion (1)
- Ground beef (1.5 lb.)
- Red enchilada sauce (.66 cup)
- Chopped green onions (8)
- Diced Roma tomatoes (2)
- Shredded cheddar cheese (4 oz.)
- Optional: Freshly chopped cilantro (as desired)

Method of Prep:
1. Use a wok or skillet to sauté the yellow onion and meat. Drain the juices and add the green onions, tomato, and enchilada sauce.
2. Once it starts to boil, simmer for about 5 minutes. Sprinkle with the salt and cheese. Continue cooking until the cheese has melted.
3. Stir in the cilantro. Serve over chopped lettuce and serving of sour cream. Add the extra carbs and enjoy.

Tips for Meal Prep:
1. If you have any leftovers, omit the cilantro, lettuce, and sour cream.
2. Wrap each portion tightly in plastic wrap and then in foil. Freeze.
3. Remove from the freezer and bake at 350° Fahrenheit until the cheese is melted, and the dinner is warmed.

Chapter 5: Meal Prep for Kids

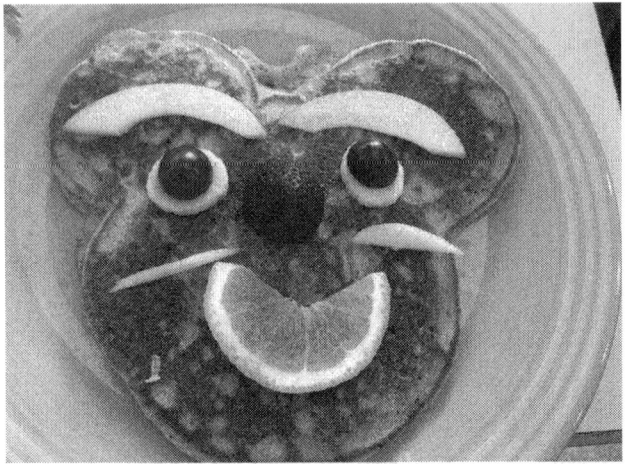

You will find these quick and easy recipes are easy to prepare in a short time!

Special Smoothie Options: Smoothies are included for children who don't always like veggies or some fruits. All that is required is a freezer- safe container or a push-up popsicle mold to make a special snack.

You can make a unique pack using 2 cups of fruit, 1 cup of optional greens, and a sliced banana. When you're ready to eat, place 1 cup of liquid into the blender (or half yogurt and half water), add the fruit, and mix. Day 2 and 4 are using the mango base with additional boosters to make it a meal.

Week 1

Day 1

Breakfast: Apple Banana Muffins

Yields Provided: 12

Ingredients for Prep:

- Baking powder (1 tsp.)
- Whole wheat flour (1.33 cups)
- Salt (.25 tsp.)
- Baking soda (.5 tsp.)
- Egg (1)
- Olive oil (3 tbsp.)
- Unsweetened applesauce (.5 cup)
- Vanilla extract (1 tsp.)

Method of Prep:

1. Set the oven temperature at 375° Fahrenheit.
2. Heavily grease a muffin tin.
3. Whisk the egg and mashed bananas. Fold in everything except the flour.
4. Lastly, stir in the flour, using caution not to overmix.
5. Portion the batter into each of the tins.
6. Bake for approximately 20-25 minutes.

Tips for Meal Prep:

1. When the muffins are done, transfer them to the countertop, leaving them in the pan for about five minutes. Arrange them on a cooling rack to thoroughly cool before proceeding.
2. Place the muffins into a freezer bag or another type of storage container.
3. Store in the fridge for about five days or freeze for later.

Lunch: Cranberry Tuna Salad

Yields Provided: 5

Ingredients for Prep:

- White tuna - packed in water (16 oz. can)
- Low-fat mayo (3 tbsp.)
- Salt and pepper (as desired)
- Light sour cream (3 tbsp.)
- Celery (.5 cup)
- Red onion (.25 cup)
- Lemon juice (1 tbsp.)
- Dried cranberries (.25 cup)
- Apple (1 diced)

Method of Prep:
1. Drain the tuna.
2. Chop the celery and mince the onion. Measure out the rest of the fixings.
3. Combine and mix all of the ingredients.

Tips for Meal Prep:
1. Place a cover on the salad.
2. Store in the refrigerator to enjoy for breakfast or brunch.

Dinner: Hawaiian Chicken Kebabs

Yields Provided: 8

Ingredients for Prep:

- Chicken breasts (1 lb.)
- Yellow & Red bell pepper (half of 1 each)
- Purple or red onion (half of 1)
- Pineapple chunks (1.5 cups)
- Pineapple (.5 cup)
- Orange (.5 cup)
- Teriyaki sauce (.25 cup)
- Salt (1 tsp.)
- Ginger (.5 tsp.)
- Onion powder (1 tsp.)
- Black pepper (1 tsp.)

- Garlic powder (1 tsp.)

Method of Prep:
1. Soak the wooden skewers in water for one hour.
2. Slice the peppers and onions into 1-inch pieces.
3. Prepare the marinade (orange juice, teriyaki, and pineapple). Marinate the chicken for one to two hours.
4. Prepare the skewers. Alternate the chicken and veggies (2 to 3 of each veggie and 3 to 4 pieces of meat).
5. Combine the spices in a small container (black pepper, salt, ginger, onion, and garlic powder). Sprinkle over the kebabs.
6. Cook on the grill (med. flame) 5 to 6 minutes on each side.
7. Take the goodies from the skewers and enjoy the feast.

Tips for Meal Prep:
1. You have two options.
2. *Option 1:* Go through step 3 to prepare the skewers,
3. Cover the skewers with foil and cook the following day.
4. Continue the recipe.
5. *Option 2:* Prepare and cook the kebabs. Remove from the skewers if desired.
6. Store in the fridge. For best results, enjoy the next day or two

Snack: Apple Pie Cookies

Yields Provided: 24

Ingredients for Prep:

- Sugar-free yellow cake mix (1 box)
- Applesauce - unsweetened (.5 cup)
- Eggs (2)
- Diced apples (1 cup)
- Cinnamon (.5 tsp.)

Method of Prep:

1. Warm the oven temperature at 375° Fahrenheit.
2. Prepare a baking tin with a silicone baking mat or a piece of parchment paper.
3. Combine all of the fixings, mixing well. Scoop out and make one-inch balls. Arrange in the pan about two inches apart.
4. Bake until they're done to your liking or about 10 to 12 minutes.

Tips for Meal Prep:

1. Prepare the cookies and let them cool.
2. Store in an airtight container until desired.

Day 2

Breakfast: Mango Smoothie Base & Oats

Yields Provided: 1

Ingredients for Prep:

- Frozen mango chunks (1.5 cups)
- Liquid: Coconut water, dairy milk, almond milk, or water (1 to 1.5 cups)
- Optional: Chia seeds (1 tbsp.)

Method of Prep:

1. Combine the fixings in a blender until creamy smooth.
2. Use these optional nutrient boosters as desired:
    a. Ground flax (1 tbsp.)
    b. Hemp seeds (1 tbsp.)
    c. Coconut oil (1 tbsp.)
    d. Avocado (¼ of 1)
    e. Goji berries (1 tbsp.)

3. Add .25 cup of oatmeal to finish the smoothie with the boosters and base.

Tips for Meal Prep:
1. Freeze the prepared smoothie.
2. The night before, you can place the container in the fridge to defrost.
3. You can also put it into a lunchbox with a straw to be defrosted for lunches or a quick treat.

Lunch: Buffalo Chicken Tenders

Yields Provided: 6

Ingredients for Prep:

- Chicken breasts (1 lb.)
- Panko breadcrumbs (1 cup)
- Flour (.25 cup)
- Eggs (3)
- Red hot sauce (.33 cup)
- Brown sugar (.5 cup)
- Garlic powder (.5 tsp.)
- Water (3 tbsp.)

Method of Prep:
1. Set the oven setting to 425° Fahrenheit. Lightly prepare a baking sheet with a spritz of cooking oil.
2. Slice the chicken into strips and pound into a ½-inch thickness for even cooking and tenderness. Toss into a zipper-type baggie along with the flour. Shake well.
3. Add the breadcrumbs in one dish and the eggs in another.
4. Place the sliced pieces of chicken in with the eggs, then the breadcrumbs. Arrange on the prepared pan. Lightly spray with a misting of cooking oil.
5. Bake 20 minutes.
6. Prepare the sauce with the rest of the fixings in a small saucepan.

Tips for Meal Prep:

1. Let the chicken strips and sauce cool completely.
2. Wrap the chicken and place it in an airtight container. Add the sauce to another dish and store both in the fridge.
3. When ready to eat, warm the fixings.
4. Prepare any veggies you want as a side dish.
5. Enjoy the tenders with the sauce and your favorite side of veggies.

Dinner: Chili & Mac 'n' Cheese

Yields Provided: 6

Ingredients for Prep:

- Cooked ground beef (.5 lb.)
- Box - your favorite Mac 'n' cheese (1)
- Red kidney beans (1 cup)
- Green, canned chili (1 can - 4 oz.)
- Grated cheddar cheese (.25 cup)
- Chili powder (2 tsp.)

Method of Prep:

1. Prepare the box of macaroni and cheese.
2. Cook the ground beef until done.

3. Combine all of the fixings and serve.

Tips for Meal Prep:
1. You can divide the leftovers into individual containers to use over the next few days or leave it in one bowl for the next dining meal.

Snack: Pumpkin Cupcakes

Yields Provided: 24

Ingredients for Prep:

- 100% Pumpkin puree (15 oz. can)
- Water (1 cup)
- Sugar-free yellow cake mix (1 box)
- Also Needed: 2 dozen muffin tins with liners

Method of Prep:
1. Set the oven temperature setting to 350º Fahrenheit.
2. Prepare the muffin tins.
3. Combine all of the fixings. Pour into the prepared cupcake holders
4. Bake until lightly browned or about 22 minutes.

Tips for Meal Prep:
1. Transfer the cupcakes to the countertop and cool on a rack.
2. When they are fully cooled, store in the fridge.

3. Freeze to use anytime.

Day 3

Breakfast: Banana Almond Pancakes

Yields Provided: 4

Ingredients for Prep:

- Banana (half of 1)
- Large egg (1)
- Cinnamon (.125 tsp.)
- Ground almond flour (1 tsp.)
- Olive oil (2 tbsp.)

Method of Prep:
1. Whisk the egg and mix with the cinnamon and flour.
2. Mash the banana using a fork and combine it with the rest of the fixings.
3. Warm the oil in a skillet. Pour the batter to the pan. Flip once during the cooking process.
4. You'll have delicious pancakes in 20 minutes from start to finish.

Tips for Meal Prep:
1. Cool thoroughly and store in freezer bags according to how many servings you will use at one time.
2. Place the frozen pancakes onto a microwave-safe dish.
3. Microwave using the high setting for 1- 1.5 minutes.
4. Garnish with your favorite toppings.

Lunch: Colored Iceberg Salad

Yields Provided: 4

Ingredients for Prep:

- Iceberg lettuce (1 head)
- Bacon (6 slices)
- Sliced green onions (2)
- Sliced radishes (6)
- Shredded carrots (3)
- Red vinegar (.25 cup)
- Minced cloves of garlic (3)
- Olive oil (.25 cup)
- Black pepper (1 pinch)

Method of Prep:
1. Prepare the bacon in a skillet until crispy. Arrange on paper towels to drain the grease.
2. Use a large-sized salad bowl or individual dishes to prepare the salad.
3. Combine the torn lettuce leaves with the black pepper, garlic, carrots, green onions, bacon, oil, vinegar, and radishes.

Tips for Meal Prep:
1. This is a great one for the kids to get healthy veggies by using delightful colors.
2. Cover with plastic lids or plastic wrap until time for lunch.

Dinner: Delicious Meatloaf

Yields Provided: 6

Ingredients for Prep:

- 93% lean ground beef (2 lb.)
- Almond flour (2 tbsp.)
- Coconut flour (2 tbsp.)
- Garlic powder (1 tsp.)
- Onion powder (1 tsp.)
- Black pepper (.25 tsp.)
- Salt (1 tsp.)
- Egg (1)
- Worcestershire sauce (1 tbsp.)
- Regular or almond milk (1 tbsp.)
- BARBECUE sauce (.5 cup + more for serving)
- Also Needed: 9x5 loaf pan

Method of Prep:

1. Warm the oven at 350° Fahrenheit. Prepare the pan in
2. Note: You can also place the loaf pan on a baking tray to prevent spillovers in the oven.
3. Whisk the salt, pepper, garlic powder, and both flours in a mixing container.
4. In another container, mix the egg, barbecue sauce, milk, Worcestershire sauce, and ground beef.
5. Combine everything and place it in the pan.

6. Bake for 45-65 minutes (depending on its thickness).
7. After it has baked for about halfway (20 min.), add barbecue sauce to the top and continue baking until the internal temperature reaches 155 Fahrenheit.
8. Serve and prepare the rest for freezing.

Tips for Meal Prep:
1. Cool thoroughly and place in a storage container and freeze for another time.

Snack: Whole Grain Banana Bread

Yields Provided: 14

Ingredients for Prep:

- Millet flour (.5 cup)
- Quinoa flour (.5 cup)
- Rice flour (.5 cup)
- Tapioca flour (.5 cup)
- Amaranth flour - brown (.5 cup)
- Baking powder (.5 tsp.)
- Salt (.125 cup)
- Baking soda (1 tsp.)
- Grapeseed oil (2 tbsp.)
- Raw sugar (.5 cup)
- Mashed banana (2 cups)

- Egg whites (.75 cup)
- Also Needed: 1 loaf pan - 5 by 9-inch

Method of Prep:
1. Lightly spray the loaf pan with a spritz of cooking oil. Sprinkle with a little flour and set aside.
2. Heat the oven temperature setting to reach 350º Fahrenheit.
3. Combine each of the dry fixings in a large mixing container - omitting the sugar.
4. Whisk the egg, mashed banana, oil, and sugar in another bowl. Thoroughly mix, adding the fixings to the loaf pan.
5. Bake for 50-60 minutes.

Tips for Meal Prep:
1. Transfer the loaf pan to the countertop to cool.
2. When cooled, place the entire loaf in a freezer bag. You can also slice and store the bread in the fridge or freezer for individual servings.

Day 4

Breakfast: Mango Smoothie Base & Greens

Yields Provided: 1

Ingredients for Prep:

- Liquid: Almond milk, coconut water, dairy milk, or water (1 to 1.5 cups)
- Frozen mango chunks (1.5 cups)
- Optional: Chia seeds (1 tbsp.)

Method of Prep:

1. Combine the smoothie fixings in a blender until creamy.
2. Use these optional nutrient boosters as desired:
   a. Hemp seeds (1 tbsp.)
   b. Ground flax (1 tbsp.)
   c. Avocado (¼ of 1)
   d. Coconut oil (1 tbsp.)
   e. Goji berries (1 tbsp.)

Tips for Meal Prep:
1. Add a scoop of protein powder with the boosters and base to finish the smoothie. Jazz it up to suit your youngster.
2. Store the smoothie in the freezer.
3. The night before, place the container in the fridge to defrost.
4. You can also add it to a lunchbox with a straw to be defrosted for a quick treat.

Lunch: Tuna Melt

Yields Provided: 4

Ingredients for Prep:

- Chunk white tuna – packed in water (12 oz. can)
- Coleslaw – packaged or homemade (1.5 cups)
- Green onion chopped (3 tbsp.)
- Mayonnaise – fat-free (3 tbsp.)
- Dijon-style mustard (1 tbsp.)
- English muffins – split in half (4)
- Cheddar cheese, reduced-fat – shredded (.33 cup)

Method of Prep:
1. Warm up the barbecue grill, broiler, or toaster oven.
2. Mix the drained tuna, coleslaw, and onions.
3. Whisk the mayo and mustard. Mix well.

4. Stir in the tuna mixture and combine well.

Tips for Meal Prep:
1. Place a lid on the tuna dish and store it in the fridge.
2. When it's mealtime, cut the muffins into halves.
3. Spread the tuna mixture on the muffins and arrange on a broiler pan.
4. Place on the rack about four inches from the burner. Broil for 3- 4 minutes.
5. Toss the cheese over the top to melt and broil for about one to two minutes.

Dinner: Loaded Bacon Mac & Cheese

Yields Provided: 4-6

Ingredients for Prep:

- Mac 'n' Cheese (1 box)
- Cooked bacon (1 cup)
- Grated Monterey Jack cheese (.25 cup)
- Grated mozzarella cheese (.25 cup)

Method of Prep:
1. Make the macaroni and cheese and prepare the bacon.
2. Combine all of the fixings to serve now.
3. Note: It is noted by some that the powdered cheese is not as tasty as the creamy options.

Tips for Meal Prep:

1. You can prepare the mac 'n' cheese and bacon but store them individually until time to serve or use.
2. It will not store well in the freezer but should be good for several days.

Snack: Banana Oatmeal Cookies

Yields Provided: 36 cookies

Ingredients for Prep:

- All-purpose flour (1.5 cups)
- Ground nutmeg (.25 tsp.)
- Salt (.25 tsp.)
- Baking soda (1 tsp.)
- Butter (.25 cup or .5 stick)
- Ripened mashed bananas (2-3 medium or 1 cup)
- Brown sugar - Firmly packed (1 cup)
- Egg (1 large)
- Applesauce (.5 cup)
- Vanilla (1 tsp.)
- Old-fashioned rolled oats (2.5 cups)
- *Optional:* Chopped nuts (1 cup)

Method of Prep:

1. Combine the nutmeg, salt, flour, and baking soda. Set aside for now.

2. Beat the butter and brown sugar in a large mixing container using the medium setting of an electric mixer until well blended. Fold in and mix the vanilla, egg, applesauce, and mashed bananas.
3. Using the low-speed setting, combine with the flour until just combined. Stir in the oats and nuts. Mix until just incorporated.
4. Place the container in the fridge for 10 minutes or up to six hours.
5. When ready to bake, just warm up the oven to 350° Fahrenheit.
6. Prepare the baking pan with some cooking spray. (Tip: Bake on a parchment paper-lined pan or silicone liner for the best results.)
7. Spoon the dough onto the tins about three inches apart and bake 15 to 17 minutes. Remove while they're still soft on the top.
8. Let them rest in the pan a few minutes before moving with a spatula to a cooling rack.

Tips for Meal Prep:
1. Make this batch any time your snacks are getting low.
2. Once they are moved to the cooling rack; cool thoroughly.
3. Store in a closed container to use later.

Day 5

Breakfast: 2-Ingredient Pancakes

Yields Provided: 12-inch pancake (1)

Ingredients for Prep:

- Eggs (2)
- Ripe banana (1)
- Cinnamon
- Vanilla

Method of Prep:
1. Mash the bananas and whisk two eggs.
2. Use some cooking spray to grease the skillet/griddle. Scrape in the batter.
3. No syrup is needed for these tasty treats. Add a little cinnamon or vanilla if desired.

Tips for Meal Prep:
1. Prepare these deliciously quick and easy pancakes.
2. You can do this the night or day before you want them.
3. Either freeze or let it chill in the fridge for a day.

Lunch: *Pear & Banana Breakfast Salad*

Yields Provided: 2

Ingredients for Prep:

- Asian pear (1)
- Banana (1)
- Lime (half of 1)
- Cinnamon powder (5 tsp.)
- Toasted pepitas (2 oz.)

Method of Prep:
1. Core and cube the pear. Peel and slice the banana. Toast the pepitas. Juice the lime.
2. Combine all of the fixings into two dishes.

Tips for Meal Prep:
1. Store in the fridge until time to serve.
2. Toss well and serve it onto serving platters for breakfast.

Dinner: *Chicken Fried Rice*

Yields Provided: 6

Ingredients for Prep:

- Cooking oil spray (2 squirts)

- Scallions (.5 cup)
- Carrots (.5 cup)
- Frozen-thawed green peas (.5 cup)
- Cooked regular or instant long-grain brown rice (2 cups)
- Garlic cloves (2)
- Egg whites (4 large)
- Soy sauce - low-sodium (3 tbsp.)
- Chicken breasts (12 oz.- ½-inch cubes)

Method of Prep:
1. Chop the green and white parts of the scallion and dice the carrots and garlic. Remove all of the skin and bones from the chicken. Scramble or cook the egg to your liking for the mixture.
2. Prepare a skillet with the spray and set the temperature to med- high.
3. Toss in the garlic and scallions to sauté for two minutes.
4. Stir in the carrots and chicken and sauté about five more minutes.
5. Fold in the prepared brown rice, cooked egg whites, peas, and soy. Sauté for about one minute.
6. Let it cool entirely.

Tips for Meal Prep:
1. Your kids will love this.
2. Cooked chicken can stay in the fridge for 3-4 days. After that, you'll need to toss it. You can also freeze it for longer prep times.

3. *Option 1:* Heat the rice using the microwave. Add a few tablespoons of broth or water per one cup of rice. Cover to create a steaming effect as it reheats.
4. *Option 2:* Stir-fry the rice: Use a sauté pan or large wok to heat canola or peanut oil using the high-temperature setting.

Snack: Apples & Dip

Yields Provided: 4

Ingredients for Prep:

- Chopped peanuts (2 tbsp.)
- Unchilled fat-free cream cheese (8 oz.)
- Vanilla (1.5 tsp.)
- Brown sugar (2 tbsp.)
- Orange juice (.5 cup)
- Apples (8 small or 4 medium)

Method of Prep:
1. Chop the peanuts well and place them in a storage container.
2. Take the cream cheese out of the fridge for about 5 minutes to soften at room temperature.
3. Combine the cream cheese with vanilla and brown sugar until smooth.

Tips for Meal Prep:
1. Store the mixture in the fridge.
2. Time to Eat: Remove the core from the apples and slice.
3. Fold the nuts into the cream cheese mixture.
4. Serve the dip with sliced apples and a drizzle of juice on top.

Day 6

Breakfast: Mango Smoothie Base & Tofu

Yields Provided: 1

Ingredients for Prep:

- Frozen mango chunks (1.5 cups)
- Liquid: Dairy milk, almond milk, coconut water, or water (1 to 1.5 cups)
- Optional: Chia seeds (1 tbsp.)

Method of Prep:
1. Combine the fixings in a blender until smooth. Store in the freezer until time to use.
2. Use these optional nutrient boosters as desired
    a. Coconut oil (1 tbsp.)
    b. Hemp seeds (1 tbsp.)
    c. Avocado (¼ of 1)
    d. Goji berries (1 tbsp.)
    e. Ground flax (1 tbsp.)
3. Add 3 ounces of tofu to the chosen fixings and mix until it's the desired consistency.

Tips for Meal Prep:
1. Freeze the prepared smoothie in a freezer bag or freezer-safe jar.

2. The night before, you can put the container in the fridge to defrost.
3. Add the frozen smoothie into a lunchbox with a straw. It will defrost by lunchtime.

Lunch: Chicken Salad

Yields Provided: 6

Ingredients for Prep:

- Shredded chicken breast (2 cups)
- Mayonnaise (1 tbsp.)
- Nonfat sour cream (.25 cup)
- Nonfat Greek yogurt (.5 cup)
- Bell pepper (2 tbsp.)
- Gala apple (half of 1)
- Garlic powder (1 tsp.)
- Dill pickle relish (1 tsp.)
- Onion powder (1 tsp.)
- Freshly cracked black pepper (.5 tsp.)
- Paprika (.5 tsp.)
- Salt (.5 tsp.)

Method of Prep:
1. Combine all of the fixings with a sprinkle of the pepper and salt as desired.

Tips for Meal Prep:
1. Prepare the salad and store in the refrigerator using a glass container with a lid.
2. Serve it any time for a snack or lunch on your choice of bread, veggies, or crackers.

Dinner: Cheesy Beef Egg Rolls

Yields Provided: 8

Ingredients for Prep:

- Egg roll wrappers (8)
- Cheddar cheese stick - cut in half (4)
- Cooked roast beef - chopped (2 cups)
- Creamy style horseradish (.25 cup)
- Frying oil

Method of Prep:
1. Warm a deep fryer or oil in a pan to approximately 350° Fahrenheit. Prepare an egg roll wrapper, placed in a diamond shape.
2. Place a small amount of horseradish sauce in the center. Lay down ¼ cup of shredded beef. Arrange a cheese stick (half) over the beef and fold in the two sides. Take the bottom point and fold it like an envelope.
3. Wet the top side of the wrapper with water along the edge.
4. Roll from the bottom to form the stick into the shape of a cigar.

Tips for Meal Prep:
1. Cool and use within a day or so. You can also freeze and prepare later.
2. Bake for 12-15 minutes at 400° Fahrenheit.

Snack: Banana Roll-Ups

Yields Provided: 2

Ingredients for Prep:

- Whole wheat bread (1 slice)
- Medium peeled banana (.5 of 1)
- Salt-free chunky peanut butter (1.5 tsp.)

Method of Prep:
1. Use a rolling pin to flatten the bread.
2. Apply the peanut butter to one side of the bread. Add the banana.
3. Roll it up and slice into three to four segments.

Tips for Meal Prep:
1. After you roll up the bananas, just store them in the fridge in a closed container.
2. Enjoy anytime.

Day 7

Breakfast: Berry Monkey Bread Cinnamon Rolls

Yields Provided: 6

Ingredients for Prep:

- Refrigerated orange rolls (2 cans)
- Berries (2 pints)
- Optional: Softened cream cheese (3 oz.)
- Basil (3 tbsp.)

Method of Prep:
1. Chop the orange rolls and scatter them onto the bottom of a greased bundt pan.
2. Sprinkle with half of the berries, and repeat.
3. You can also press a dollop or two of cream cheese in the dough and berries with a sprinkle of basil.
4. Bake for 20 minutes. Wait a few minutes and turn it over and out.
5. Drizzle with the orange spread if you are using it the same day.

Tips for Meal Prep:
1. If these are for prep, wait on adding the spread until it's time to eat.

2. Leave the rinsed berries in a container also until mealtime.

Lunch: Strawberry Sandwiches

Yields Provided: 4

Ingredients for Prep:

- Stevia or favorite sweetener (1 tbsp.)
- Softened cream cheese - low-fat (8 oz.)
- Grated lemon zest (1 tsp.)
- Whole wheat English muffins (4 toasted)
- Sliced strawberries (2 cups)

Method of Prep:
1. Slice the strawberries. Set the low-fat cheese out to soften. Grate the lemon.
2. Use a food processor and combine the stevia, cream cheese, and lemon zest.

Tips for Meal Prep:
1. Once combined, cover with foil or plastic wrap.
2. When it's breakfast time, toast the muffins.
3. Use a butter knife to spread the cheese mixture onto the toasted muffin halves. Add the berries and serve.

Dinner: Air-Fried Parmesan Chicken

Yields Provided: 4

Ingredients for Prep:

- Chicken breasts (2)
- Reduced-fat mozzarella cheese (6 tbsp.)
- Seasoned breadcrumbs (6 tbsp.)
- Olive oil/melted butter (1 tbsp.)
- Marinara sauce (.5 cup)
- Grated parmesan cheese (2 tbsp.)
- Cooking spray (as needed)

Method of Prep:
1. Warm the Air Fryer at 360° Fahrenheit for nine minutes. Chop the chicken in half to make four servings.
2. Combine the parmesan and breadcrumbs in one dish. In another dish, melt the butter. Lightly brush the butter over the chicken and dip in the mixture.
3. When the fryer is hot, just add two of the pieces in the basket and spray a layer of oil over the top of the chicken. Cook for six minutes and flip each piece. Chop each piece with 1 tablespoon of sauce and 1.5 tablespoons of the cheese.
4. Cook three more minutes and set aside to prepare the other two.
5. Repeat the process. Serve and enjoy or store for later.

Tips for Meal Prep:
1. Prepare the chicken and let it cool.
2. Store in a wrapper of foil.
3. Serve for one to two days and freeze at that time for the best results.

Snack: Baked Pumpkin Pie Egg Roll

Yields Provided: 4

Ingredients for Prep:

- Pumpkin puree (.75 cup)
- Greek yogurt (.25 cup)
- Pumpkin pie spice (1 tsp.)
- Brown sugar (2 tbsp.)
- Egg roll wrappers (4)
- Cooking spray
- Cinnamon
- Fat-free Cool-Whip

Method of Prep:
1. Set the oven temperature to 350° Fahrenheit.
2. Whisk the pie spice, brown sugar, pumpkin, and yogurt –mixing well.
3. Spread about ¼ cup of the pumpkin mixture in the middle of the wrapper.
4. Fold the bottom corner and run a line of water across the rest of the sides to act as glue. Prepare and close each of the rolls.
5. Arrange the rolls on a greased baking sheet, pizza stone, or parchment-lined pan.
6. Give the tops a spray of the cooking oil and bake until crispy (11 to 13 min.).

Tips for Meal Prep:
1. This super easy recipe is great anytime.

2. Let the cookies cool and store in an airtight cookie jar for later.

Week 2

Day 8

Breakfast: Overnight Oats with Bananas & Walnuts

Yields Provided: 1

Ingredients for Prep:

- Ground cinnamon (.25 tsp.)
- Low-fat or nonfat milk (.5 cup)
- Rolled oats (.5 cup)
- Mashed ripe banana (1)
- Chopped walnuts (2 tbsp.)
- Optional: Sweetener of choice as desired
- Also Needed: 1 mason jar

Method of Prep:
1. Fill the mason jar with the oats, cinnamon, banana, and walnuts.
2. Pour in the milk and place it in the fridge.

Tips for Meal Prep:
1. Let it sit overnight while you sleep or about 8 hours.
2. When serving, add more milk as desired.

Lunch: Heirloom Tomato & Cucumber Toast

Yields Provided: 1

Ingredients for Prep:

- Persian cucumber (1)
- Heirloom tomato (1 small)
- Olive oil (1 tsp.)
- Dried oregano (1 pinch)
- Black pepper and salt (to your liking)

For Serving:
- Low-fat whipped cream cheese (2 tsp.)
- Whole Grain Crispbread or another favorite (2 pieces)
- Balsamic glaze (1 tsp.)

Method of Prep:
1. Dice the cucumber and tomato.
2. Combine all of the fixings except for the cream cheese and glaze.

Tips for Meal Prep:
1. Store the prepared mixture in a closed container until ready to serve.
2. Smear the cheese on the bread, and add the mixture (step 1).
3. Top it off with the balsamic glaze and serve.
4. Note: Increase the ingredient portions to suit your needs.

Dinner: Drumsticks with Apple Glaze

Yields Provided: 4

Ingredients for Prep:

- Apples (2)
- Molasses (.25 cup)
- Ground ginger (.5 tsp.)
- Apple butter (.25 cup)
- Salt (.5 tsp.)
- Freshly cracked black pepper (.25 tsp.)
- Lemon - juiced (half of 1)
- Chicken drumsticks (4 skin-on or skinless)

Method of Prep:
1. Core and slice the apple into 8 pieces. Sprinkle using the lemon juice.
2. Combine all of the components for the marinade. Add the drumsticks to the mixture. Marinate in the fridge for 15 minutes.

3. Warm the oven broiler. Prepare the broiler pan with foil. Arrange the drumsticks in the pan and broil for 12 to 15 minutes. Turn a couple of times and baste with the marinade.
4. Serve with sliced apple wedges.

Tips for Meal Prep:
1. Cool the chicken and add it into freezer bags for storage unless you will be eating it in the next day or two.
2. Wait to slice the apple until serving time.

Snack: Pumpkin Cookies

Yields Provided: 6

Ingredients for Prep:

- Whole wheat flour (2 cups)
- Baking soda (1 tsp.)
- Coconut sugar (1 cup)
- Old-fashioned oats (1 cup)
- Pumpkin pie spice (1 tsp.)
- Egg (1)
- Melted coconut oil (1 cup)
- Pumpkin puree (15 oz.)
- Roasted pumpkin seeds (.5 cup)
- Dried cherries (.5 cup)

Method of Prep:
1. Warm the oven to reach 350° Fahrenheit.
2. Prepare a baking tin with a sheet of aluminum foil.
3. Combine all of the fixings in a mixing container.
4. Mix well and shape into medium cookies.
5. Place each one on the baking tin.
6. Bake for approximately 25 minutes.

Tips for Meal Prep:
1. Move the pan to a cooling rack before storing or serving.
2. Enjoy whenever you want a healthy treat.

Day 9

Breakfast: Pineapple Oatmeal

Yields Provided: 4

Ingredients for Prep:

- Chopped walnuts (1 cup)
- Cubed pineapple (2 cups)
- Old-fashioned oats (2 cups)
- Nonfat milk (2 cups)
- Grated ginger (1 tbsp.)
- Eggs (2)
- Stevia or your favorite sweetener (2 tbsp.)
- Vanilla extract (2 tsp.)
- Also Needed: 4 ramekins

Method of Prep:
1. Set the oven temperature at 400° Fahrenheit.
2. Combine the oats with walnuts, pineapple, and ginger. Stir well and divide into the ramekins.
3. In a mixing container, combine the eggs with the milk, vanilla, and sweetener. Empty the egg mixture over the oats.
4. Arrange the ramekins in the oven and set a timer to bake for about 25 minutes.

Tips for Meal Prep:
1. Serve when ready or cool for storage.
2. Cover the ramekins with plastic wrap or foil and place in the refrigerator until it's mealtime.
3. Remove the wrap. Pop it into the microwave for 30 seconds with a splash of milk if needed. Serve.

Lunch: Baked Sweet Potatoes

Yields Provided: 3

Ingredients for Prep:
- Sliced onion (1)
- Sweet potatoes (3 diced)
- Freshly cracked black pepper & salt (.5 tsp. each)
- Cinnamon (5 tsp.)
- Olive oil (2 tbsp.)

Method of Prep:
1. Warm a skillet on the stovetop and pour in the oil. After it's heated, toss in the sliced onion and sauté for one to two minutes.
2. Set the oven temperature to 355° Fahrenheit.
3. Combine the potatoes with the onion and the remainder of the fixings.
4. Set a timer to bake for 30 to 35 minutes. Serve and enjoy!

Tips for Meal Prep:
1. Cool and store in the fridge for 2-3 days.
2. Warm in a 350° Fahrenheit oven.

Dinner: Lean Cheeseburgers

Yields Provided: 2

Ingredients for Prep:
- Whole-wheat hamburger buns - with seeds (4)
- 95% lean ground beef (1 lb.)
- Quick-cooking oats (2 tbsp.)
- Steak seasoning blend (.5 tsp.)
- Low-fat cheese - ex. cheddar or American (4 slices)
- Optional: Lettuce leaves & tomato slices

Method of Prep:
1. Split the burger buns in half.
2. Dump the oats into a plastic zipper-type baggie and securely seal. Squeeze out all of the excess air and use a rolling pin to crush the oats until they're a fine texture.
3. Mix the oats with the beef and steak seasoning. Shape into four - ½-inch patties.
4. Have the charcoal grill prepared until the coals are ash covered.
5. Place a lid on the grill to cook for 11 to 13 minutes, or you can use the medium heat setting on a gas grill and cook for 7 to 8 minutes. The thermometer inserted horizontally into the center should read 160° Fahrenheit.
6. Prepare the bun with lettuce and tomato if you're using it and top it off with a burger and a slice of cheese.

7. Close the sandwich and serve.

Tips for Meal Prep:
1. Follow all of the steps to step six.
2. Let the burgers cool thoroughly and wrap in plastic wrap. Place in freezer bags for storage.

Snack: Chocolate Pudding

Yields Provided: 4

Ingredients for Prep:
- Nonfat milk (2 cups)
- Salt (.125 tsp.)
- Cornstarch (3 tbsp.)
- Sugar (2 tbsp.)
- Cocoa powder (2 tbsp.)
- Vanilla (.5 tsp.)
- Chocolate chips (.33 cup)

Method of Prep:
1. Whisk the cornstarch, cocoa powder, salt, and sugar together. Stir in the milk.
2. Cook using the medium heat setting until it starts to boil and thicken.
3. Transfer to the countertop. Stir in the vanilla and chocolate chips.
4. Serve and chill until set using a layer of plastic wrap over the top of the bowl.

Tips for Meal Prep:
1. So easy, just prepare and scoop into individual dishes until you are ready to eat them.

Day 10

Breakfast: Cinnamon-Apple French Toast

Yields Provided: 4

Ingredients for Prep:

- Liquid egg whites (1.33 cups)
- 1% milk (1 cup)
- Eggs (4)
- Cinnamon (2 tsp.)
- Apples (2)
- Low-calorie bread (8 slices)
- *Also Needed*: 9x13 casserole dish

Method of Prep:
1. Peel and dice the apples. Grease the baking dish with cooking spray. Prepare the oven temperature to 350° Fahrenheit.
2. Use a microwavable dish to combine and cook the cinnamon and apples for three minutes.
3. Line the baking dish using bread slices and a layer of cooked apples.
4. Whisk the egg whites and milk. Pour over the bread.
5. Bake 45 minutes.

Tips for Meal Prep:
1. Let the mixture thoroughly cool.
2. Use a layer of aluminum foil or plastic wrap to cover the baking dish.
3. Refrigerate overnight.
4. When you're ready to eat, set the oven temperature at 350° Fahrenheit.
5. Discard the cover of the baking dish.
6. Bake until set and lightly browned.
7. Transfer the dish to the stovetop for 10 minutes.
8. Serve with your favorite toppings.

Lunch: Leftover Turkey Noodle Soup

Yields Provided: 4

Ingredients for Prep:
- Turkey stock – low-sodium canned/homemade (6 cups)
- Bay leaf (1)
- Garlic cloves (2)
- Carrot (1 cup)
- Onion (.75 cup)

- Celery (.75 cup)
- Salt (as desired)
- Freshly cracked black pepper
- Fresh parsley (.25 cup)
- No-yolk egg noodles (3 oz.)
- Leftover shredded turkey (8 oz. - 2 cups)

Method of Prep:
1. Fill a large soup pot with the turkey stock.
2. Dice the carrot, garlic, onion, and celery. Mince the garlic.
3. Add the bay leaf, celery, onion, carrots, salt, and black pepper to your liking. Simmer until the vegetables are softened (10-15 min.).
4. Chop and toss in the parsley, shredded turkey, and noodles. Simmer for about five minutes. Discard the bay leaf and serve.

Tips for Meal Prep:
1. Chill the soup and pour it into four individual containers.
2. Serve as needed over the next day or two.

Dinner: Honey Grilled Chicken

Yields Provided: 2

Ingredients for Prep:

- Margarine (2 tbsp.)
- Minced garlic (1 clove)
- Chicken breast (4 halves)
- Honey (.33 cup)
- Lemon (1 juiced)

Method of Prep:
1. Prepare the grill using the medium heat setting.
2. Use the medium heat setting on the stovetop to melt the margarine. Toss in the minced garlic and simmer slowly for two minutes. Whisk the juice and honey and spread half over the breasts.
3. Spritz the grill with oil. Arrange the chicken on the grate. Cook for 5-8 minutes per side. Baste with the rest of the sauce at the end of the cooking cycle.
4. The chicken will be firm with clear juices when poked with a fork.

Tips for Meal Prep:
1. Cool the chicken and place into individual or containers of veggies for a complete meal option.

Snack: Cranberry & Apple Dessert Risotto

Yields Provided: 4

Ingredients for Prep:

- Fat-free milk (3.5 cups)

- Apple (1)
- Dried cranberries (.5 cup)
- Arborio rice (.5 cup)
- Butter (1 tbsp.)
- Apple cider (1.5 cups)
- Salt (1 dash)
- Light brown sugar (2 tbsp.)

Method of Prep:
1. Measure and add the dried cranberries into a bowl of water. Wait for them to plump.
2. Combine the salt, cinnamon, and milk in a saucepan. Once it is hot, transfer the pan to the countertop to steep.
3. Melt the butter in another pan. Add the sliced/diced apple. Stir often until most of the juices are absorbed. Stir in the sugar/milk mixture.
4. Cook until the rice has a creamy texture. Discard the cinnamon stick and drain the cranberries.
5. Stir in the risotto. Serve warm.

Tips for Meal Prep:
1. Cool and scoop into four containers for a quick on the go snack.

Day 11

Breakfast: Oatmeal & Blueberry Muffins

Yields Provided: 12

Ingredients for Prep:

- Unsweetened almond milk (1 cup)
- Canola oil (1 tbsp.)
- Oats (1.5 cups)
- Baking soda (.5 tsp.)
- Salt (.5 tsp.)
- Baking powder (1 tsp.)
- All-purpose flour (.66 cup)

Method of Prep:
1. Use a blender to pulse the oats and soak in the milk for a minimum of 30 minutes.
2. Set the oven temperature to 400° Fahrenheit.
3. Prepare the muffin tins.
4. Whisk the baking soda, salt, baking powder, canola oil, vanilla extract, honey, and applesauce. Mix well.
5. Fold in the brown sugar, soaked oats, and flour. Mix and divide into the prepared tins.
6. Bake about 24 minutes until the tops are nicely browned.

Tips for Meal Prep:
1. Take the muffin tin out of the oven.
2. Set out on the countertop.
3. Once cooled, store them in a plastic bag, seal at room temperature for up to three days.

Lunch: *Ravioli Lasagna*

Yields Provided: 6-8

Ingredients for Prep:
- Frozen ravioli (1 lb.)
- Pasta sauce (24 oz.)
- Frozen chopped spinach (8 oz. pkg.)
- Fat-free ricotta (15 oz.)
- Minced garlic (1 tsp.)
- Mozzarella (2 cups - shredded)
- Also Needed: 9x13 pan

Method of Prep:
1. Break up the frozen spinach into a small bowl and mix in the garlic and ricotta.
2. Pour a thin layer of sauce over the bottom part of the pan.
3. Lay down the first layer of ravioli, top with half the spinach mixture, 1/3 of the red sauce, then ½ cup of mozzarella. Repeat this layer again.
4. Top with remaining ravioli, red sauce, and mozzarella.

Tips for Meal Prep:
1. Eat it Now or Prep to Freeze: Set the oven at 375° Fahrenheit. Place a layer of foil over the pan and bake for 30 minutes. Discard the layer of foil and continue baking an additional ten minutes until golden and bubbly. Serve.
2. Cool thoroughly and cover with plastic wrap, pressing down to remove as much air as possible, then cover with foil. Label with the date and contents before freezing.
3. Baking from Frozen: Remove the plastic and foil, and cover again with foil. Warm the oven to 375° Fahrenheit. Set a timer and bake for one hour. Remove the foil and bake for ten minutes more minutes until golden, bubbly and all the pasta is cooked through.

Dinner: Ground Pork Loaf

Yields Provided: 4

Ingredients for Prep:
- Red onions (1 small)
- Garlic (2 cloves)
- Olive oil (1 tbsp.)
- Lemon - juiced and zested (1)
- Cherry tomatoes (1-pint)
- Black pepper (as desired)
- Basil (1 tbsp.)
- Low-sodium tomato paste (2 tbsp.)
- Low-sodium vegetable stock (.5 cup)

Method of Prep:
1. Pour the water into a skillet and let it heat up.

2. Mince the garlic. Chop the onions, tomatoes, and basil. When hot, toss in the onion and garlic. Cook slowly for about five minutes.
3. Stir in the tomatoes, stock, lemon juice and zest, tomato paste, black pepper, and the pork. Stir well and cook for 15 minutes.
4. Garnish with the basil and serve when ready.

Tips for Meal Prep:
1. Allow the meat to totally cool.
2. Portion into the chosen freezer container.
3. Defrost and use it as needed.

Snack: Applesauce

Yields Provided: 3-4

Ingredients for Prep:

- Granny Smith apples (1 lb.)
- Water (1 cup)
- Lemon juice (1 tbsp.)
- Sugar (.5 cup)

Method of Prep:
1. Peel, core, and chop the apples.
2. Fill a large pot of water using just enough to cover the apples.
3. Simmer the apples until softened or for about 20 minutes. Add them to a blender or food processor.
4. Pour in the lemon juice and sugar. Pulse until well combined.

5. Add the mixture back into the pot and simmer 4-5 additional minutes.

Tips for Meal Prep:
1. Cool thoroughly and scoop into individual bowls for a quick and healthy on-the-go snack.

Day 12

Breakfast: Cantaloupe Blueberry Breakfast Bowl

Yields Provided: 2

Ingredients for Prep:

- Whole cantaloupe (1)
- Blueberries (1 cup)
- Cottage cheese (1.5 cups)
- Chopped pecans (.25 cup)
- Hemp seeds (2 tbsp.)

Method of Prep:
1. Wash and pat dry the cantaloupe; slice in half.
2. Chop the pecans and add with the hemp seeds in a small container.
3. Store the cantaloupe with a layer of plastic wrap.

Tips for Meal Prep:
1. Time to Serve: Scoop a ¾ cup serving of the cottage cheese into each half.
2. Garnish both portions with the pecans/seed mix and blueberries.
3. Serve and enjoy it immediately.

Lunch: Pizza Logs

Yields Provided: 8

Ingredients for Prep:
- Egg roll wrappers (8)
- Pizza sauce - your healthy option (8 tsp.)
- Italian seasoning (1 tsp.)
- Light mozzarella string cheese sticks (4 - cut into halves)
- Turkey-pepperoni slices (24)

Method of Prep:
1. Warm the oven to reach 425° Fahrenheit.
2. Lightly mist a large baking tray using a spritz of cooking oil spray and set aside.
3. Prepare a dish of water as a fingertip dish.
4. Arrange each egg roll wrapper on a flat surface with the corner facing toward you.
5. Spread 1 tsp. of sauce across the center of the wrapper, leaving 0.5-inch on each side.
6. Sprinkle Italian seasoning, a row of 3 pepperoni slices, and half of a cheese stick.
7. Fold the bottom corner over the fixings and roll. Fold the side corners in and tuck them as you give the filled section another roll.
8. Dampen the edges of the remaining corner of the wrapper. Finish rolling the filled log to close and place on the baking tray.
9. Arrange the wrapped log on the baking sheet. Continue with the remainder of the fixings.
10. Once they're all wrapped and ready on the baking tray, lightly spritz the tops using a portion of cooking oil spray.

11. Bake for 10 to 14 minutes. Flip them over about halfway through the cooking process.

Tips for Meal Prep:
1. Cool and keep in the refrigerator for a few days for the most flavorful results (if they last that long).

Dinner: Lemon Chicken

Yields Provided: 2

Ingredients for Prep:

- Lemon (1)
- Breasts of chicken (2)
- Oregano (1 pinch)
- Olive oil (1 tbsp.)
- Salt & Pepper (to your liking)

Method of Prep:
1. Discard the bones and skin from the chicken. Squeeze juice from the lemons over the chicken.
2. Sprinkle using pepper and salt.
3. Use medium heat to warm up the oil in a skillet on the stovetop. Cook the chicken. As it is cooking, sprinkle with oregano and additional pepper or salt as desired.
4. Poke it with a fork. It's done when the juices in the center of the chicken run clear.

Tips for Meal Prep:
1. Portion into freezer bags and defrost as a quick base for dinner.

Snack: Lemony Banana Mix

Yields Provided: 4

Ingredients for Prep:
- Strawberries (5)
- Banana (4)
- Lemons (2)
- Coconut sugar (4 tbsp.)

Method of Prep:
1. Juice the lemons and slice the strawberries into halves. Peel and chop the bananas.
2. In a mixing bowl, combine all of the fixings.
3. Toss well and serve cold.

Tips for Meal Prep:
1. Serve over the next couple of days.
2. Store in a covered container or individual dishes.

Day 13

Breakfast: Cherries & Oats

Yields Provided: 6

Ingredients for Prep:

- Water (6 cups)
- Almond milk (1 cup)
- Cinnamon (1 tsp.)
- Old-fashioned oats (2 cups)
- Vanilla extract (1 tsp.)
- Cherries (2 cups)

Method of Prep:
1. Remove the pits and slice the cherries.
2. Combine all of the fixings in a small pot.
3. Bring the pot to a boil using the medium- high heat setting.
4. Cook the mixture for 15 minutes and divide it into serving containers or in one dish.

Tips for Meal Prep:
1. Wait for the oatmeal cool to touch (about one hour).
2. Cover tightly and place in the fridge.

3. If using individual jars for oatmeal storage, microwave for two to three minutes until hot.

Lunch: Turkey & Pear Pita Melt

Yields Provided: 1

Ingredients for Prep:

- Sliced pear (1)
- Deli turkey – low-sodium (3.5 oz.)
- Mixed greens (1 cup)
- Shredded cheddar cheese (1 tbsp.)
- Large whole wheat pita (half of 1)

Method of Prep:
1. Slice the pear and rinse the greens.
2. Stuff the pita with the turkey, cheese, and pears.
3. Place in a toaster oven if you have one, or use the main oven.
4. When warm, add the greens to the hot pita and enjoy the remainder of the pear slices on the side of the dish.

Tips for Meal Prep:
1. Prepare the pita, but don't toast it until it is time to eat.
2. Store in the fridge until mealtime.

Dinner: Pork Chops & Apples

Yields Provided: 4

Ingredients for Prep:
- Low-sodium chicken stock (1.5 cups)
- Pork chops (4)
- Black pepper (as desired)
- Yellow chopped onion (1)
- Minced garlic cloves (2)
- Chopped thyme (1 tbsp.)
- Cored & sliced apples (3)
- Olive oil (1 tbsp.)

Method of Prep:
1. Heat the oven until it reaches 350° Fahrenheit.
2. Pour the oil into a pan. Set the temperature on medium-high.
3. When hot, add the pork chops and sprinkle with the pepper.
4. Cook for five minutes per side.
5. Add the garlic, onion, lime, apples, and the stock.
6. Toss well and add the mixture to a baking dish. Set a timer and bake for 50 minutes.
7. Serve when ready.

Tips for Meal Prep:
1. Prepare the dish until ready. Set aside to thoroughly cool.
2. Store in a sectional container or individual container and pop into the freezer.

Snack: Delicious Apple Pie

Yields Provided: 8

Ingredients for Prep:

For the Crust:
- Dry rolled oats (1 cup)
- Ground almonds (.25 cup)
- Whole wheat pastry flour (.25 cup)
- Packed brown sugar (2 tbsp.)
- Water (1 tbsp.)
- Canola oil (3 tbsp.)

For the Filling:
- Frozen apple juice concentrate (.33 cup)
- Tart apples (6 cups or 4 large)
- Cinnamon (1 tsp.)
- Quick-cooking tapioca (2 tbsp.)

Method of Prep:
1. Heat the oven to reach 425° Fahrenheit.
2. Prepare the Pie Crust: Combine the dry fixings in one mixing bowl and the dry in another. Combine the two until a dough is formed. Blend together until the dough sticks together. You may need more or less water.
3. Press the dough into a nine-inch pie plate. Set aside.
4. Prepare the Filling: Peel and slice the apples. Mix all of the fixings. Let it stand for about 15 minutes. Stir and place into the pie crust.

5. Bake for 15 minutes at 425° Fahrenheit, reducing the heat for the last 40 minutes at 350° Fahrenheit.

Tips for Meal Prep:
1. You have about two days to enjoy your pies unchilled at room temperature.
2. If the pie has been sliced, place them into a container and loosely cover loosely using plastic wrap. The pie will keep for another two to three days in the fridge.

Day 14

Breakfast: Tropical Breakfast Pie

Yields Provided: 4

Ingredients for Prep:

- Granulated sugar (.5 tsp.)
- Unsweetened shredded coconut (2 tbsp.)
- Refrigerated biscuit dough (7.5 oz.)
- Fresh pineapple (1 cup)
- *Also Needed*: 8-inch-square casserole dish

Method of Prep:
1. Warm up the oven in advance to 350° Fahrenheit.
2. Lightly coat the casserole dish with a splash of cooking spray. Break apart the dough into ten portions and slice into quarters.
3. Load a zipper-type bag with the sugar and coconut. Shake and add the dough bits. Shake gently, but thoroughly to coat.
4. Place the biscuits into the dish and garnish with the diced pineapple.
5. Bake for 25 minutes.

Tips for Meal Prep:
1. Transfer to the counter to cool before placing it in the refrigerator.

2. Serve yourself whenever you need a quick and healthy breakfast dish.

Lunch: Baked Macaroni with Red Sauce

Yields Provided: 6

Ingredients for Prep:
- Diced onion (.5 cup)
- Whole-wheat elbow macaroni (7 oz.)
- Spaghetti sauce - reduced-sodium or homemade (15 oz.)
- Extra-lean beef (.5 lb.)
- Parmesan cheese (6 tbsp.)

Method of Prep:
1. Set the oven to 350° Fahrenheit. Spritz a casserole baking dish with cooking oil spray.
2. Sauté the onions and beef in a frying pan until the onion is fragrant. Drain the grease out of the pan.
3. Fill a pot with water and prepare the pasta until tender or about 10 to 12 minutes. Empty the mixture into a mesh colander to drain.
4. Combine the pasta with the meat and add the sauce. Stir and scoop into the prepared dish. Bake for 25 to 35 minutes.
5. Serve and enjoy each serving with 1 tablespoon of the cheese.

Tips for Meal Prep:
1. Properly stored in closed containers, homemade pasta, and the sauce will last for 2 to 3 days in the fridge.
2. Freeze it in heavy-duty freezer bags.

Dinner: BARBECUE Ranch Chicken Bites

Yields Provided: 4-6

Ingredients for Prep:

- Ranch dressing (.66 cup)
- BARBECUE sauce (.33 cup)
- Chicken breasts (2 lb.)
- Optional: Finely chopped fresh chives (1 tbsp.)
- Skewers (10 - 9 to 12-inch)

Method of Prep:
1. If you are using wooden skewers, soak in water for at least 15 minutes. Prepare a rimmed baking sheet using a sheet of foil and spritz with a misting of cooking spray.
2. Pour the ranch dressing and BARBECUE sauce in a large mixing bowl. Stir to combine. Transfer half to a small serving bowl, cover, and refrigerate. Remove the skin and bones from the chicken, cut it into 1-inch chunks, and add it to the remaining sauce. Toss to combine.
3. Marinate for about half an hour on the countertop or cover and refrigerate for up to 24 hours. (The ideal time is about 2 hours. At 24 hours, the chicken is very tender but starts to break down slightly.)
4. When ready to cook, arrange a rack 4 to 5 inches from the heating element and warm the oven to broil.
5. Thread the chicken onto the skewers, 6 to 7 pieces per skewer. Place the skewers (not touching) on the baking sheet. Broil until charred in spots and

cooked through, or about 8 minutes. Top with chives, if using, and serve with the reserved sauce for dipping.

Tips for Meal Prep:
1. After the chicken is prepared, either store in the fridge for 3-4 days or put into individual freezer bags until needed.

Snack: Wacky Chocolate Cake

Yields Provided: 6

Ingredients for Prep:
- Whole wheat pastry flour (3 cups)
- Unsweetened cocoa powder (3 tbsp.)
- Sugar (1 cup)
- Salt (.5 tsp)
- Baking soda (2.25 tsp.)
- Vinegar (2 tbsp.)
- Vanilla (1 tbsp.)
- Hot water (2 cups)
- Canola oil (.5 cup)

Method of Prep:
1. Warm up the oven to reach 350° Fahrenheit.
2. Likely spritz a baking dish with cooking oil spray.
3. Whisk the baking soda, salt, sugar, and cocoa powder.
4. Stir in the oil, vinegar, and vanilla.

5. Slowly pour in the water as you whisk the mixture for about 2 minutes.
6. Dump the batter into the baking dish and set a timer to bake for 30 minutes.
7. When cool, slice into 18 squares and serve.

Tips for Meal Prep:
1. Cool the cake and store it in a closed container.
2. It should be good for three days.

Chapter 6: Delicious Snacks Dips & Spreads

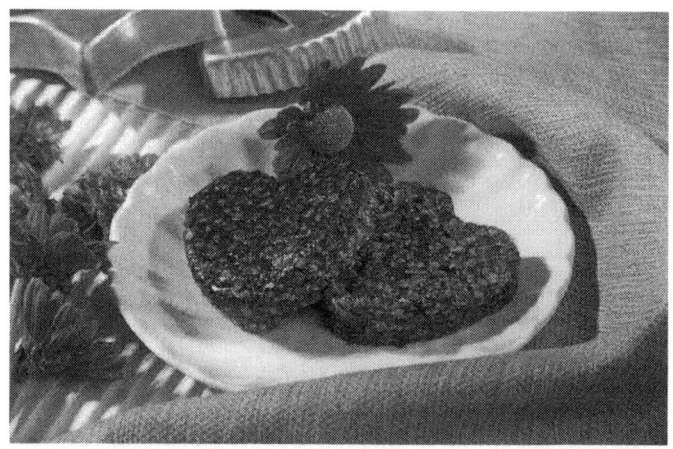

Black Bean Brownies – Vegan

Yields Provided: 12

Ingredients for Prep:
- Black beans (1.5 cups)
- Unsweetened applesauce (.25 cup)
- Blackstrap molasses (.25 cup)
- All-purpose flour (.25 cup)
- Unsweetened cocoa powder (.33 cup)
- Salt (.5 tsp.)
- Baking powder (.5 tsp.)
- *Also Needed*:
- 8x8 casserole dish
- Cooking spray
- Food processor or blender

Method of Prep:
1. Set the oven in advance to 375° Fahrenheit. Spray the dish with the spray.
2. Drain and rinse the beans and add them to the blender. Pulse until fairly smooth. Dump into a container with the molasses and applesauce. Stir.
3. Sift in the salt, flour, cocoa powder, and baking powder. Mix well.
4. Pour into the prepared dish and bake 35 minutes.
5. Perform the toothpick test for doneness. If it's clean when inserted into the center of the brownies, it's done.

Tips for Meal Prep:
1. Let the brownies cool after they are done.
2. Make a double batch; store one and freeze one!

Breakfast Cookies

Yields Provided: 12 Cookies

Ingredients for Prep:

- Rolled oats (2 cups)
- Large bananas (2 mashed)
- Chocolate chips (.75 cup)

Method of Prep:
1. Warm the oven to 350° Fahrenheit.
2. Stir the oats and bananas until they are thoroughly combined.

3. Stir in chocolate chips.
4. Roll the cookies into 2-inch balls, and then flatten to make the cookie shape.
5. Bake on a parchment paper-lined cookie sheet for 12 minutes.

Tips for Meal Prep:
1. Cool thoroughly and store in closed containers until ready to eat.

Chocolate Biscotti

Yields Provided: 15

Ingredients for Prep:
- Large egg (1)
- Monk fruit sweetener or erythritol (.25 cup)
- Stevia concentrated powder (.25 tsp.)
- Softened butter (.25 cup)
- Vanilla extract (.5 tsp.)
- Almond flour (1.75 cups)
- Xanthan gum (.25 tsp.)
- Unsweetened cocoa (.5 cup)
- Baking soda (.5 tsp.)
- Sea salt (.25 tsp.)
- Cinnamon (1 tsp.)
- *Optional:* Sugar-free chocolate chips
- *Optional:* Chopped nuts

Method of Prep:

1. Set the oven to reach 325° Fahrenheit.
2. Mix the butter with the egg, stevia, granular sweetener, and vanilla.
3. In another container, sift or whisk all the dry fixings and mix until well incorporated.
4. Combine the wet and dry fixings, stirring as you go. Chocolate chips or nuts can be mixed in at this time.
5. Prepare the ball of dough. Arrange the dough ball on a layer of parchment baking paper, silicone baking mat or cookie sheet. Shape the dough into a long flat log.
6. Bake for approximately 18 to 20 minutes. Transfer from the oven and lower the heat setting to 275° Fahrenheit. Cool for about 10 minutes. Slice into thin strips about .5-inch wide.

Orange Cream Cheese Cookies & Nuts

Yields Provided: 18

Ingredients for Prep:

- Softened butter (.75 cup)
- Eggs (3)
- Coconut flour (.5 cup)
- Baking powder (1.5 tsp.)
- Monk fruit sweetener (.75 cup)
- Baking soda (.25 tsp.)
- Sugar-free dried cranberries (.25 cup)
- Macadamia nuts chopped (.5 cup)
- Dried grated orange zest (1.5 tsp.)

Method of Prep:
1. In a mixing container, beat the sweetener with the eggs and butter until well combined.
2. Whisk or sift the coconut flour, baking powder, and soda. Beat on the low setting or with a spoon until fully mixed.
3. Fold in the berries, orange zest, and nuts.
4. Shape into rounds and arrange on the cookie sheet.
5. Arrange the cookies a minimum of one inch apart for baking on a parchment-lined cookie sheet. Press each mound down slightly to flatten.
6. Bake at 350° Fahrenheit until edges have started to brown or for eight to ten minutes.

Tips for Meal Prep:
1. Cool on a cooling rack.
2. Enjoy right out of the fridge for a week, or they can be frozen for longer storage.

Peanut Butter Bites

Yields Provided: 2 bites

Ingredients for Prep:
- Rolled oats (1.5 cups)
- Natural peanut butter - for nut-free use sunflower seed butter (.5 cup)
- Honey or maple syrup (3 tbsp.)

Method of Prep:
1. Add the oats to a food processor or blender. Blend until oats reach a flour consistency.

2. Next, add the peanut butter and honey or maple syrup. Process until the fixings are well combined and come together to form a dough ball. You may need to scrape the sides once or twice.
3. Roll into round bites – about a scant tablespoon per bite. If the dough isn't holding together, add one to two tablespoons more of the peanut butter.
4. If the dough starts to stick to your hands, oil them with coconut oil or cooking spray.

Tips for Meal Prep:
1. Store the *Peanut Butter Bites* in an airtight container in the fridge for up to 2 WEeks.

Tag-along Cookies Copycat Girl Scout™ *Cookies*

Yields Provided: 12

Ingredients for Prep:

- Vanilla wafer cookies (12)
- Chocolate chips (.5 cup)
- Creamy peanut butter (3 tbsp.)
- Coconut oil (.25 tsp.)

Method of Prep:
1. Spread the peanut butter on the wafers and place them on a parchment paper-lined cookie tin.
2. Place the chocolate chips in the microwave at 15-second intervals until melted. Add a splash of coconut oil to make the chips smoother.
3. Dip the wafers into the chocolate to cover and place it on the paper-lined pan.

Tips for Meal Prep:
1. Cool thoroughly and place it in the fridge to set.
2. Cover and eat as desired.

3 Ingredient Reese's Fudge

Yields Provided: 24

Ingredients for Prep:
- Vanilla frosting - not fluffy (1 container)
- Mini Reese's Pieces (10 oz. bag)
- Peanut butter cups (10 oz.)

Method of Prep:
1. Discard the foil wrapper from the frosting and microwave the container for 30 seconds.
2. Add the peanut butter chips in another container and microwave for one minute.
3. Stir it all together and toss in about ¾ of the bag into the mixture.
4. Grease the baking tin and add the fudge.

Tips for Meal Prep:
1. Before slicing into squares for storage, be sure it is thoroughly cooled (about 30 minutes).

Movie Night Popcorn Galore

These are a sure way to enjoy movies on a budget! Just choose the desired flavors.

Prepare the popcorn in advance and combine the chosen topping from these:

Birthday Cake Popcorn

Yields Provided: 4

Ingredients for Prep:
- Melted white chocolate chips (1 cup)
- Biscoff spread (1 tbsp.)
- Betty Crocker ™ candy sprinkles (2 tbsp.)
- Popcorn (8 cups)

Method of Prep:
1. Melt the chocolate chips and mix in the Bischoff spread.
2. Drizzle over the prepared popcorn and top with the sprinkles.
3. Cool before serving.

Caramel Apple Popcorn

Yields Provided: 10

Ingredients for Prep:

- Popped popcorn (12 cups)
- Brown sugar (1 cup)
- Light corn syrup (.25 cup)
- Salt (.5 tsp.)
- Baking soda (.5 tsp.)
- Vanilla (1 tsp.)
- Cinnamon chips (1 cup)
- Toffee bit (1 cup)
- Whole pecans (1 cup)
- Dried apple chips (1 cup)
- Butter (1 tbsp.)

Method of Prep:

1. Place the brown sugar, light corn syrup, salt, and butter in a microwave-safe bowl.
2. Microwave for about 1 minute, just until the butter is melted, then stir together until well mixed.
3. Return to the microwave and cook for 2 minutes, stir, then cook for an additional 2 minutes.
4. Add the baking soda and vanilla to the caramel. Stir until well mixed.
5. Place your popped popcorn in a large bowl and drizzle the caramel over the popcorn.
6. Sprinkle the cinnamon chips, toffee bits, pecans, and dried apple chips over the popcorn. Toss lightly. Allow cooling before serving.

Chocolate Coffee Peanut Butter Pretzel Popcorn

Yields Provided: 4

Ingredients for Prep:

- Popcorn (8 cups)
- Instant coffee grounds (.5 tbsp.)
- Crushed peanut butter pretzels (.5 cup)
- Chocolate bars - melted (2 bars/4 oz.) or Dark chocolate chips (1.5 cups)

Method of Prep:
1. Melt the chocolate and stir in the grounds of coffee.
2. Drizzle and toss over the popcorn with the pretzels.
3. Let the chocolate harden (room temp) before serving.

Cool Ranch Popcorn

Yields Provided: 4

Ingredients for Prep:
- Melted butter (.25 cup)
- White cheddar mac & cheese powder (2 tbsp.)
- Dry ranch dressing mix (2 tbsp.)
- Smoked paprika (.5 tsp.)
- Popcorn (8 cups)

Method of Prep:
1. Drizzle the prepared butter over the popcorn.
2. Whisk and sprinkle with the spice combo (paprika, cheddar & ranch powder).
3. Toss gently and serve.

Sriracha Popcorn

Yields Provided: 4

Ingredients for Prep:
- Melted butter (.25 cup)
- Sriracha (2 tbsp.)
- Garlic (1 clove)
- Popcorn (8 cups)

Method of Prep:
1. Mince the garlic and melt the butter.
2. Whisk the garlic, Sriracha, and butter to pour over the popcorn.
3. Enjoy immediately.

Dips & Spreads

Baked Potato Dip

Yields Provided: 8

Ingredients for Prep:
- Crispy crumbled turkey bacon (2 strips)
- Chives (1 tbsp.)
- Shredded 2% cheddar sharp cheese (.33 cup)
- Onion powder (.125 tsp.)
- Black pepper (.125 tsp.)
- Garlic powder (.125 tsp.)
- Salt (.125 tsp.)
- Fat-free sour cream (1 cup)

Method of Prep:
1. Brown the bacon until it's crispy and combine with the rest of the fixings.
2. Cool in the refrigerator for a minimum of one hour.

Tips for Meal Prep:
1. Be sure to let the dip cool completely.
2. Store in the refrigerator.
3. Serve with a tray of tasty veggies.

Italian Basil Pesto – Vegan

Yields Provided: 8 Servings - 2 tbsp. each

Ingredients for Prep:

- Tightly packed basil leaves (1 cup)
- Garlic cloves (2 large)
- Lemon juice (1 tbsp.)
- Lemon zest (1 tsp.)
- Toasted pine nuts (2 tbsp.)
- Olive oil (1 tbsp.)
- Water (.25 cup)
- Sea salt and freshly cracked pepper (to your liking)
- *Also Needed*: Food processor

Method of Prep:
1. Toss the pine nuts, lemon juice and zest, basil, and garlic into the processor. Blend until smooth, yet fairly chunky.
2. Pour in the oil and water to process until almost smooth.
3. Remove and place in a serving dish with a sprinkle of salt and pepper to your liking.
4. Stir and let the flavors blend for about ½ hour before serving.

Tips for Meal Prep:
1. Prepare the pesto as described.

2. Pour the mixture into a mason jar and serve any time.

Jalapeno - Bacon & Corn-Cheese Dip

Yields Provided: 3

Ingredients for Prep:
- Parmesan cheese (.25 cup)
- Shredded cheddar cheese (2 cups)
- Softened cream cheese (8 oz.)
- Drained corn (2 cans - 15 oz. each or as desired)
- Diced jalapenos (.25 cup)
- Bacon strips (8 cooked and crumbled)

Method of Prep:
1. Set the oven temperature to 400° Fahrenheit.
2. Prepare a cast iron skillet with a portion of cooking spray.
3. Combine all of the fixings, mixing well, and add to the pan.
4. Bake 20 minutes and serve.

Tips for Meal Prep:
1. Prepare the mixture for the dip and let it cool.
2. Store in the fridge in an airtight dish.
3. Serve as a delicious snack.

Pea Guacamole with Tortilla Chips

Yields Provided: 1

Ingredients for Prep:

- Avocado (¼ of 1 medium)
- Frozen green peas (.25 cup - thawed)
- Fresh lime juice (2 tsp.)
- Chopped uncooked red onion (2 tsp.)
- Cilantro (1 tbsp. - chopped)
- Table salt (.125 tsp.)
- Fresh tomatoes (1 tbsp. - chopped)
- Chips (7)

Method of Prep:

1. Use a blender or mini food processor to puree the lime juice with the peas and avocado.
2. Once it's smooth, stir in the onion, salt, and cilantro.

Tips for Meal Prep:

1. Store in the fridge until needed.
2. Serve with a portion of cilantro, onion, and tomato. Serve with a side of chips.

Spiced Smoky Red Pepper Dip

Yields Provided: 8 Servings /.25 cup each

Ingredients for Prep:
- Roasted red peppers - packed in water (32 oz.)
- Walnut oil (2.5 tsp.)
- Smoked variety paprika (1.25 tsp.)
- Finely chopped garlic (1 medium clove)
- Ground cumin (.5 tsp.)
- Table salt (.25 tsp.)
- Fresh oregano or chopped parsley (1 tbsp.)

Method of Prep:
1. Rinse and drain the peppers.
2. Puree all of the fixings, except for the oregano or parsley, in a blender or food processor.

Tips for Meal Prep:
1. Store in a glass container until time to serve.
2. Garnish with fresh herbs and serve.

Conclusion

I hope you have enjoyed your new collection of recipes in the *Meal Prep Cookbook for Beginners*. I hope it was informative and provided you with all of the tools you need to achieve your goals, whatever they may be.

The next step is to prepare a list of the cooking equipment and ingredients you will need to get started using your new techniques for meal prep. The suggestions provided were tested by the pros and are some of the easiest ones you will discover if you search the Internet. The guesswork is removed with the detailed instructions.

Index of Recipes

Chapter 3: Simple Meal Prep Week 1:

Day 1:

Breakfast: Avocado & Egg Breakfast Lunch: Beef Soup

Dinner: Mediterranean Whitefish Snack: Avocado Hummus Snack Jars

Day 2:

Breakfast: Broccoli Cheddar Egg Muffins Lunch: Apples with Almonds & Figs Salad Dinner: Pork Chops with Creamy Sauce Snack: Bacon Cheddar Cheese Crisps

Day 3:

Breakfast: Gluten-Free Roasted Grapes & Greek Yogurt Parfait Lunch: Tomato & Olive Salad

Dinner: Chicken and Asparagus Pan Dinner Snack: Bacon Knots

Day 4:

Breakfast: Spinach Muffins Lunch: Arugula Salad

Dinner: Jalapeno Popper Burgers Snack: Peanut Butter Power Granola

Day 5:

Breakfast: Greek Yogurt Pancakes Lunch: Tomato Soup

Dinner: Turkey Sloppy Joes Snack: Fried Queso Fresco

Day 6:

Breakfast: Omelet Waffles

Lunch: Chicken-Apple-Spinach Salad Dinner: Apricot BARBECUE Chicken Snack: Veggie Egg Cups

Day 7:

Breakfast: Banana Oat Pancakes Lunch: Ham Salad

Dinner: Baked Chicken Fajita Snack: Mini Crustless Quiche

Week 2:

Day 8:

Breakfast: Veggie Egg Scramble Lunch: Asparagus Soup Dinner: Asian Glazed Chicken Snack: Veggie Snack Pack

Day 9:

Breakfast: Spinach - Feta & Egg Breakfast Quesadillas Lunch: Salmon Vegetable Frittata

Dinner: Thai Peanut Chicken Snack: Beef & Cheddar Roll-Ups

Day 10:

Breakfast: Breakfast Bowls Lunch: Chili Con Carne Dinner: Cajun Chicken Snack: Fruit Snack Pack

Day 11:

Breakfast: Carrot Muffins Lunch: Classic Stuffed Peppers Dinner: Cilantro Lime Chicken

Snack: Avocado Hummus Snack Jars

Day 12:

Breakfast: Buckwheat Pancakes Lunch: One-Tray Caprese Pasta Dinner: Shrimp Taco Bowls

Snack: Vanilla Cashew Butter Cups

Day 13:

Breakfast: Corn & Apple Muffins Lunch: Smoked Sausage & Orzo Dinner: Chicken & Broccoli Snack: Protein Sack Pack

Day 14:

Breakfast: Veggies & Eggs

Lunch: Starbucks™ Protein Bistro Box

Dinner: Sweet & Sour Meatballs

Snack: Ham – Swiss & Spinach Roll-Ups

Chapter 4: Keto Diet

Week 1:

Day 1:

Breakfast: Almost McGriddle Casserole Lunch: Caesar Salmon Salad

Dinner: Chipotle Roast

Snack: Peanut Butter Protein Bars

Day 2:

Breakfast: Jalapeno Cheddar Waffles Lunch: Chicken 'Zoodle' Soup Dinner: Chicken Nuggets

Snack: Blueberry Cream Cheese Fat Bombs

Day 3:

Breakfast: Baked Green Eggs

Lunch: Mushroom & Cauliflower Risotto Dinner: Chili Lime Cod

Snack: Coffee Fat Bombs

Day 4:

Breakfast: Vegan Gingerbread Muffins Lunch: Spicy Beef Wraps

Dinner: Asparagus & Chicken Snack: Mocha Cheesecake Bars

Day 5:

Breakfast: Egg Loaf

Lunch: BARBECUE Pork Loin Dinner: Short Ribs

Snack: Delicious No-Bake Coconut Cookies

Day 6:

Breakfast: Spinach Quiche Lunch: BLT Salad in a Jar Dinner: Buffalo Chicken Burgers

Snack: Spice Cakes

Day 7:

Breakfast: Morning Hot Pockets Lunch: Greek Salad

Dinner: Buffalo Sloppy Joes Snack: Brownie Muffins

Week 2:

Day 8:

Breakfast: Avocado Eggs Lunch: Tuna Salad

Dinner: Bacon & Shrimp Risotto Snack: Pumpkin Pie Cupcakes

Day 9:

Breakfast: Tomato & Cheese Frittata Lunch: Beef & Pepperoni Pizza Dinner: Chicken & Green Beans Snack: Amaretti Cookies

Day 10:

Breakfast: Blueberry Pancake Bites Lunch: Buffalo Chicken Burgers Dinner: Roasted Leg of Lamb

Day 11:

Breakfast: Blueberry Essence Lunch: Italian Tomato Salad Dinner: Bacon Cheeseburger

Snack: Strawberry Cream Cheese Bites

Day 12:

Breakfast: Pancakes & Nuts Lunch: Pulled Pork for Sandwiches

Dinner: Shrimp Alfredo Snack: Coconut Macaroons

Day 13:

Breakfast: Cinnamon Smoothie Lunch: Pita Pizza

Dinner: Roasted Chicken & Tomatoes Snack: Pecan Turtle Truffles

Day 14:

Breakfast: Bacon Cheese & Egg Cups Lunch: Caprese Salad

Dinner: Enchilada Skillet Dinner

Chapter 5: Meal Prep Recipes for Kids
Week 1:

Day 1:

Breakfast: Apple Banana Muffins Lunch: Cranberry Tuna Salad Dinner: Hawaiian Chicken Kebabs Snack: Apple Pie Cookies

Day 2:

Breakfast: Mango Smoothie Base & Oats Lunch: Buffalo Chicken Tenders Dinner: Chili & Mac 'n' Cheese

Snack: Pumpkin Cupcakes

Day 3:

Breakfast: Banana Almond Pancakes Lunch: Colored Iceberg Salad Dinner: Delicious Meatloaf

Snack: Whole Grain Banana Bread

Day 4:

Breakfast: Mango Smoothie Base & Greens Lunch: Tuna Melt

Dinner: Loaded Bacon Mac & Cheese Snack: Banana Oatmeal Cookies

Day 5:

Breakfast: 2-Ingredient Pancakes Lunch: Pear & Banana Breakfast Salad Dinner: Chicken Fried Rice

Snack: Apples & Dip

Day 6:

Breakfast: Mango Smoothie Base & Tofu Lunch: Chicken Salad

Dinner: Cheesy Beef Egg Rolls Snack: Banana Roll-Ups

Day 7:

Breakfast: Berry Monkey Bread Cinnamon Rolls Lunch: Strawberry Sandwiches

Dinner: Air-Fried Parmesan Chicken Snack: Baked Pumpkin Pie Egg Roll

Week 2: Meal Prep Recipes for Kids

Day 8:

Breakfast: Overnight Oats with Bananas & Walnuts Lunch: Heirloom Tomato & Cucumber Toast Dinner: Drumsticks with Apple Glaze

Snack: Pumpkin Cookies

Day 9:

Breakfast: Pineapple Oatmeal

Lunch: Baked Sweet Potatoes

Dinner: Lean Cheeseburgers

Snack: Chocolate Pudding

Day 10:

Breakfast: Cinnamon-Apple French Toast

Lunch: Leftover Turkey Noodle Soup

Dinner: Honey Grilled Chicken

Snack: Cranberry & Apple Dessert Risotto

Day 11:

Breakfast: Oatmeal & Blueberry Muffins Lunch: Ravioli Lasagna

Dinner: Ground Pork Loaf Snack: Applesauce

Day 12:

Breakfast: Cantaloupe Blueberry Breakfast Bowl Lunch: Pizza Logs

Dinner: Lemon Chicken Snack: Lemony Banana Mix

Day 13:

Breakfast: Cherries & Oats Lunch: Turkey & Pear Pita Melt Dinner: Pork Chops & Apples Snack: Delicious Apple Pie

Day 14:

Breakfast: Tropical Breakfast Pie Lunch: Baked Macaroni with Red Sauce

Dinner: BARBECUE Ranch Chicken Bites Snack: Wacky Chocolate Cake

Chapter 6 Delicious Snacks – Dips & Spreads

- Black Bean Brownies – Vegan
- Breakfast Cookies
- Chocolate Biscotti
- Orange Cream Cheese Cookies & Nuts
- Peanut Butter Bites
- Tagalong Cookies Copycat Girl Scout ™Cookies
- 3 Ingredient Reese's Fudge

Movie Night Popcorn Galore
- Birthday Cake Popcorn
- Caramel Apple Popcorn
- Chocolate Coffee Peanut Butter Pretzel Popcorn
- Cool Ranch Popcorn
- Sriracha Popcorn

Dips & Spreads
- Baked Potato Dip
- Italian Basil Pesto – Vegan
- Jalapeno-Bacon & Corn-Cheese Dip
- Pea Guacamole with Tortilla Chips
- Spiced Smoky Red Pepper Dip

Emotional Eating

Complete Guide to Lose Weight and Build a Joyful Relationship with Food Through Mindfulness-Based Eating Solutions — Stop Compulsive Overeating, Sugar Addiction, and Eating Disorders

by ALAN DIETER

© **Copyright 2019 by Alan Dieter - All rights reserved.**

The content contained within this book may not be reproduced, duplicated or transmitted without direct written permission from the author or the publisher.

Under no circumstances will any blame or legal responsibility be held against the publisher, or author, for any damages, reparation, or monetary loss due to the information contained within this book. Either directly or indirectly.

Legal Notice:

This book is copyright protected. This book is only for personal use. You cannot amend, distribute, sell, use, quote or paraphrase any part, or the content within this book, without the consent of the author or publisher.

Disclaimer Notice:

Please note the information contained within this document is for educational and entertainment purposes only. All effort has been executed to present accurate, up to date, and reliable, complete information. No warranties of any kind are declared or implied. Readers acknowledge that the author is not engaging in the rendering of legal, financial, medical or professional advice. The content within this book has been derived from various sources. Please consult a licensed professional before attempting any techniques outlined in this book.

By reading this document, the reader agrees that under no circumstances is the author responsible for any losses, direct or indirect, which are incurred as a result of the use of the information contained within this document, including, but not limited to, — errors, omissions, or inaccuracies.

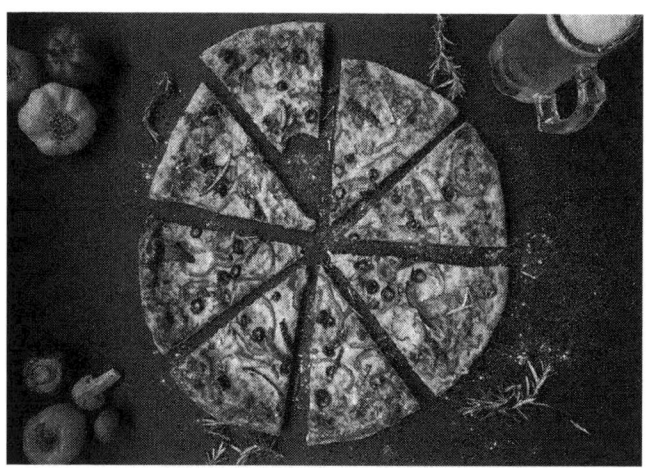

Table of Contents

Introduction 587
Chapter 1: What Is Emotional Eating? 588
What Is Emotional Eating? 588
Physical Causes 589
Mental Causes 590
Physical Symptoms 591
Mental Symptoms 591
Chapter 2: Mental Health and Physical Health 593
Mental Health and Poor Eating Habits 593
Bad Physical Health and Poor Eating Habits 594
Poor Mental Health Leads to Poor Physical Health 595
Poor Physical Health Leads to Poor Mental Health 596
How to Improve Physical Health 597
Chapter 3: Addictions 598
What Causes Food Addictions? 598
Combatting Food Addictions 599
What Causes Sugar Addictions? 601
Combatting Sugar Addictions 602
Seeking Professional Help for Addictions 603
Chapter 4: Setting Goals 604
Determining the Proper Way to Treat Your Body 604
Setting Goals 606
Specific 606
Measurable 606
Achievable 607
Relevant 607
Time-Based 607
Planning Those Goals 607
Prioritizing Goals 607
Setting Goals 608
Starting a Journal 608
Seeking Help from Others 608
Easing into Better Habits 608
Trying Challenges 608
Slightly Changing Routines 609
Chapter 5: Mindset 610

- Mindset for Achieving Goals 610
  - Developing a "Change" Mindset 610
  - Developing a Detail-Oriented Mindset 610
  - Developing a "Constructive Criticism" Mindset 611
  - Developing a "Progress" Mindset 611
  - Mindset for Staying Motivated Despite Obstacles 611
  - Adopting a Disciplined Mindset 612
  - Rewarding Oneself 612
  - Penalizing Oneself 612
- Mindset for a Healthier Body 613
  - Developing a "You Are What You Eat" Mindset 613
  - Developing a "Fitness" Mindset 614
  - Developing a "Work-Life Balance" Mindset 614
  - Developing an Overall Positive Mindset 614
- Mindset for a Healthier Mind 615
  - Taking Care of Oneself 615
  - Surrounding Oneself with Other People 615
  - Being in an Environment in Which One Thrives In 616
  - Mindset for Avoiding Addiction 616
  - Recognizing When Help Is Needed 617
  - Having a Balance Between Cutting Oneself Slack and Staying Motivated 617
  - Not Giving Up Along the Way 617
  - Staying Motivated 617
- **Chapter 6: Mindfulness 618**
  - What Is Mindfulness? 618
  - Mindfulness for Food Cravings and Compulsive Overeating 619
  - Incorporating Mindfulness into Your Life 620
  - Learning How to Enjoy Your Food 621
  - Freeing Oneself of Distractions 621
  - Focusing on Hunger 622
- **Chapter 7: Intuitive Eating 623**
  - How to Eat Intuitively and Implement Intuitive Habits 624
  - Intuitive Eating Effects 626
- **Chapter 8: Detoxing 628**
  - What Is a Sugar Detox? 628
  - How to Sugar Detox 629
  - Benefits of Sugar Detoxes 630
  - Detoxing Tips 631
- **Chapter 9: Taking Care of Your Mental Health 633**
  - Becoming More Aware of Your Emotions 633
  - Learning What Makes You Happy 635
  - Improving Your Self-Talk 636
  - Practicing Self-Care 637
  - Loving Yourself 638
  - Practicing Self-Respect and Self-Compassion 639
- **Chapter 10: Repairing Your Relationship with Food 640**
  - Signs of an Unhealthy Relationship with Food 640
  - Building a Healthy Relationship with Food 641
  - Loving Food Without Overeating 642
  - Learning to Value Health 643
- **Chapter 11: Eating Disorders 645**
  - Types of Eating Disorders 645
  - Anorexia Nervosa 645
  - Bulimia Nervosa 646
  - Binge Eating Disorder 646
  - Avoidant Restrictive Food Intake Disorder 646
  - Rumination Disorder 646
  - Unspecified Feeding or Eating Disorder 647
  - Purging Disorder 647
  - Night Eating Syndrome 647
  - Other Specified Feeding and Eating Disorders 647
  - Causes of Eating Disorders 647
  - Genetics 648
- Personality 648
- Trauma 648
- Coping Mechanism 648
- Outside Influences 648

Overcoming Eating Disorders 649
Listening to Yourself 649
Learning to Love and Accept Yourself 649
Seeking Help 649
Understanding the Causes and Symptoms 650
Chapter 12: Tips and Tricks 651
Little Ways to Improve Your Health 651
Drinking More Water 651
Exercising 651
Having Time for Yourself 652
Tips for Healthier Eating Habits 652
Eating More Fruits and Vegetables 652
Lessening Your Sugar and Salt Intake 653
Choosing Healthier Options 653
How to Be Happier Overall 653
Adjusting Your Sleep Schedule 653
Cleaning Up Your House 653
Undergoing Social Media Detox 654
Expressing Gratitude 654
Managing Poor Eating Habits 654
Listening to Your Body 654
Reducing Your Food Stock 654
Reducing Distractions While Eating 655
Regulating Your Portions 655
Having an Eating Schedule 655
Conclusion 656

Introduction

Congratulations on purchasing *Emotional Eating,* and thank you for doing so!

The following chapters will discuss a variety of topics—all relating to how you can improve your eating habits and overall health. You will be able to have more control over your emotional eating habits and start implementing healthy habits. You will be able to understand your physical and mental health better and take care of yourself.

You will learn what emotional eating is. It is important to understand the physical and mental causes of emotional eating, as well as some of the physical symptoms of it. It is also crucial to understand what physical and mental health entails. Your mental health can have a great effect on your eating habits. Poor physical health can also lead to poor eating habits. Similarly, one's physical health will affect one's mental health (and vice-versa). You must understand how you can improve your physical health. Food and sugar addictions are important to understand, as well as how to combat them. Setting goals is important so that you may treat your body properly. Thus, you must know how to plan, set these goals, achieve these goals, and ease into better habits.

There are several mindsets to understand—a mindset for achieving goals, staying motivated, having a healthier body, avoiding addiction, and having a healthier mind. Mastering mindfulness can help with food cravings, compulsive overeating, and enjoying your food. Understanding intuitive eating and how to implement it can have numerous positive effects on the body. Detoxes are great to learn about. Sugar detoxes are important to understand and implement, as there are many benefits.

You will learn about how to take care of your mental health by becoming more aware of your emotions, learning what makes you happy, improving your self-talk, practicing self-care, loving yourself, and practicing both self-care and self-compassion. You will also learn how to repair your relationship with food. It is important to know what the signs of an unhealthy relationship with food are, how to build a healthy relationship with food, how to love food without overeating, as well as how to learn to value your health. You will learn about eating disorders—the signs, symptoms, causes, and types of them. Additionally, you will learn how to overcome eating disorders. Finally, you will receive some additional tips and tricks about how you can improve your health overall, how to adopt healthier eating habits, how to be happier and healthier, as well as how to manage poor eating habits.

There are many topics covered, as the emotional eating is a larger-scale problem than simply fixing your diet. Mental health is what drives emotional eating, and overall physical health may be improved. When you improve your mental health, you will be able to begin establishing healthier habits for yourself and value yourself even more. This will allow you to be more motivated to take care of yourself and your health. It is also crucial that you understand the causes of your actions. If you can identify the source of your issues, you will be able to understand yourself more. Understanding why you do what you do will really help you to improve your habits. You can better prevent certain habits of yours from occurring.

There are plenty of books on this subject on the market—thank you again for choosing this one! Every effort was made to ensure it is full of as much useful information as possible. Please enjoy it!

Chapter 1: What Is Emotional Eating?

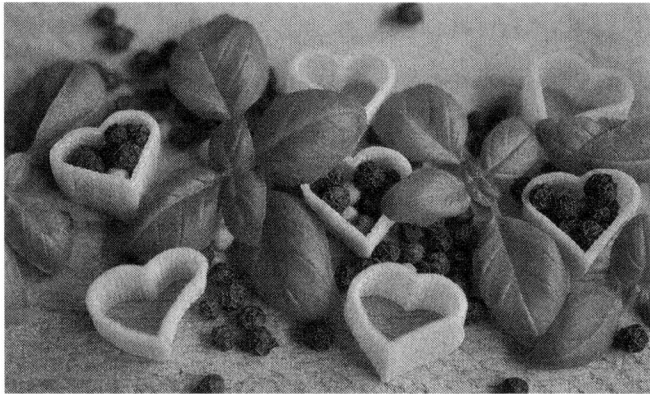

We are often cautioned not to give in to emotional eating. It is tempting to alleviate any physical or emotional pain with delicious foods to distract oneself from these issues. Food is necessary for life, and humans have developed more and more ways to enjoy food. Whether that be from eating out at restaurants to sweet treats to purchase from the store, eating has become a hobby for many. It is an enjoyable activity that increases one's happiness. However, emotional eating is widely regarded as a bad habit. It could also have serious consequences for the individual. It is crucial to understand what emotional eating is, what may cause one to eat emotionally, and what may happen to the body when one does eat as a result of their emotions. By understanding these, the individual may recognize what they are doing to their body, as well as why they may want to stop doing so to improve their health.

What Is Emotional Eating?

Of course, we all treat ourselves to an unhealthy snack every once in a while. There may be times where one uses food to make themselves feel better. This is normal. For those with a sore throat due to a cold or such, a popsicle or ice cream might be a nice treat to ease the throat. After a gym session, it may be necessary to refuel and consume food with protein in it. These are examples of normal eating habits. An occasional treat from time to time is okay. However, when it turns into an addiction, a bad habit, or a way of maintaining one's mental health, it can become a problem. If one relies on food (especially unhealthy food) to maintain their happiness, and they develop a dependency on food, this can prove extremely harmful.

On the other hand, emotional eating may be caused by the opposite. Some may feel the need to reward themselves with food constantly. If individuals find themselves motivating themselves by means of food, this may be a sign of an unhealthy relationship with food. Although it is normal to occasionally celebrate with food (i.e., birthdays, holidays, etc.), there is a point where one is making too many excuses for their unhealthy habits. For instance, one may motivate themselves at work by eating a sweet every time they complete a task. This can lead to a strong dependency on food and a subsequent unhealthy relationship with food. The person has become reliant on food for their daily tasks.

There are several signs of an emotional eater. One may eat because they are simply bored. One may eat out of negative feelings such as anger, sadness, loneliness, frustration, or others. One may also eat as a way of coping with stress. Eating out of positive emotions may also be a sign of an emotional eater. Eating as a response to emotions and situations is not healthy. It is important to understand that any unnecessary excess of food is unhealthy, especially when it occurs often. If a person eats until they have stuffed themselves every time or simply eats "for fun" instead of when they are hungry, this is another sign of an unhealthy relationship with food. There may be addictions associated with certain foods or types of foods as well, which is also unhealthy. If one feels guilty or embarrassed about food and feels the need to hide their eating habits, this is also a sign. There may be other, not-so-obvious signs of an emotional eater. These people tend to hide their problems from others and suppress their emotions. They may also choose to not engage in normal activities that they used to enjoy. They may feel poorly about their bodies and create a cycle that causes further guilt and unhealthy habits. These people may also have higher stress levels and fail to understand or execute healthy coping mechanisms. It may be more common in those who live "at the moment," as food only serves as a temporary cure.

Physical Causes

So, what causes one to eat emotionally? Of course, there is the mental aspect of it. One will eat based on their emotions. However, there are several other reasons that one may have the tendency to eat based on their emotions or when certain situations occur in their lives.

One cause may lie in a false hunger or an actual physical hunger that may be cured. The individual should learn the difference between physical hunger and emotional hunger. Physical hunger occurs when the body needs more fuel to power its processes. The body will signal that it needs food, typically by either a stomach that feels empty or by means of stomach growls. The body may also feel weak or out of energy. One may feel shaky or lightheaded. This hunger will be resolved by eating food. This hunger must also not be confused with the craving of a certain food. Cravings may also be satisfied when that certain food is consumed, yet physical hunger may be satisfied with any food. The individual may not be certain whether they are actually hungry or just desire food out of boredom, emotions, or any mental aspects. It is important to listen to the body instead of the mind. It is also crucial to eat when one is hungry and stop when one is full. Emotional eating may also result in stuffing oneself, which is not necessary or healthy. By training one's body to eat when they are hungry and eat the perfect amount to satisfy that hunger, a healthier relationship with food will be developed. This may be fine-tuned by training oneself to listen to their body's cues and be more in tune with their body.

One may also genuinely feel physically hungry very often. This excessive hunger can result from poor eating habits and further unhealthy habits. This can be due to a number of reasons. If a person does not consume a proper amount of protein, fiber, or fat, they will not stay full for long. Additionally, one who consumes too many refined carbohydrates will not stay full for long. An improper amount of sleep may also result in poor appetite control, as a proper amount of sleep is needed to regulate one's ghrelin (appetite-stimulating hormone) levels. The individual may also simply be dehydrated (either by too little water or too much alcohol). Both hunger and dehydration have similar physical feelings, and they can be confused quite easily. For this reason, it is important to drink water constantly throughout the day. One may try drinking water when they are hungry to test if it is true hunger or simply dehydration. Exercise also plays a huge role in one's hunger. More energy is used; therefore, more is needed to fuel the body. This may also lead to overeating, as one may justify their habits by exercising more to allow themselves to eat more. Although it is important to drink a lot of water, one may experience more hunger with a primarily liquid-based diet. This is due to the faster digestion of liquids than solids. There may also be medical reasons for the increased hunger, such as medication or a medical condition or disease that one may have.

Mental Causes

A huge aspect of emotional eating is the emotional and mental aspect of it. Humans, throughout time, have developed more of a liking to food. Instead of working for it and using it as fuel for one's body, it has become a source of entertainment, a meaning of socializing, and a hobby to enjoy. Each day, new recipes are concocted, restaurants are built, and food items are stocked in stores. This cultural revolution that celebrates food has led to serious consequences for humans. The tasting festivals, holiday gatherings, and other food-related events all celebrate delicious food and lead to an association between food and happiness.

For those who struggle with their mental health, feel stressed, or otherwise have less control over their emotions, food serves as an escape from negativity. Because it's associated with happiness, it can also be used as a sort of bribe to motivate one or as a means of celebration. This association between food and happiness can take a toll on one's health. Some may use it as a way to literally and figuratively fill the hole in their stomach and heart, respectively. It serves as a way to comfort one and to incur positive emotions.

This process becomes cyclical, as the individual will most likely feel guilty for consuming an excess of food unnecessarily. This guilt may cause further shame and negative emotions, which will lead to the further consumption of food to cope with these emotions, leading yet again to guilt and shame. This overall will affect one's perception of themselves and lead to poorer mental health.

The negative emotions that one feels that will cause them to eat emotionally can result from a number of factors. Those that struggle with depression, anxiety, and the like may eat as a way of coping with their mental struggle. Some may simply eat when they have a tough day at work. They may deal with heartbreak or relationship issues by turning to food. It may be caused by financial stress. There are many reasons that one may feel emotionally unwell and turn to food to aid their emotional well-being.

One may also eat more often because of poor eating habits, which can cause the brain to think that one is hungry even when they are not. For instance, one who eats while distracted will not mentally register the food that they are putting into their bodies. The brain will not truly consider the food that was consumed, as it was focused elsewhere. The same goes for those who eat their food too quickly. The brain does not have time to register the amount of food that was consumed in such a short period of time. There may also be individuals that don't associate certain foods with fullness. For instance, one may view a certain food as simply a snack and feel the need to eat more to make up for the food that they didn't previously consume. Those with high-liquid diets can experience this more frequently, as the meal may be mentally regarded as just a beverage as opposed to a full meal, despite any additives that may reside in it. One may also have no other hobbies or pleasures to look forward to. Perhaps the person neglects themselves from others and doesn't make plans that excite them. The person may feel bored with their job. Food may be the only source of happiness in their life. If one goes too long without eating, they may also subject themselves to improper eating habits, as they will eat whatever they can get their hands on. There is also the possibility of "oh well." Perhaps someone slipped up in their diet and thinks that they have already messed up, so why not just continue? This can lead to a domino effect and a continued pattern of poor eating. Instead of going back to their diet, the person will continue the bad eating because they slipped up once and think that continuing won't hurt them anymore. However, one must be able to have an overall healthy relationship with eating and should care about what they are putting into their bodies. After all, food is the source of energy for animals and must be the proper source of energy to help the body run most effectively.

Physical Symptoms

It's no surprise that emotional eating will take a toll on the body. Of course, there will be mental consequences, too. However, the body will not be able to function as well under this sort of treatment from the individual. Overeating and the consumption of unhealthy foods can lead to many consequences and side effects for the emotional eater. Because they are eating not out of hunger but due to triggers (whether that be emotional or situational), the individual is not treating their body the best that they can. Additionally, overstuffing oneself may lead to additional side effects and health issues.

Those who overeat may experience nausea. This is due to eating a large quantity of (typically unhealthy) food at once, especially if it is much more than normal. The individual will experience nausea and may have stomach pain, diarrhea, and other digestive issues occur. One may also feel bloated frequently and may even feel tired as a result of the extra work that their digestive system must undergo to digest the larger amount of food that they consume.

Another common consequence of emotional eating is weight gain. This can lead to obesity and being overweight, which can cause anything from muscular and skeletal problems to heart issues. It can lead to diabetes, high blood pressure, and fatigue. This is, of course, caused by regular emotional eating. It will be more severe with those who frequently overeat as a result of emotional eating. For instance, someone who binges each time they are stressed (and becomes stressed quite often) will see a more apparent weight gain than one who only rarely eats based on their emotions. However, emotional eating will take a toll on the body, regardless. It is an unhealthy relationship for one to have with food. It is also typical for one to eat foods that are high in carbohydrates, sugar, and calories when they are stressed. These foods are lower in nutritional value and can hinder one's bodily performance. It may lead to lethargy and an inability to function as well, especially when performing cardiovascular activities and exercises.

Mental Symptoms

Although the body will suffer from emotional eating, one's mental health will also suffer. Because it is used as a way to cope with emotions, one may develop an inability to otherwise cope with their emotions and any stress that they may experience. As a result of turning to food for comfort and relief, the person may abandon other and healthier ways of treating their mind and body better.

One may also develop negative thoughts and feelings as a result of their emotional eating. For instance, one may feel guilty about their habits. They may also feel guilty about their health and body as a result of the way they treat themselves. This can lead to poor self-confidence and even the withdrawal of oneself from social situations. This neglect can further lead to loneliness, causing even greater stress, sadness, and anxiety. Emotional eating has a domino effect in that it furthers problems that further other problems. This can even lead to other mental health issues such as depression.

Emotional eating can truly hurt the individual. It is triggered by emotions or situations, whether those are positive (using food as a reward) or negative (using food to procure happiness). It can be caused by a variety of emotions and by a sense of false hunger. Emotional eating can cause one's mental health to decline. It may also cause one's physical health to decline. Overall, emotional eating causes many consequences and is the result of poor health.

Chapter 2: Mental Health and Physical Health

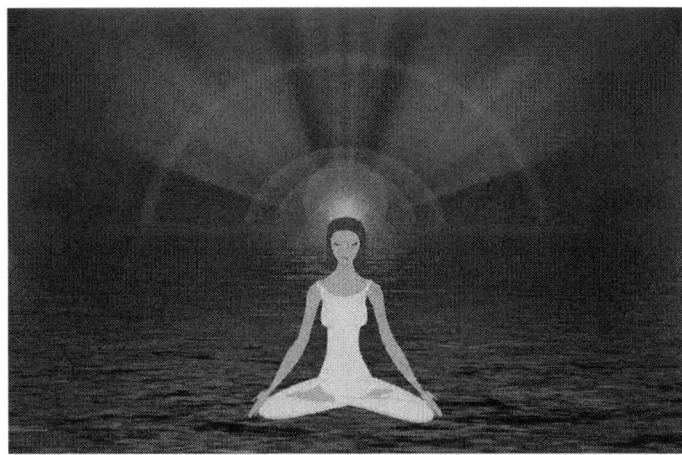

Mental and physical health are closely related. When one has great mental health, their physical health tends to be greater. When one's mental health suffers, one's physical health tends to suffer, too. One with greater physical health tends to have greater mental health. Similarly, one with poor physical health tends to suffer from poor mental health. Negative emotions and overall poor mental health can lead to hunger and the tendency to overeat and simply eat poorly. Poor physical health can also contribute to hunger and poor eating habits. It is also important to maintain one's physical health to improve one's mental health. It is also important because one's physical and mental health influences their hunger and digestion, and it further helps one's overall health. Taking care of oneself is more than just diet and exercise, although those are two crucial aspects of the individual's health.

Mental Health and Poor Eating Habits

Mental health or negative emotions have a strong connection with proper eating habits and hunger. Hunger can cause mental health issues, and poor mental health can contribute to a false sense of hunger due to some sort of emptiness that one experiences. Poor mental health can also lead to additional poor eating habits and a poor relationship with food.

For those who don't have access to nutritious food or who struggle to have sufficient funds to support the purchase of an adequate amount of sustainable food, food insecurity can result. They will become hungry and produce more cortisol, which causes the person to become stressed. In the long-term, this can be linked to depression, anxiety, and further mental disorders. It can even lead to suicidal thoughts, especially in teens. Hunger can lead to a lack of concentration, which can make it much more difficult to pay attention, leading to further frustration, as one will struggle to focus. Studies have concluded that those with food insecurity issues are much more likely to experience mental health issues than those who do not struggle with food insecurity. This link between food insecurity and mental health highlights the importance of consuming the right amount of the proper foods to feed oneself. By not doing so, one is hurting their mental health.

For those who fail to feed their body the proper amount of the right type of food, further issues can result. The individual will feel stressed and lethargic, leading to greater sadness, frustration, or overall dissatisfaction with their health. These negative emotions can lead to further poor habits, as the person will cope with these emotions by eating more foods that lack the nutrition they need. When one does not receive enough food, they will feel weak and have less motivation. This can lead to a cause of poor mental health, as one will not enjoy activities that they normally would. They may lack the energy or motivation to do what they love typically. Additionally, one who puts improper foods into their body will feel guilt and shame. This will cause them to think of themselves poorly and develop further issues that need to be coped with. If they continue to cope with these issues in an unhealthy manner, however, they will further their issues.

These issues can be multiplied in mothers and youth. There are typically more mothers that struggle with food insecurity as a result of the financial obligations that they must meet. For those who are pregnant, this is very harmful to their developing baby, which must be given the proper nutrients to develop in a healthy manner. It is also important for the mother, whether pregnant or not, as they must keep their energy up to support their child. Mothers must maintain their mental health to be able to support their child properly, yet this can be difficult if faced with food insecurity. As the children grow, they may struggle to pay attention in school and focus on their studies.

Bad Physical Health and Poor Eating Habits

In addition to affecting one's health, poor eating habits can take a toll on the body. One's physical health can suffer as a result of hunger and other poor eating habits. Studies have found links between hunger and health issues such as high blood pressure, heart disease, and diabetes.

It can greatly affect children, who need a proper amount of food to develop healthily. In children, development can be slowed or hindered as a result of hunger. It can also cause health issues such as asthma and anemia. It can also cause issues with kidneys, vision, and nerves. Food insecurity has been found to be linked with obesity, which can lead to many health issues itself, such as heart disease, high blood pressure, and musculoskeletal issues. Children who are malnourished experience slowed brain development as well as slower development of their muscles and bones. This can also weaken the body's immune system. Those who are malnourished will also have health issues with their teeth, gums, and skin. Food insecurity in children can occur, and it typically involves compromises being made. Instead of receiving the right amount of healthy food, children may be forced to eat less food than they need to thrive. They may also have to compromise when it comes to the nutritional value of their food. Because it often costs more for nutrition-packed food, children may have to eat unhealthy foods in order for their parents to be able to afford to keep them fed.

Pregnant mothers can really suffer from malnutrition. Not only will their babies struggle to develop properly, but they will feel weak from the lack of food in their bodies. Pregnant mothers need to be nourished even more while pregnant to ensure that they and their babies are healthy. Babies of malnourished mothers tend to have a lower birth weight, which can lead to long-term development issues.

Those who are hungry for short periods of time will certainly feel the short-term effects of hunger. One's stomach will growl, they may feel lethargic and weak, and they may also feel empty. One may even start shaking or develop a headache. Those who are hungry will feel their bodies give them signs that it is time to eat. For those who go hungry for the long-term, more serious effects will occur. The individual may become "immune to eating." They may be hungry but not wish to eat. If they do eat, they may even become sick from that. They will also experience other symptoms from not eating. They may struggle to sleep and feel tired constantly. It will be harder to stay focused. Malnutrition will lead to further fatigue and dizziness. It can also lead to a weakened immune system, subjecting the individual to an increased risk of sickness. The individual may also become infected more easily. Ear infections are more common in those who are malnourished and hungry. More frequent infections can lead to the development of diseases in those who experience food insecurity.

Poor Mental Health Leads to Poor Physical Health

Those who are mentally sound tend to feel more motivated to do what they love and to take care of themselves. One who is mentally stable will find it easier to set a proper eating and exercise routine for themselves and will be able to stick to it. Those who struggle with their mental health will have a harder time staying motivated to take care of themselves. They may also find it more difficult to stick to their goals and treat themselves the way they should. Those who have low self-confidence or self-worth may find it more difficult to treat themselves well. One who has low self-worth (perhaps as a result of low self-confidence) will not see themselves as worth taking care of, and they may neglect healthier habits in favor of less healthy habits. One with low self-confidence may withdraw from certain situations. They may feel embarrassed about their health and as a result, will not wish to go to the gym or exercise outside (or anywhere others may see them). They may also begin to slowly neglect themselves from others and avoid social situations when possible. This can lead to further unhealthy habits and worsen one's mental health. Those with depression and anxiety may also avoid social situations and treat themselves badly for similar reasons. Those who don't keep active will experience physical health issues and may not be as motivated to eat well as a result of already doing harm to their physical health.

There is a very real link between physical and mental health. Those with poor mental health are more likely to make unwise decisions when it comes to their physical health. Those with mental health issues are less likely to stay physically active. The main cause is a lack of motivation. Those with poor mental health are also more likely to develop poor and unhealthy eating habits. They may skip meals, overindulge, choose options that aren't the most nutritional, or eat very quickly. Those who struggle with mental health may find themselves starving themselves or not having a large appetite. Individuals with less-than-optimal mental health may also have a greater dependency on tobacco and alcohol. Those with mental health issues are more likely to develop smoking and drinking habits, which are typically used as ways to cope with their troubles. For those affected by stress, psoriasis may develop and present itself on the skin.

It has been found that those with mental health issues have shorter lifespans as a result of both suicide and physical health issues that arise as a result of their mental health issues. Their respiratory and circulatory systems suffer as a result of additional stress that is placed on their body from internal struggles. When one experiences difficulties with their mental health, they tend to be less likely to seek help for their issues. They don't feel the need to take care of themselves as much and will skip on routine checkups that would be able to detect health concerns before it is too late.

Poor Physical Health Leads to Poor Mental Health

Those with poor physical health will increase the likelihood of having poor mental health. Those with physical health problems are likely to feel less self-confident. They will not feel as confident doing activities that others wouldn't have a problem with. They recognize that they may not take the best care of their bodies. This can lead to feelings of guilt and shame about one's body and the way they treat it. Those individuals may also feel less socially included. They may withdraw themselves because of their condition, whether that be staying home to rest (due to fatigue), avoiding situations that involve physical activity (because of an inability to keep up with others), or neglecting themselves from others (as a result of embarrassment). Regardless of the reason, social withdraw can lead to serious mental health issues. One will feel lonely and will not get the socialization that they need to remain mentally sound.

Physical health issues can also cause one to feel stressed. They may feel overwhelmed by the severity of their situation, the costs associated with it, or treatments that they must undergo. For those that receive a diagnosis of a health issue, the mental reaction could be even worse than the physical issue itself. The individual may feel stressed about possible lifestyle changes that they must make. Perhaps they must change their diet or exercise routine. No matter the reason, the individual may experience more stress and anxiety from the situation. If the diagnosis is for a serious health issue, they may become worried or depressed due to the severity of the situation.

Certain physical issues have serious mental health effects. Those with heart disease are much more likely to develop depression. These individuals may feel more stressed and less at ease because of their condition. Additionally, they may seek proper physical treatment for their problems and think that it is adequate. They often fail to consider, though, how important treatment is for their mental health issues as well. They may focus primarily on their physical issues and neglect their mental issues in the process. Many individuals check on their physical health regularly, yet it is not as common to stay in tune with how one's mental health is. Most doctors fail to consider how one's mental health is when they are considering how healthy they are overall. One may feel physical pain. This is a constant reminder for that individual to seek help and receive treatment. Mental health isn't as obvious, however. Although one may experience metaphorical pain, they are less likely to seek proper treatment when they feel any sort of mental issue arise in themselves.

Those who receive an inadequate amount of sleep also subject themselves to a great number of mental health issues. They are more likely to feel fatigued and unmotivated as a result. They may also develop emotional instability as a result of an improper amount of energy that is needed for the individual to function.

How to Improve Physical Health

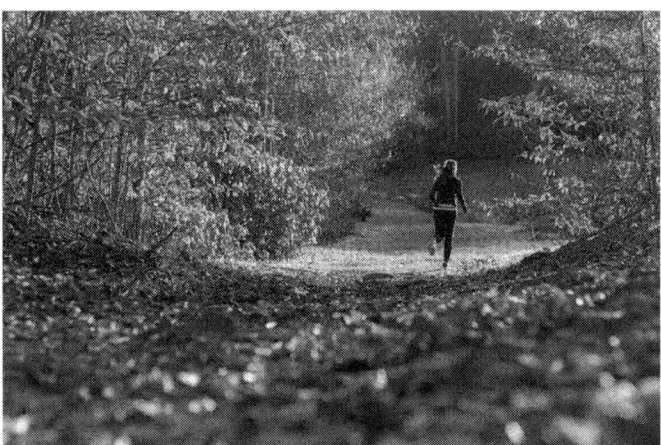

Commonly, it is said that one should "eat healthily and exercise" to be healthy. Of course, this is true. However, there is more to it than just this. One must exercise the proper amount so that they are working their body enough while also getting the rest that they need. They should also do the right types of exercise. It is important for one to practice cardiovascular exercises for improved heart health. It is also important to practice strength exercises to build the strength of one's muscles and bones so they may move more freely without trouble. One must also develop proper eating habits. This includes getting the proper amount of the right foods to fuel one's body. It also entails eating at the right times so that the individual is fueled throughout the day. They must also avoid processed foods and foods that lack proper nutrition as much as possible.

It is important that one drinks enough water. The best solution is to avoid sugary drinks and to get the proper amount of water for one's weight, height, age, and activity level. This will vary from person to person, and there are online calculators available, as well as the advice of a doctor. It is also crucial for the individual to receive a proper amount of sleep. This will also vary from person to person, although it is mostly based on one's age. Receiving too much and too little sleep will both negatively affect one's body.

When an individual does fail to take care of their physical health, their mental health will suffer. On the other hand, an individual who neglects their mental health will experience physical health issues. Similarly, one who is hungry and has poor eating habits will experience both physical and mental health problems. These issues are all closely related, and one will affect the other. There are several ways to improve one's physical health, which will also work to improve that individual's mental health. By improving both of these, the individual is making it easier for themselves to be able to develop proper eating habits.

Chapter 3: Addictions

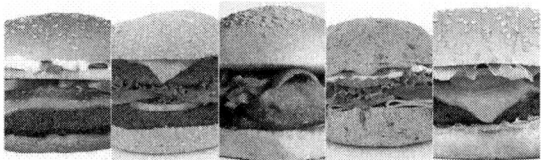

Many addictions can occur in individuals. Addictions can result in anything. Some may be addicted to a hobby they have, such as running or watching television. Addictions can start out as a passion for a certain activity, yet they can turn unhealthy once it becomes an obsession for the individual. There can be "healthy" and "unhealthy" addictions. For instance, one may be addicted to running. This is highly regarded as a healthy activity, yet it can be unhealthy if it becomes excessive and is harmful to the individual. People can develop an addiction to alcohol or to drugs, which can lead to serious damages to their physical health. It is also possible to become addicted to certain foods or to food as a whole. This can lead to several consequences for the individual, yet it can be overcome. It is important to understand the causes of these addictions.

What Causes Food Addictions?

When one is addicted to food, they have an uncontrollable impulse to eat. They don't eat to live—they live to eat. It is typically a response to an emotional or situational trigger. Although the body depends on food for its survival and uses it as fuel, those who are addicted to food typically become dependent upon a certain type of food. This can be especially detrimental to the body if the food is unhealthy, such as sweets, chips, or certain grains. This addiction can occur similarly to how one will develop a dependency on cigarettes or alcohol. The brain will depend on the release of chemicals (like dopamine) that the food allows them to have. When one eats the food, it satisfies this craving for it and will release dopamine, making the individual happy. It is pleasurable to the body. The lack of this food (whether the person has yet to eat it or does not have access to it) can lead to serious distress and will cause desperation for this food. Until one satisfies their craving, their body will yearn for that food.

Research suggests, however, that food addictions differ from substance addictions such as cigarettes or alcohol. This is because these are substance addictions. The properties in these substances are addictive themselves. However, food can be a behavioral addiction. Eating becomes a regular habit, and even a hobby, for some individuals. Although it is important to eat enough food to maintain one's energy, there is such a thing as an excess of food, especially when that food lacks nutritional value.

There are certain foods that one is more likely to become addicted to. The most common foods are high in sugar, fat, and starch. Foods such as chips, French fries, sweets, and white bread are the most common foods to become addicted to. These foods taste good and satisfy one's craving. They also tend to be lower in nutritional value, which can further one's health issues. These foods, known as highly palatable foods (which are high in sugar, fat, and salt), are more likely to trigger the sections of the brain that addictive drugs do. They trigger the same reward and pleasure parts of the brain that those drugs do. Consuming such foods will trigger chemical releases that lead to pleasure in people. Because of this happiness associated with eating such foods, individuals with food addictions want more so that they may experience that pleasurable sensation again. This feeling of happiness might cloud one's ability to perceive fullness and satisfaction with what they have already consumed. This leads to a loss of control and a subsequent need to frequently consume such foods and feel the pleasure associated with it.

There are several signs that one may have a food addiction. One may have obsessive food cravings that are uncontrollable and may even interfere with the individual's daily life. They may experience obsessive thoughts about food that interferes with their ability to concentrate until they consume such food. They may have binging episodes or eat compulsively. They may try to stop overeating but find themselves unable to. It may be hard to control portion sizes and the frequency of eating. This can even take a toll on their social life and finances. They may try to hide food from others or feel embarrassed and guilty when eating. They may also depend on food for their emotional well-being. It is also possible that the individual will have lower self-confidence and self-worth. They may try to restrict themselves from eating and starve themselves after a binging episode. They may try to exercise compulsively to make up for their binging. They may even force themselves to vomit after an episode of overeating occurs.

Combatting Food Addictions

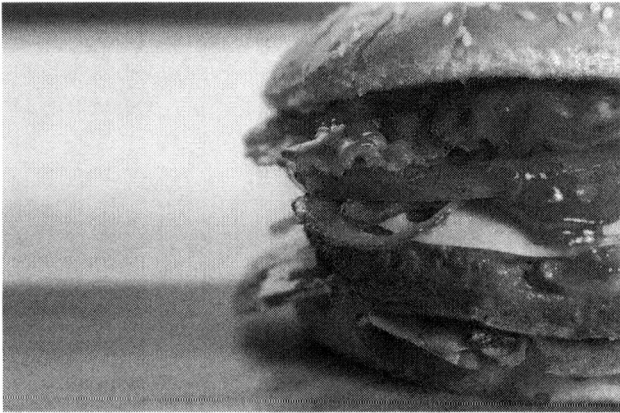

If left untreated, those with food addictions can face several consequences. They may have food interfere with their daily lives. It may be difficult to concentrate until they satisfy their craving and give in to their addiction. They may need to leave events in order to satisfy their craving. It can interfere with one's social life and any romantic, family, or friendly relationships. If one begins to build their day around food, this can really become troublesome, as they must give in to their craving and potentially ignore other scheduled events. It may harm one's work or academic life if it impairs cognitive function. Food addictions can further lead to health issues. One may become overweight or obese as a result of their addiction and the potential to overeat. Although not all with food addictions are overweight, it can occur as a result. Some may have a metabolism that allows them to eat more than necessary without any weight gain. Some may also self-induce vomiting or excessively exercise to attempt to counteract the excess of food that they consume.

It is important to combat food addictions, as they can deteriorate one's physical and mental health. There are several ways to do so. Before seeking professional help, one may try to make small changes to improve their lifestyle and the situation of their addiction. One may try to replace their unhealthy foods gradually with better alternatives. For instance, one may replace candy with berries. This will still allow for one to enjoy the sweetness of the food, yet there will be greater nutritional value in it. There are many small switches to make. Another is with beverages. Instead of consuming sweetened beverages, one may gradually incorporate water into their diet. Soda is crucial to replace. The individual may gradually incorporate more water and less sweetened beverages into their diet. They may also reduce the caffeinated and alcoholic beverages that they consume, replacing those with water as well. It is important to drink the right amount of water every day. There are certain eating habits that may also prove highly beneficial to those with food addictions. For instance, one may start gradually replacing meals at restaurants with home-cooked meals. They may focus more on their food and less on other distractions. By eating slowly and truly registering everything that they are eating, the individual may develop a greater sense of self-awareness. The individual may also schedule their meals and stick to it. Some may prefer much smaller meals throughout the day, while others prefer three sustainable meals. This is up to personal preference and the advice of one's medical professional. While shopping, it is important to stick to one's grocery list. It can be tempting to weave in and out of the aisles out of the grocery store. There are also many tempting sales (such as buy one get one free). When shopping, one should also eat before. By sticking to the grocery list, the individual may be more aware of what they are putting into their bodies and make wiser choices regarding what will be accessible to them in their homes. The pantry and refrigerator will be filled with more favorable options. It is also possible for one to track every food that they consume. There are many digital applications to track one's calories and macronutrients. It will greatly help one to realize what exactly it is that they are putting into their bodies and how it is for their health. This can help with portion sizes and for understanding what certain foods will do to the body.

While adjusting one's eating habits can greatly help, there are other ways to allow one to make better decisions about their eating habits. By receiving enough sleep, one will not feel the need to supplement their diet with unnecessary foods to make up for their lack of energy. Exercising on a regular basis will encourage one to take care of their body further so that their progress is not lost. However, one must appropriately fuel up for their workouts and avoid the mentality of allowing themselves to overeat because they exercised. It is also important that the individual makes strides towards improving their mental health, as this can lead to the need to eat emotionally in the first place. By reducing stress and developing healthier ways to deal with their emotions, the individual will help themselves greatly.

What Causes Sugar Addictions?

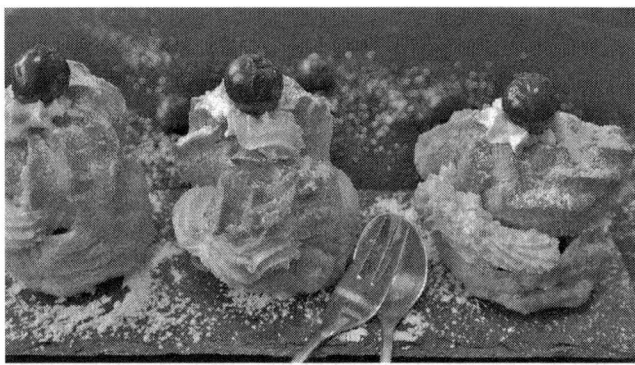

These days, sugar is added to almost everything. Seasonal beverages at coffee shops are loaded with sugar. Desserts line the aisles at grocery stores. Soda has become a social drink. There are even food items with sugar that one wouldn't even expect! It's tough to avoid sugar, as it's in almost everything. Most people consume way beyond the recommended amount of sugar each day. One may even develop an addiction to sugar, making it even harder to avoid. The individual may develop an emotional or psychological dependence on sugar, causing their body to "need" it. It makes it even harder to avoid when one eats mostly processed foods and refined grains, which create additional sugar once digested. This is one way that it may be more difficult for one to recognize their sugar addiction. Sugary foods like donuts and ice cream are more apparently filled with sugar. However, those with a sugar addiction may crave more than just sweets; refined carbs are a common addiction of those with a sugar addiction because of the glucose produced when those refined carbs are metabolized. Although sugar can occur naturally in many foods, such as fruit, an excess of sugar (especially added sugar) can prove harmful to the body. For this reason, sugar addictions should be dealt with appropriately. One must first recognize what causes an individual to develop an addiction to sugar.

After consuming sugar, one will likely experience a "sugar high." This is a spike of energy in the body that allows one to combat possible fatigue that they may feel. It is typically accompanied by a rise in one's happiness as a result of the dopamine that is released after one consumes sugar. Sugar has often been compared to addictive drugs such as cocaine. Those who overindulge in sugar will also increase their chances of diabetes, obesity, and heart disease.

There are several types of people that may be more at risk for developing a sugar addiction. Those with anxiety, depression, and increased stress levels may be more tempted to reach for sugary foods to increase their happiness and suppress any negative emotions. Those who struggle with constant fatigue may also be more likely to reach for sugar due to the endorphins that are released and the subsequent increase in one's energy. They will use sugar to cope with their emotions and depend on it to maintain their energy levels. When this dependency occurs, one has developed an addiction to it.

There are several signs that one may be addicted to sugar. They may fill their diet with sugar-rich foods and experience frequent cravings for such foods. They will emotionally eat foods that are rich in sugar to cope with certain emotions or situations that may occur in their lives. They may even have binging episodes involving sugary foods and find it hard to control themselves around sugar. This can lead to mental consequences such as feeling helpless or having poor self-esteem and self-worth.

Combatting Sugar Addictions

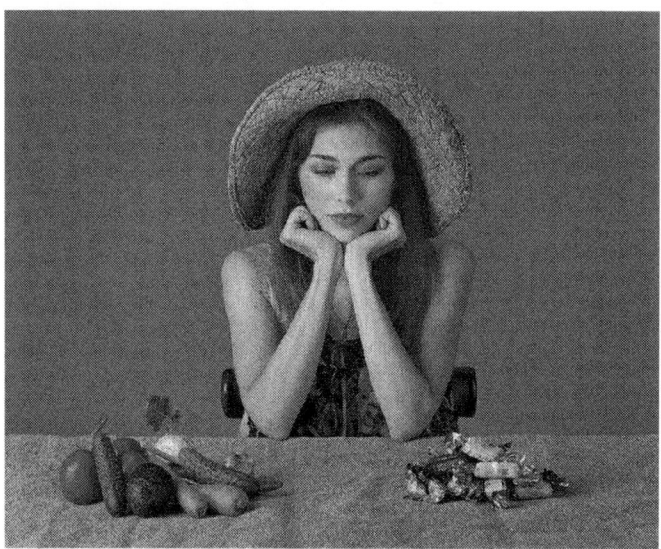

There are several ways to break free from sugar addiction. Once one recognizes that they have a sugar addiction, they may take steps towards helping themselves to overcome that addiction. Before seeking professional medical help for sugar addiction, one may consider easier remedies that they can do themselves. It can be difficult to break an addiction, but there are ways to help one to overcome that addiction more easily.

One may gradually replace their sugary favorites with healthier alternatives. Replacing refined carbohydrates for whole-grain options is a quick and simple switch. Instead of snacking on chips and other salty snacks, one may find popcorn that is natural and doesn't have added sugar or sodium. It is important to gradually replace any sugary beverages in one's diet with water. By making small switches here and there gradually, it will be easier for one to develop proper eating habits without relapse. It is important not to cut out all sugar completely right away. This will only lead to a later binge of the food and a loss of motivation. By gradually switching one's diet to be healthier, it will make it much easier for the individual to transform their diet into one that is more sustainable. Products must be researched, however. Some food products claim to be "healthy" but just contain alternatives to sugar that are worse than sugar itself. For this reason, one must inspect the ingredients before purchasing the product. When in doubt, it is better to go for more "whole" foods. This way, the individual knows just what they are putting into their bodies. If one can't pronounce an ingredient in the product, it may not be the best chemical to put in the body. It's best to know just what one is eating. For instance, an apple is simply that: an apple. When one purchases cheesy puffs, however, this can get more complicated. There are many more ingredients, most of which are unknown to the general population. It's better to be aware of what is going into the body.

One quick and easy fix is not to surround oneself with tempting foods. This can quickly be done by cleaning out one's pantry and refrigerator and ridding oneself of the foods that are not nutritionally sufficient. However, one must not bring in new foods that will cave in to their addiction. By setting a proper shopping list and sticking to it, this can be done more easily.

By sticking to an eating plan, one may combat their sugar addiction. Instead of eating out, one may make food at home. It's wise to prepare meals ahead of time. This way, there's food that is already made. The excuse of eating out for convenience can't be used. This also helps with preparing foods that are based on what's best for the body, not the taste buds. When one is hungry, they are more likely to eat foods that are not the best for them nutritionally. This eliminates that issue.

Seeking Professional Help for Addictions

If there have been several steps taken to attempt to combat the addiction, but no results are seen, it may be time to seek professional medical help for the addiction. Although this may be costlier and take extra time, it is necessary if the individual has put in the effort to combat their addiction themselves but is unable to take control of their bodies and food cravings. Otherwise, they face serious health consequences, especially if left untreated for a long period of time. There are several ways that one may seek help and receive treatment for their food or sugar addiction.

One may try cognitive-behavioral treatment (CBT). This helps to identify thought patterns and change them to create a new coping mechanism for the individual that doesn't involve eating. One may try medication for their mental issues. It is also a possibility to try solution-focused therapy. This aims to find solutions for triggers of overeating and emotional eating. Trauma therapy may be used for those who eat as a result of past trauma. One may use eating as a coping mechanism for this trauma, and they should seek help for coping with that trauma and any emotions associated with it. One may seek the help of a nutritional counselor or dietary planner, who may create an individualized plan for the person and come up with meals that they may eat each day in order for them to be nutritionally satisfied.

There are also 12-step programs, which involve meetings with others who share the addiction to food. This can help one to feel less lonely and meet others that also struggle with their issue. Typically, one will receive a sponsor to truly help them to develop a plan to combat their addiction. There are also commercial treatment programs, which may cost more but will still offer beneficial information and effective solutions to those who struggle with food addiction. One may also visit a psychiatrist to discuss their issues and receive medication that will help them to feel better and eliminate the need for using food as a coping mechanism.

When one experiences emotional troubles, they need a way to cope with those issues. For those that turn to food, addictions to certain foods or sugary foods can become quite common. There are several ways to recognize and treat these addictions. One may first try to solve their problems themselves. If that is ineffective, though, they may need to seek professional help for their addiction.

Chapter 4: Setting Goals

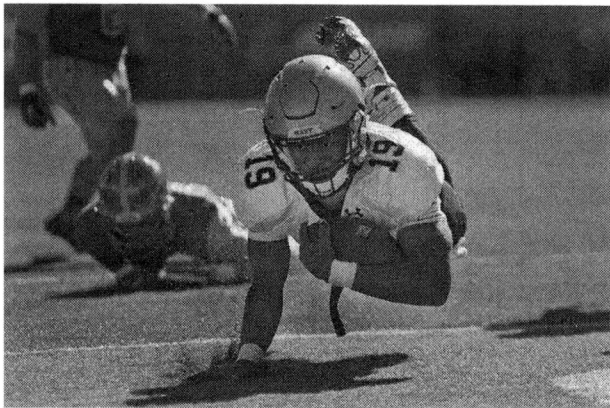

It's always important to set goals. It's crucial to constantly set goals to improve oneself and work towards being happier and healthier. It is especially important to set goals regarding health. Everyone gets off the path to success once in a while, and it is important to constantly check in to ensure that the proper steps are taken to maintain the best body and mind possible. By being more aware of which aspects of one's self can be improved, it will be easier to work towards being the best person possible.

Determining the Proper Way to Treat Your Body

Before setting goals, one must determine which aspects of their health that they wish to most improve. It may help to keep a log of one's daily activities and the foods they consume (as well as water that they drink). This will help put into perspective what improvements must be made to help with the individual's health. There are several aspects that the individual may make improvements to. Of course, diet and exercise are common ways to improve one's health, yet other aspects should also be considered to maximize the individual's health.

One aspect that may be improved upon is improving the types of foods that one puts into their body. They may limit themselves to only consuming certain foods on holidays or birthdays. This goal will depend on the person, as some individuals will have more improving to do than others. For instance, one that consumes seven donuts a week may try to first dwindle that number down to one per week, eventually having only a few per year or cutting that out altogether. There may be a certain type of food that the individual wishes to reduce in their diet or replace it with another food. They may also wish to incorporate more nutritious foods into their diet. There are several food-related goals. One may wish to adopt a vegan, vegetarian, or plant-based diet. They may wish to switch from refined grains to whole grains. They may also wish to switch to healthier fats.

In addition to improving the types of foods that one eats, they may also wish to set goals for their eating habits. For instance, portion sizes may have to be reduced. It may also be wise to set a schedule to stick to regarding meals to eliminate binging episodes and excessive snacking. One may also set goals regarding eating with fewer distractions and taking more time to eat so that their brain properly registers the foods that they will consume. The individual may also set the goal of not eating past fullness.

For many, fitness is also a common category in health-related goal-setting. There are different ways to set goals regarding fitness. One may wish to exercise for a certain amount every week. They may wish to set goals in a specific activity, such as running for 3 miles at 6 mph without stopping (or running a 6-minute mile). They may also wish to visit the gym a certain amount of times per week. It may involve an event, such as running a 5k. There may also be a certain category for the exercise, such as incorporating more cardio or more strength into workouts. Fitness goals may even be as simple as improving one's posture. This can help muscles to be healthier. They may even set simple goals such as walking or biking instead of driving or using the stairs instead of an elevator.

Along with diet and exercise, the individual may wish to aim for a healthier weight or slimmer waist size. A doctor should be consulted to determine the ideal weight based on the person.

Sleep is very important. Without proper sleep, one is more likely to develop poor eating habits and suffer mental health issues. One may wish to set a schedule for their sleep, such as going to bed at 10 each night and waking up at 5 each morning. They may also set a goal for the number of hours of sleep every night. One may also make the goal of sleeping through the night, which may be accomplished by consulting a medical professional and taking supplements. The individual may also set goals for their nightly routine, making sure to unwind before bed and reducing poor nightly habits.

Water is also an important goal to set. One typically will set goals increasing the amount of water they drink on a daily basis so that they consume the proper amount. This may also involve replacing other beverages with water.

One may wish to set goals regarding the elimination of poor habits. One may wish to eliminate or reduce the amount of tobacco or other drugs that they use. This can help reduce the risk of lung cancer (for smokers) and decrease potential health problems. Another goal may be to eliminate or reduce the amount of alcohol that the individual consumes. This may also be replaced with water to ensure that the individual is staying hydrated and not consuming unnecessary beverages. One may choose to limit the number of drinks they consume or how often they drink.

Social goals are important to set to ensure that one's mental health stays in check. If the individual has found themselves neglecting themselves from others, it may be time to set some social goals. Perhaps the individual wishes to make plans with friends at least once per week. They may set the goal of finding two clubs to join or an organization to volunteer with and sticking to that. They may set a number of times per month that they wish to volunteer or attend meetings. They may also set goals to spend more time with family members. This may also involve technology goals. Perhaps one wishes to cut out or reduce social media usage in favor of face-to-face socialization. They may also wish to reduce the amount of time that they spend on certain devices.

One may also set mental goals. This will help to keep one's emotions more stable, and their mental health will be improved as a result. One may wish to practice gratitude by writing in a journal each day. The individual may also set the goal of relaxing for a certain time each day or week. It is important to take time for oneself. This can be done by going for walks, reading, meditating, writing, creating, or whatever else is relaxing. One may also set spiritual or religious goals to attend services, pray, or learn more about one's faith. This can also help.

One may also set medical goals. They may wish to regularly visit a therapist, dentist, doctor, or other medical professional regularly and stick to their appointments.

Setting Goals

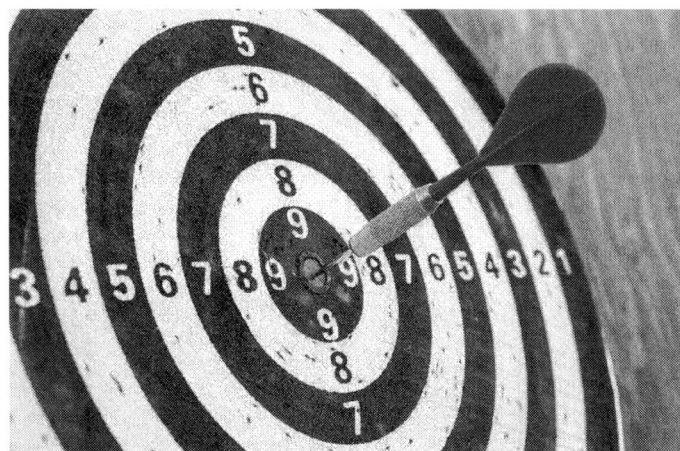

There is a certain way to set goals for oneself. Although many set the goal of "being healthier," what does this mean? It's hard to determine if one has met that goal because it is not clearly defined. Once the individual has determined what aspects of their health that they would like to improve, they must set proper goals accordingly. These goals must be strong objectives that will allow the goal-setter to monitor their progress towards achieving these goals. These goals must be SMART, which is an acronym for being specific, measurable, achievable, relevant, and time-bound.

Specific

The goal must be specific. This means that it must be clear and well-defined what exactly the goal is. This will make it easier for both the individual and any others that will encourage that individual to take steps towards achieving that goal. The individual should know what they are doing, how they would like to impact themselves, and what the action is. For instance, instead of setting the goal of simply losing weight, the individual may wish to lose 10 pounds by replacing sugary foods with more nutritional options and by visiting the gym.

Measurable

The goal must be measurable. Instead of simply saying that one will visit the gym, they can set the goal of visiting the gym for an hour three days a week. This allows the individual to measure if they are making progress towards their goal.

Achievable

The goal must be achievable. Although losing twenty pounds in a week may sound great to some, this is not realistic, nor is it healthy. Going to the gym for two hours, seven days a week, is also not realistic or healthy, as rest is needed. Time, supplies, and health should be considered when setting goals that are realistic.

Relevant

The goal must be relevant. This means that the goal should have importance to the individual. Otherwise, it will be difficult to find the motivation to work towards that goal. For instance, one that wants to incorporate more cardiovascular exercises into their routine but hates running should not set the goal of running three miles each morning. They may instead choose to focus on another exercise, such as dancing, biking, or swimming. Goals should be exciting. The individual should look forward to improving themselves and working towards their goal. Otherwise, it will be quite easy to abandon the goal set.

Time-Based

The goal must be time-based. Otherwise, it is hard to measure them, and there will be room to slack off. If one's goal is to lose 24 pounds in the next year, it can be much easier to work towards. This makes splitting the goal easy. Instead of looking at it as losing a total of 24 pounds, the individual can see it as losing only 2 pounds per month, which does not sound as difficult. By splitting the goal into smaller goals based on the time period, it will be easier to measure and not seem as overwhelming as looking at the whole goal.

Planning Those Goals

It's one thing to come up with the goals for one. However, it is important to truly take action and plan how to go about accomplishing those goals. There are several ways to do so. There are also ways to make it easier to accomplish those goals and to find additional motivation to work towards those goals. The individual may prioritize their goals, split them up, start a blog or journal, accomplish goals in a group, or even seek professional help for working towards their goals.

Prioritizing Goals

The individual should prioritize their goals. This is important to ensure that they are working towards what is most important to them. This step may also involve eliminating goals that are irrelevant or unimportant. It may also involve combining certain goals. For instance, instead of eating better and exercising more, the individual may set the goal of losing weight by eating better and exercising more. Typically, it is best to stick to one to three goals. It's difficult to keep track of more than this, and it makes it easier to place greater importance on achieving these goals.

Setting Goals

When setting goals, it's important to split them up. This will make it much easier and realistic to go about achieving. For instance, if one wishes to run 40 miles in a month, they may instead look at it as (assuming that a month has four weeks) ten miles per week. They may further split that up and run 2 miles 5 days per week. Two miles seems much more achievable than forty. Goals may be split up into smaller daily, weekly, or even monthly goals. If the goal is measurable, this should be quite easy to accomplish, and the progress towards achieving that goal will be easy to track.

Starting a Journal

One way to make accomplishing goals easier is to start a journal or log. This will make it simple to track progress and even write how one feels about their goals. It can help with maintaining motivation. It's a great way to remind oneself why they are working towards this goal. These can also be used as a scheduling tool to help the individual to come up with a plan for their goals. They may combine this with prioritizing to determine what is important and use the goal-splitting to write a plan.

Seeking Help from Others

One may also seek help from others. It is really beneficial when one sets goals with others. That means that all people involved may hold each other accountable, encourage each other, and remind each other why these goals are important. They may find a friend to go to the gym with or otherwise be active with. They may have each person living with them start eating healthier foods. The individual may join a club for those with similar goals. They may even seek the help of a professional in guiding them to success. The professional will have more knowledge about proper goals and how to achieve them.

Easing into Better Habits

There are many ways to make small changes that will have a big impact on one's life. Of course, one can make progress towards their goals each and every day. They may split up their goals and tackle a portion daily, working towards the bigger goal and making their body the healthiest they can. However, there are many small changes that one may make to improve their health. These small habits can have a great effect on a person's body, mind, and overall health. By incorporating these habits into one's lifestyle, they are truly helping themselves.

Trying Challenges

One fun way to go about making healthier choices is to try challenges. There are many 30-day challenges out there, most of which have a schedule to follow each day and are already planned out. These usually involve doing a bit each day or starting a new habit and sticking to it for thirty days. By committing for thirty days, the individual is training their brain to think of the new habit as normal. It also allows the individual to follow a plan that already has goals that are split up and easier to follow. These goals are also measurable.

These challenges can be for anything. They may even be for a different length of time (such as a week). By looking at the goal as a fun challenge instead of a goal to work towards, it will be more fun and seen as a sort of game to play. The individual may set a goal to do yoga, meditate, go without eating certain foods or drinks, drink enough water, only have three meals per day, or do a certain exercise a certain way. These are all small habits to make one healthier and to improve their body and mind.

Slightly Changing Routines

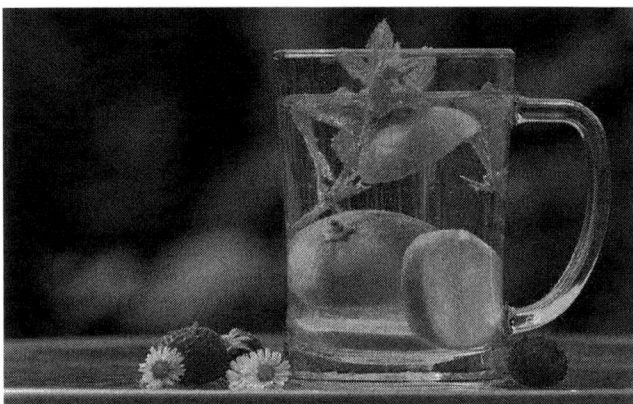

Another great way to incorporate healthy habits is by slightly changing morning and night routines. For instance, one may choose to have a glass of lemon water within thirty minutes of waking up every morning. They may also reserve a certain time, such as eight a.m., for exercising for an hour. By starting off the morning on the right foot, the individual is setting themselves up for success. This will start the day off well and motivate the individual, as they have already accomplished something at the beginning of their day. Nighttime routines are also important, as this is a way to unwind and prepare the individual for sleep. One great habit is shutting off all electronics an hour before bed. Setting a sleep schedule, creating a skincare routine, reflecting, setting goals for the next day, and reading are all great habits to incorporate into one's nighttime routine.

Setting goals are crucial for improving one's health. It is important to know what goals to set, how to set them, how to accomplish them, as well as how to incorporate healthier habits into one's life. By following these steps, the individual is setting themselves up for success in achieving their health-related goals in life.

Chapter 5: Mindset

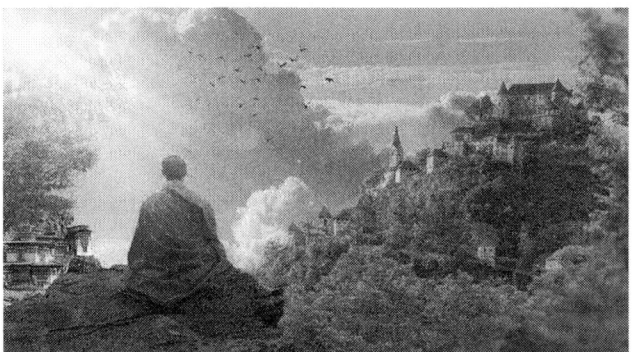

Adopting the proper mindset is crucial for one's success. Without the proper mindset, the individual will not have the motivation to work towards and achieving their goals. It is important to have the proper mindset for achieving goals so that they may work towards them. There is a certain mindset necessary for remaining motivated when one gets hit with issues to face. One must adopt the right mindset to avoid unhealthy addictions. There is a proper mindset for improving one's physical health and having a healthier body. The proper mindset is also necessary for better mental health and a healthy mind.

Mindset for Achieving Goals

When one wishes to take steps towards achieving their goals, a certain mindset must be adopted. It is crucial that one sticks to their goals and works towards them every day. To do so, certain aspects regarding one's mindset may need some tweaking to help them to achieve their goals.

Developing a "Change" Mindset

The first mindset adjustment is to change. In order to better oneself, change is necessary. This may be difficult for some. Some individuals stay with jobs that they don't enjoy despite knowing that better options are available because they settle for what's comfortable to them. In order to achieve one's goals, however, a change must be made. Whether that's a change in routine, scheduling, or behavior, change is necessary to work towards achieving a goal. One must recognize that change, although it may be nerve-wracking at first, is beneficial and should be viewed as advancement towards becoming a better person.

Developing a Detail-Oriented Mindset

It's also important to develop a detail-oriented mindset. When working towards goals, it's important to take into account every action that is taken and what may be improved upon. This will really help one to track progress towards achieving goals. It will also help the individual to know what exactly it is that they want. When one becomes clearer about what their goal is and why they have set it, it will be easier to work towards. This will also help with scheduling exact ways to make progress towards the goal and will help when the individual is recording their daily progress.

Developing a "Constructive Criticism" Mindset

Another mindset that must be adopted is the constructive criticism mindset. If working towards a goal, the individual must already be aware that some change must be made in their life. Although it isn't always enjoyable to be criticized, it is necessary to use constructive criticism to one's advantage. This means taking it from both others and from oneself. When crafting the goals to accomplish, one must realize what it is that they need to improve about themselves. They must also be willing to hear what others see, as this will give an outsider's perspective. This can also be helpful while working towards those goals. One must constantly check in with themselves and determine if there is any way that they may be able to achieve their goals more efficiently and effectively. It takes a strong person to be able to acknowledge that they may be slacking off with working towards their goals. However, the sooner that it is recognized, the sooner the individual may go back to working towards their goals and bettering themselves.

Developing a "Progress" Mindset

The final mindset that is important for achieving goals is that progress is just as important as achieving the goal. Often, people adopt an "all or nothing" mentality. This can prove detrimental, as progress is what drives results. It is still helpful even if a person only slightly improves their health. Many smaller changes lead to a great change and an improvement in health.

Mindset for Staying Motivated Despite Obstacles

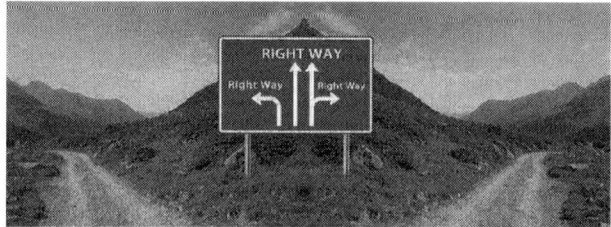

There are several adjustments that are beneficial to one's mindset when trying to stay motivated despite obstacles. There will always be inconveniences that arise or negative influences that hinder one's performance. For instance, holidays may be a time that can be tempting to cave in to overeating tendencies. When one is sick and has a sore throat, they may be tempted to binge on ice cream. Friends may want to go out to eat and go drinking. These are all ways that the individual may be swayed towards making a choice that they wouldn't make otherwise.

Adopting a Disciplined Mindset

To remain motivated, one must adopt a disciplined mindset. They must be able to practice self-control. It is okay to give in to unhealthy choices every once in a while. Although it would be ideal for eating perfectly nutritious meals all the time, this is not realistic. One must enjoy themselves every so often. However, this shouldn't be taken too far. Perhaps the individual has chosen to allow themselves one cheat meal per week. This is adequate, provided that they remain disciplined. Although it's fine to eat that meal out and choose foods that wouldn't usually be consumed, the individual shouldn't overstuff themselves or eat beyond what they should. They must remain disciplined and stick to their original plan.

Rewarding Oneself

It is important to reward oneself. When progress has been made, it is important to recognize that and to celebrate one's success. Every step forward should be viewed as progress towards achieving the goal. However, the individual shouldn't stop and celebrate every tiny bit of progress that is made in a way that will interfere with other goals. They must also not give up or stop just because they have made progress. Even though progress is good, the individual should keep working towards their goal.

Penalizing Oneself

Along with rewarding oneself, it is crucial to adopt the proper mindset concerning punishing oneself. It is not beneficial to punish oneself for making mistakes or for getting off track with one's goals. It is important to acknowledge that the mistake has been made, determine why that mistake was made, and determine how to avoid making the same mistake in the future. However, one should not punish themselves for making a mistake; imperfection is inevitable. The individual must move on. Similarly, the individual should not "domino" once they make a mistake. One should not abandon their goals as a result of one mistake. For instance, one may eat fries on a day where they shouldn't (perhaps they've already had their unhealthy foods for the week and reached their capacity). Although this decision may not have aligned with their goals, they shouldn't have the mindset of not caring. Often, people will do so and think they've already made a mistake. What's the harm in making more mistakes? It's already been messed up. They will then proceed to drink soda, have a cheeseburger, and go back to the same pre-goal mindset. However, this should not be the case. When a mistake has been made, the individual should go right back to their goals. They should not stray farther off the path, as this can lead to further damage and possible abandonment of the goals altogether.

Mindset for a Healthier Body

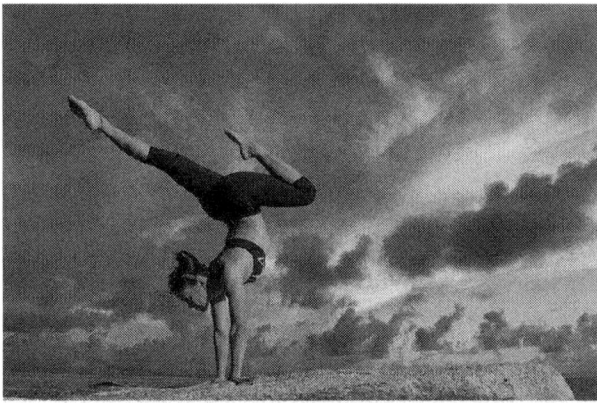

One must adjust their mindset for a healthier body. To achieve a healthier body, one must have a passion for improving their physical health. This is crucial for success. Although one may enjoy eating potato chips and watching television all day, the individual with a proper mindset will be able to take care of themselves properly and have the motivation to help themselves to become better. There are a few factors to adjust when changing one's mindset.

Developing a "You Are What You Eat" Mindset

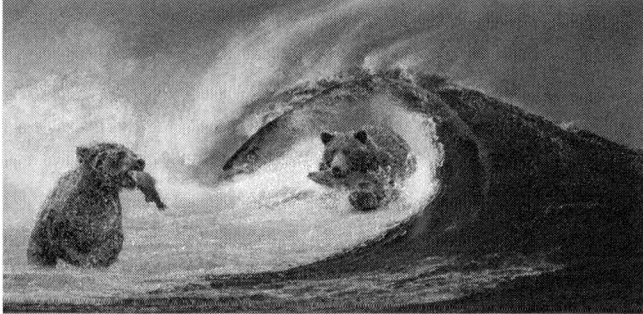

One must first consider the "you are what you eat" mindset. Although this is a common phrase that is typically not given much meaning, it is very true. If one consumes healthy, nutritional foods, their body will be healthy and full of nutrition. If one does not watch the health of the foods they consume, their body will not be healthy. It is important to understand the reasoning for eating well. What an individual puts in their body will directly affect their health. By not caring about one's diet, the individual is increasing their risk of a number of health problems. This can cause short-term and long-term issues for that individual and for their health.

Developing a "Fitness" Mindset

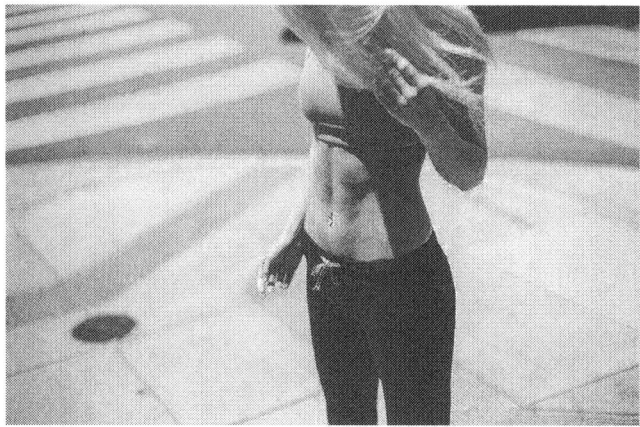

A similar mindset is necessary regarding fitness. Although it may be easy to avoid exercising, it is highly beneficial for the individual to exercise. The individual's fitness level also directly corresponds to their health. One who eats well but doesn't exercise is missing half of the equation and will be unable to unlock their full potential. It is important to stay in motion so that the individual may move properly, especially into older age.

Developing a "Work-Life Balance" Mindset

Another mindset to adopt is that rest is just as important as work. Although it isn't okay to use sleep as an excuse for not watching one's health, the individual must ensure that they are receiving a proper amount of sleep each night. This will help to allow the body to rest from exercise. It will also help the individual to have the proper amount of energy and not to eat to make up for that lost energy. Getting too much sleep is also just as bad as receiving too little sleep. The individual must place a high value on sleep, as it is necessary for one's health.

Developing an Overall Positive Mindset

An overall positive mindset is required for those who wish to have a healthy body. Although there may be many "what if" questions, the individual should have a positive outlook and believe in themselves. Mistakes are inevitable. What matters not is if mistakes are made, they will be. It matters more about how the individual handles themselves after they make a mistake. One may also be tempted to think of negative things when reflecting on their past. Although there may have been mistakes made, the individual must think about the future and how to improve it. They should not dwell on their past mistakes; they are working towards improving their present and future selves. An "everything happens for a reason" mindset is also beneficial when it comes to a healthier body. Some that are overweight or obese may think that they "weren't blessed" with an ideal body. They may think that they are meant to live in the body that they have. By approaching it from an "everything happens for a reason" mindset, the individual may see that there is hope for them. They had that body, and now, it is time to improve that body. By improving themselves so greatly, the individual will have an even greater appreciation for their new body and all of the great progress that they made. There will be a great appreciation for all of the hard work that went into the formation of their newer and better selves.

Mindset for a Healthier Mind

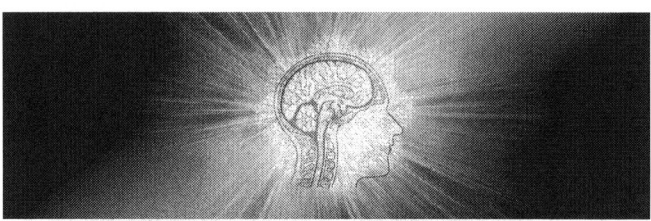

Those who want to be healthier overall must also realize that the mind is just as important as the body. Although it is important to pay attention to physical health, mental health can be just as important (if not, more important). This is because one's mental health directly affects one's physical health. If one is not in the right mindset, they will not work towards improving their physical health and may feel a barrier separating them from their current self to an improved version of themselves. Often, when people speak of health, physical health is what first comes to mind. However, individuals must not neglect mental health, as it shapes who they are. If one's mental health is inadequate, they will not have the motivation to take care of their physical health. They will not have the motivation to work towards their goals and improve themselves, as they will be stuck in the negative emotions that they are feeling.

Taking Care of Oneself

Another important mindset switch regards taking care of oneself. Society constantly seems to force individuals to put everything before themselves. Mothers must put their children before themselves. Giving is more important than receiving. It's important to put in the effort with friends even if they do not put effort into themselves. Although this is a great mindset to have, as it is kind and will be appreciated, one must also watch their own health. It's okay to take time for oneself. It's okay to spend money on oneself. It's okay to indulge in a treat once in a while. There are many ways to pamper oneself, and it should not be an activity to feel guilty about. It is necessary to take time to be alone and relax. When a stressful situation occurs, it is important to step back from the situation and take time to deal with it in a healthy manner. When one does not do so, unhealthy coping mechanisms surface, one of which is emotional eating.

Surrounding Oneself with Other People

In order to improve one's mental health, the individual should also recognize that it is crucial to surround themselves with the proper people. It is okay to distance the self from those who don't make them the best person possible. People that bring negativity into the individual's life should not be given that power. The people that one surrounds themselves with should encourage them to be the best possible person that they are. They should motivate the individual to make progress towards their goals in life.

Being in an Environment in Which One Thrives In

It is also crucial for the individual to reside in an environment that they thrive in. If one does not take care of their surroundings, they will constantly feel overwhelmed and find it difficult to focus on themselves. One way to make this happen is by having a clean environment that is free of distractions or any negative influences. A person's home and workspace should be kept clean in order to maximize their productivity and to improve their mental health. This may also involve creating a "safe space." This is a place that the individual may visit when they need time to be quiet, reflect, and take time to themselves. This may be a room, a favorite place to visit, or simply a chair to read in. No matter where it is, the individual should find the space that best suits them for this purpose. This will really help to improve the individual's mental health, as they will be able to cope better by visiting this space. This is a much healthier way to deal with any stress or issues that may come up in the individual's life. It will allow them to find peace and quiet. Instead of eating emotionally, for example, the individual may take time in this space.

Mindset for Avoiding Addiction

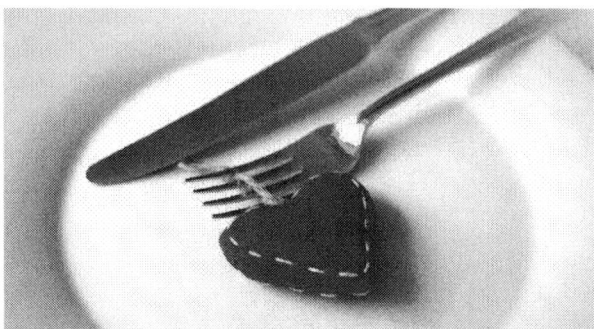

For those with addiction, a certain mindset must be adopted. It is crucial to overcome addiction, as it can take a serious toll on one's health. When overcoming addiction, one must have a positive mindset and be willing to change themselves. It will be difficult, and the individual must be willing to overcome obstacles to rid themselves of the addiction and to help to be a better person. They must also avoid addiction in the future and discipline themselves well enough to prevent relapse from occurring. This is possible with the proper mindset.

Recognizing When Help Is Needed

The individual must be able to recognize when help is needed. Although independence is important, they should not look to others as ones to depend on. Others are there to support and help. It is one's own goals that they are working towards. Sometimes, it is truly beneficial to seek the help of others. The individual must be able to motivate themselves, although they must also recognize when it would be more beneficial to seek the help of others. Perhaps a professional is needed to guide the individual towards their goals. Perhaps it would be beneficial to have a friend or group that shares similar goals. This individual may find it beneficial to receive motivation from others and be able to discuss their progress or exchange tips with others on ways to reach their goals.

Having a Balance Between Cutting Oneself Slack and Staying Motivated

There must be a balance between cutting oneself slack and staying motivated. Although it is important to be able to allow oneself to make mistakes without punishing themselves or becoming overly frustrated, it is also important to not let everything slide. There must be a distinction between trying and actually doing. One must not reward themselves when they have not worked towards their goals. Simply trying is not enough; you must actually put in the effort and make progress towards your goals.

Not Giving Up Along the Way

Similarly, when working towards your goals, it is important not to let the past get in the way. Perhaps a certain strategy has not worked. Perhaps you have tried every diet out there, every workout routine possible. You've joined groups, started a journal, or a number of other attempts. Everyone works differently. Although certain strategies may not have led you to accomplish your goals in the past, it is important to keep making an effort. You must not give up just because you messed up once. Everyone has their own way of motivating themselves. There are thousands of possible ways to better your health. If you've tried dozens of ways, there are still thousands out there waiting for you to try. This mindset is crucial to your success.

Staying Motivated

Those with goals must adopt the proper mindset for achieving such goals. There is also a certain mindset necessary for remaining motivated despite possible obstacles in the way. If one wishes to have a healthy body, one must adopt the proper mindset. Similarly, one who desires improved mental health must also adopt the proper mindset. A proper mindset is also required for those wishing to overcome and prevent future unhealthy addictions for themselves.

Chapter 6: Mindfulness

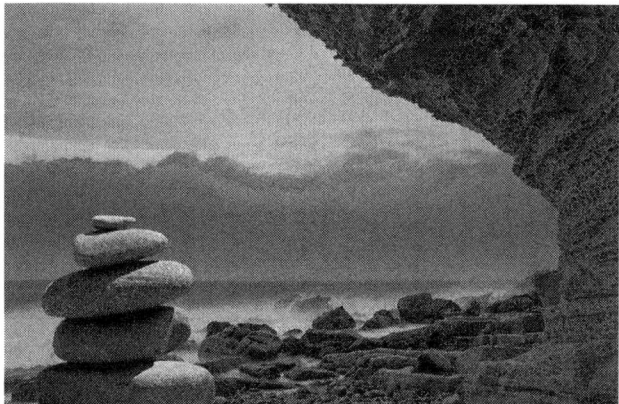

Practicing mindfulness can be beneficial for the body and mind. One that practices mindfulness will be more aware of their emotions and their hunger. One may practice mindful eating to solve certain issues. One may use mindfulness to prevent themselves from giving in to food cravings. Mindfulness may also be used to help one struggling with compulsive overeating. Practicing mindfulness will allow one also to learn how to enjoy the food that they eat. This can help one to overcome certain food addictions and to prevent compulsive overeating. Mindfulness will additionally help one's mental and physical health to be improved.

What Is Mindfulness?

Mindfulness is all about being aware. It means that the mind is aware of what's happening and what is occurring in the surrounding environment. Oftentimes, especially with the increase of dependence upon technology, we are distracted. There are constant messages to read, people to talk to, and places to be. However, it is important to live in the moment and check-in with oneself. We must learn to live in the present instead of dwelling on the past or worrying about the future. This will truly help improve one's physical and mental health.

Mindfulness is about relaxing, not reacting. Stress can lead to overwhelming emotions, yet we must take time to ourselves and listen to our bodies. No matter what is going on, it is important to take time to unwind and listen to your body. It's important to know how you are truly feeling physically and mentally. If there is something bothering you, being mindful will help you to pinpoint what it is that's bothering you. It is important to practice mindfulness at least every once in a while to tune in to your feelings and emotions. This will allow you to treat your body properly.

One common way to practice mindfulness is through meditation, although there are many ways that one may practice mindfulness. It is possible to write down one's feelings, perhaps in a journal, to truly understand what's going on. One may choose to talk to someone, whether that be a friend or a professional. This is a great way to see what's on the mind and what may need to be fixed. One may also choose to have some quiet time to themselves. They may go for a walk, simply sit down, or do whatever it takes for them to have some time to themselves.

It isn't difficult to practice mindfulness. Although many choose to add meditation to their mindfulness exercises, mindfulness may be practiced anywhere by anyone. It doesn't require great change; it simply involves taking the time to be more aware of oneself and one's thoughts. It may also provide those who practice it with several benefits. One will reduce the stress in their life, have more motivation, see their goals more clearly, and gain insight into one's mind. It will also help one to become more aware of their thoughts and increase one's ability to focus on themselves and on others. It may also make certain issues clearer that the individual would have missed otherwise.

Mindfulness for Food Cravings and Compulsive Overeating

Mindfulness can help with a number of issues, some of which are food cravings and compulsive overeating. When one practices mindfulness, they may occupy their mind with topics other than that of cravings. This provides short-term memory with a distraction, therefore interrupting cravings. When practiced in the long-term, mindfulness can work to eventually stop cravings and prevent them from occurring in the future. Mindfulness has been found to help with addictions to food, drugs, and alcohol. This is a method to try for those struggling with cravings and addictions.

Cravings result from an intense desire at the moment to fulfill some "need." For instance, one may have an intense craving for food. This craving will typically subside if the individual waits it out. However, cravings can be so intense that the individual can't wait; they must give in and fulfill their craving. If one practices mindfulness, however, they may be able to recognize that this craving is only temporary and is not caused by any logical reason. It is simply the body wanting what it can't have. It is especially helpful if the individual recognizes that this craving is not something that they need. This can be particularly true for highly unhealthy cravings, such as foods high in sugar, salt, and fat. Cravings may result from a particular emotion or situation that triggers it. If the individual can pinpoint the origin of this craving, they may help themselves more. For instance, the individual may reflect on their feelings and determine that they are feeling stressed. Instead of giving in to their craving of a dozen donuts, they may realize that they are stressed and do an activity that relieves such stress instead.

Mindfulness may also be used for compulsive overeating. Instead of continuing to shove food in your mouth, you may be more mindful. It is necessary to get used to the feeling of when you are full so that you may understand when it is time to stop eating. During meals, take the time to register how you are feeling. When you are full, don't continue eating. Perhaps listen to your body and determine why you think you should continue eating. Is it a feeling of guilt? Perhaps you don't want to waste food. If this is the case, develop a smart and easy way to save food. Perhaps you don't even realize that you are full because you eat without thinking. This is why it's crucial to check in with yourself throughout the meal to determine if you are eating to fuel your body or if you are eating mindlessly. This is important to determine so that you may prevent yourself from overeating. When you are mindful, you will be more aware of how your body feels. You will be able to determine if you are full. If so, you will know when it's the proper time to stop eating.

Incorporating Mindfulness into Your Life

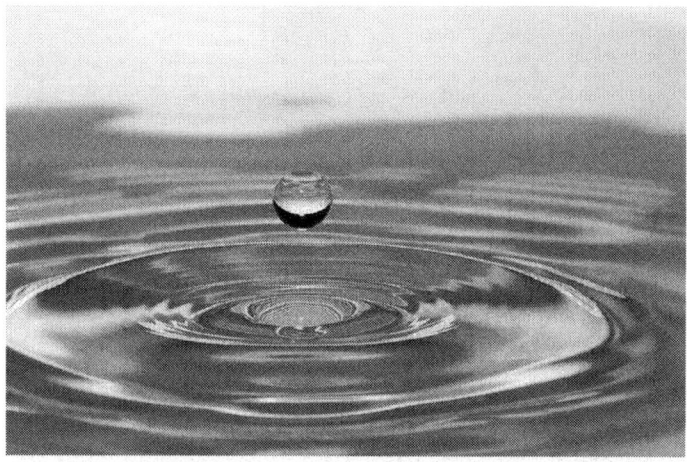

When one thinks of mindfulness, they may imagine the stereotypical meditator—burning a candle, legs crossed, soothing music, eyes closed, and maybe even humming. Although meditation is a great way to practice mindfulness and train the body to relax while the mind focuses; this is not the only way that one may practice mindfulness. There are several exercises and strategies for becoming more mindful. It doesn't have to be difficult to start with, and there are many options so that anyone may enjoy the process of becoming more mindful and having a more relaxed and focused mind.

To be mindful, one must be quiet and listen to their body. There are many apps out there that allow one to enjoy guided mindfulness sessions. This is a simple way for a beginner to start their mindfulness journey without having to worry about learning to guide themselves; they must simply listen to the guide. There are also many videos on the Internet with guided mindfulness sessions. This is a great way for a beginner to start. For an Internet-free option, one may choose just to sit and breathe. This can be for an extended period of time or simply a couple of minutes. While breathing, the individual should focus on their breath and be aware of their body's reaction to that breath. If the mind wanders, the individual should bring it back to their breath. This has the greatest benefit when the individual truly carves out their time for this experience. Otherwise, they will feel rushed and unable to focus on being mindful. Mindfulness can't be rushed. Instead of viewing it as something that must be done before moving on with the day, it must be viewed as an important part of the day. This will give it greater importance.

One may practice mindfulness while they eat. This means paying attention while one is eating. One may practice mindfulness while walking and focus on the movement of their body and their surroundings. One may practice mindful breathing, really focusing on the effect of breathing on the body. Connecting with the senses every once in a while is another way to be mindful. The individual may focus on what they are seeing, smelling, touching, tasting, hearing, and feeling at the moment. Mindful listening is crucial for both gaining knowledge and building better relationships. Instead of focusing on one's surroundings or on anything but the present, the individual should listen to the speaker and what they have to say. Full listening is much more mindful than thinking of what to say next or letting the mind wander to other topics. Taking little pauses throughout the day is also a great way to be mindful of the little things in life. One may also pause to consider their current thoughts and emotions. One may also take mindful showers and baths, truly enjoying the sensation of water on the skin. Yoga is a great way to be mindful, as it teaches the individual to focus on their breathing while being aware of the body. Of course, a very common way to practice mindfulness is by meditating.

Learning How to Enjoy Your Food

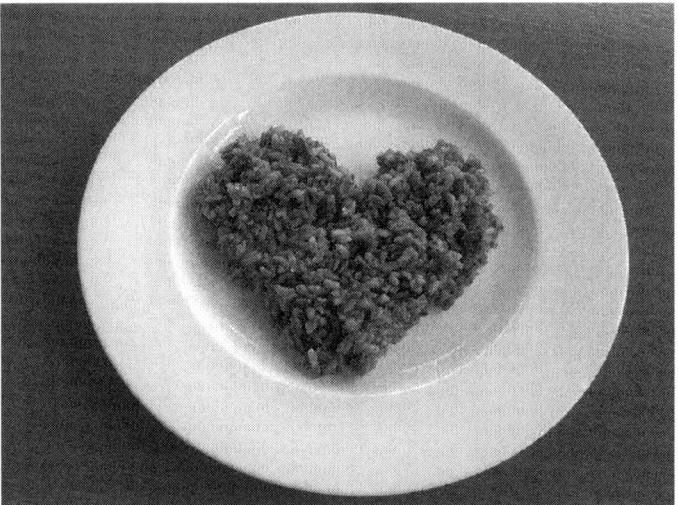

One who eats mindfully can really help themselves. Mindfully eating can keep one fuller for longer, reduce cravings, prevent overeating, and simply help the individual to enjoy their food and mealtime in general. It helps one to take control of their eating habits.

Freeing Oneself of Distractions

While eating, one should free themselves of distractions. Often, we eat while on our phones, watching television, or otherwise while distracted. One who eats mindfully will rid themselves of distractions and instead focus on the present. This means truly taking the time to appreciate the look of the food, the smell of the food, and the taste of the food. One will begin to view food as a blessing, something that is truly worth appreciating. When we don't take the time to appreciate our food truly, the brain won't register it. This is a common reason for overeating. We don't realize how much food we are putting in our bodies, so we keep putting more in. Instead of doing this, it is crucial to register every bite that we take and to really think about the food as we eat it.

Focusing on Hunger

Another way to eat mindfully is to focus on hunger. One should only eat when truly hungry. This means paying attention to the body's hunger cues. Instead of eating for fun or when one is bored, one should only eat when they are truly hungry. Listening to the body's cues will help with this. Additionally, one should only eat until they are full. Overstuffing oneself is an easy way to overeat. This can be prevented by really listening to the body's cues and determining when it is time to stop. The body will no longer give hunger cues.

Before eating, one should pay attention to their emotions. Are they eating as the result of a certain emotion, or is it due to hunger? One should notice how they feel about eating, too. Is there anxiety regarding eating? While eating, one should remain focused on their feelings and how the food makes them feel. What are the effects of food on the body and mind? The foods that one eats should not make them feel guilty or anxious, and they should make the body feel good. A person experiencing guilt or anxiety about the foods they consume or noticing a negative impact on their body and mind should make a dietary change to improve how they feel.

Mindfulness can prove highly beneficial for individuals. Mindfulness is the practice of being quiet and paying attention to one's mind and body. It can help with one's eating habits. It can help those who struggle with compulsive overeating or with hard-to-handle food cravings. It is quite easy to incorporate mindfulness into one's life, and there are several ways to do so. One may also try mindful eating, which is becoming more aware of their food while they eat. Practicing mindfulness is helpful for the body.

Chapter 7: Intuitive Eating

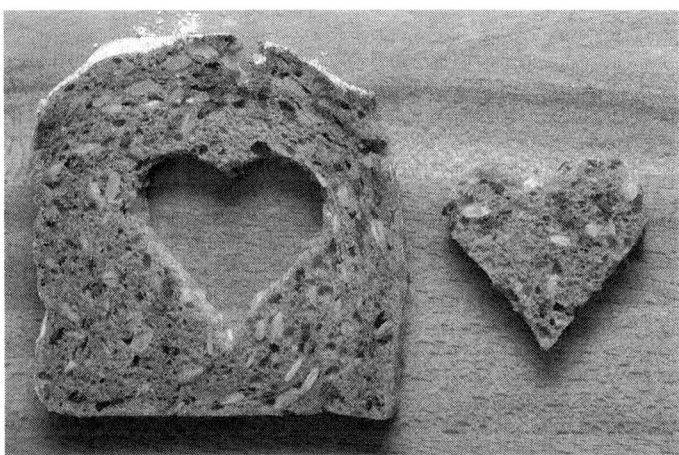

Intuitive eating is another way to improve one's health. It is important for one to understand what intuitive eating is so that they may incorporate it into their life. One may also learn how to practice intuitive eating to improve their health. There are certain intuitive habits that one may also begin to improve their health. It is important that one also sets intuitive goals to maximize their potential as a person. There are many benefits of intuitive eating, and there are several positive effects that it will have on the person who practices eating intuitively.

What Is Intuitive Eating?

Intuitive eating and mindful eating are often used interchangeably, yet their functions and practices differ. Mindful eating is being aware of the whole eating experience. It requires one to focus on their food and their feelings. However, intuitive eating relies more on one's intuition. One must really pay attention to the gut instinct they have. They must learn to eat for physical reasons instead of emotional reasons. This really relies on one's ability to understand their internal hunger and satiety cues. Although mindfulness can assist with understanding these concepts, one must rely on their intuition to really feel this. Mindfulness is the process of understanding how to use these concepts. Intuitive eating is the concept itself and may be used alongside mindfulness.

Intuitive eating is not about restricting oneself to a certain diet. It's not about counting calories, weighing yourself every day, or worrying about macros. In fact, those may actually contribute to overeating and emotional troubles. When doing this, one is just disconnected from themselves. They think more about numbers than how they actually feel. Although they may have an ideal waist size, look fit in photographs, or weigh their ideal weight, they may not be truly happy.

Intuitively eating requires the individual to pay attention to their hunger, not their boredom. It teaches people not to feel guilty about enjoying themselves and eating their favorite food. This helps to promote emotional wellness. It's important to not think about the numbers or any foods that make one feel guilty. It is more about listening to the body, which is the natural way to eat and live. It relies on internal cues as opposed to external cues. This will help the individual determine how much they should eat, what foods their body needs, and when to eat. On the other hand, those who undergo a diet are likely to be unhappy. They will restrict themselves to eating certain foods. When this occurs, they are likely to crash at some point. While dieting, people are following what works for others' bodies. However, each individual's body differs. Everyone has different wants and needs, and those must be fulfilled differently for each person. People may eat certain foods because they're generally regarded as "good" or "healthy," but it is important to eat what makes the body feel good. One should let go of any anxiety or grief over certain foods and find out what really helps to provide them with energy and happiness.

How to Eat Intuitively and Implement Intuitive Habits

To eat intuitively, one must abandon the "dieting" mentality. One must learn to not focus on weight loss or on numbers in general. They must not feel guilty for their lack of progress towards losing weight. You may have books or magazines with dieting tips; get rid of them. Diets are just fads. They contribute to gaining weight more often than losing weight. Rid yourself of dieting influences. If you follow any dieting pages on social media, unfollow them. Take control of your life instead of letting diets take control of your life. Surround yourself with positive messages regarding health and food. Cut out any negative people in your life that bring you down. Instead, surround yourself with positive health influences. Stop trying to chase after diets with the same results. Start out fresh and reset your body and mind.

Truly listen to your body's sense of hunger. This is a naturally-occurring process that signals when it is time to eat. Eating is necessary for life. It is necessary to keep your energy up. You must be able to really learn when your body needs to be refueled. Much like a car's gas light may go on, your body will start to send you apparent signals when it must be refueled. If you ignore these signals, your body will respond. As time passes, your body will become more desperate for food and begin craving some foods. You may also feel the need to binge or otherwise overeat to compensate for this prolonged hunger. By feeding yourself at the proper time, you are allowing your body to be fueled properly.

Similarly, you should understand the concept of fullness. You shouldn't feel obligated to eat when you don't want to or need to. You should also not feel guilty for leaving any food uneaten. Listen to your body and understand when you are full and have had enough. It is also important to distinguish between fullness and satisfaction. You may be full but not satisfied. Often, we will crave a certain food and will still be "hungry" until we finally eat that food. Instead of listening to our bodies, we will usually try to "feed" that craving other foods. The body, however, will still be hungry because it is not satisfied. Satisfying that craving can often prevent one from this overeating that occurs, and it will usually take less food to satisfy yourself.

You must also make peace with all the food. Eating one donut won't take you from a healthy weight to obesity. When you restrict yourself to certain foods, your body will crave the off-limits foods even more. You may feel trapped and will feel guilty about consuming any of the "taboo" foods. By disallowing oneself to have certain foods, you will feel deprived and begin developing deep cravings for these foods. When you do finally consume that food, you will likely overeat and feel guilty once more. You should not categorize foods into what is good or bad. This will only lead to guilt. Eating should be an enjoyable experience, yet it can become an activity that causes anxiety when one labels their food or criticizes themselves.

With intuitive eating, one must also pay attention to their emotions. Emotional eating occurs as a result of these emotions. Instead of coping with emotions using food, you should find another and healthier way to handle these emotions. Although the food may help with emotions, it may not be such a great idea. Often, it won't actually help. It is just a temporary distraction for a bigger issue. It is also really unwise to use eating as one's primary coping mechanism. There should be a variety of ways to help yourself feel better.

Reject vanity. With intuitive eating, one is focusing on how their body feels. If you only care about how your body looks, you may not even be truly healthy. You should not criticize your body or dislike yourself. A healthy body comes along with intuitive eating and exercise. However, one should not change their habits purely out of vanity purposes. It is important to recognize how much it matters to treat your body well. You're only given one body in your life, so you must honor it.

The same is true for exercise. Not all of us are supposed to be (or want to be) bodybuilders. It's okay if you don't like running. You should build a fitness routine that you like. That way, you'll enjoy exercising and will even look forward to it! This means that working out will become a fun activity instead of seeming like a chore. You should also pay attention to how exercising makes you feel. This is why to do it. You will have more energy, you may sleep better, and you will have more motivation.

Intuitive eating is all about abandoning the typical ways that one loses weight. You don't have to follow a certain diet. There's no "perfect" workout routine. It's all about you. It's about what you like. It's about what makes you feel good. You should pay attention to your body and how everything you do makes you feel. Although there are certain foods out there that are higher in nutritional value, you should go off of how you feel. Are the foods you eat satisfying? Are the foods you eat tasty? Of course, you may want to try putting more nutritious foods into your diet. However, you shouldn't do so because you feel obligated to or because you would feel guilty otherwise. It should be because you want to. It should be because you feel good after eating them. You must also recognize that your diet as a whole is what matters. Over time, your diet should make you feel good. It isn't all or nothing. Having some French fries or soda here and there is okay. Allow yourself to love what you eat and not feel so guilty about what you eat.

Intuitive Eating Effects

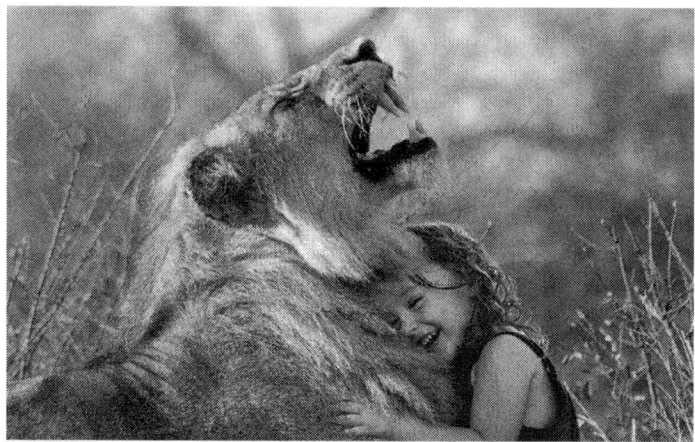

Intuitive eating has a number of positive effects on the body. It will lead to higher self-esteem and better body image. This is because instead of being fixated on your weight, waist size, or the foods that you eat, you will pay attention to how you feel. You will feel good and therefore know that you're treating your body well. You will feel much better about yourself after intuitive eating than you could ever feel with any diet or exercise routine. You'll follow the right path for your body, not the path that someone else created for themselves.

You will feel more satisfied with life. In general, you'll learn how to pay attention more to what you really want in life. In addition to your physical health, you will know what makes you happy and what doesn't. This will help you to feel much better about your life. The idea of not feeling guilty for doing what others are doing will truly help you to be more satisfied with your life. You'll stop comparing yourself to others and paying attention to numbers. Life will be more about how you feel, and if you're happy, not what others think it should be.

You will become more optimistic. In addition to feeling more satisfied with life, you will feel happier overall because you are doing what you like. You won't pay attention to negativity. You'll be surrounding yourself with those who are also positive and optimistic. Life will be more about enjoying yourself instead of following someone else's blueprint. You will view life as something that you are excited about, not something you should be better at.

Intuitive eating will greatly help your mental health. You will become better at coping and will develop better coping mechanisms for your emotions. This will also lead to a lower rate of emotional eating.

Those who implement intuitive eating also see physical results. Lower body mass indexes have been found with those who eat intuitively. It works! The right body will come with emotional eating. Those who eat intuitively also notice higher HDL cholesterol levels and lower triglyceride levels. Those who eat intuitively will also decrease their amount of cravings and decrease the likelihood of overeating. Because one will learn how to fill and satisfy their body, they won't feel the need to compensate by bingeing or by overeating in any way, giving in to cravings.

It is important to understand intuitive eating. Implementing it can have great effects on the body. There are several ways to implement intuitive eating into your life. You will be able to recognize when you are hungry and when you are full. Your physical and mental health will both receive a boost from intuitive eating. It can be combined with mindfulness and mindful eating to help your body to become the best that it possibly can. Your mental health will also receive a boost, and you will become much happier with yourself and with your life. Intuitive eating is truly beneficial for one's health.

Chapter 8: Detoxing

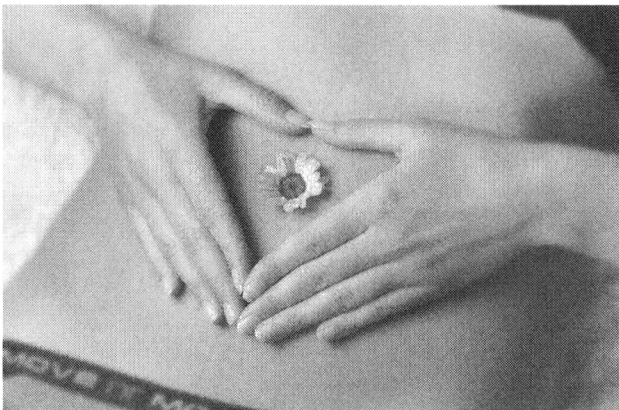

We've all heard of detoxing. It's used to rid the body of toxins and as a way to reverse any damage that we've caused to it. It's typically the result of one feeling unhappy with the way their body feels. They seek a solution to that nasty feeling and go on a detox as a result. There are many ways to detox and many foods that one may seek a detox from. Typically, one thinks of a juice cleanse when they hear the word detox. This is not the only way to detox, however.

What Is a Sugar Detox?

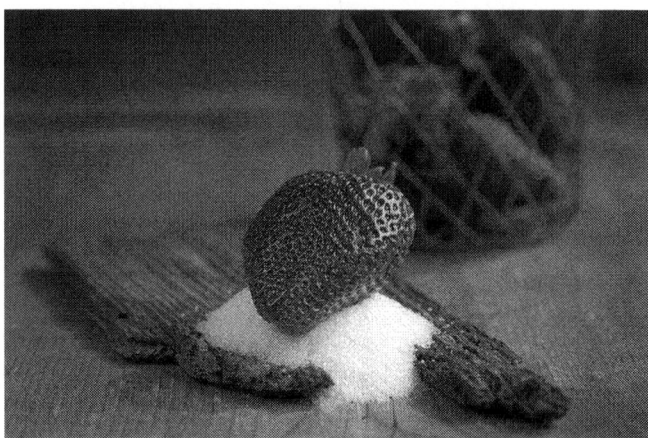

One way to cut one's sugar intake is to go on a sugar detox. This is when you cut out sugar for a certain period of time, and your body learns how to survive without it. It isn't easy for many, as we are surrounded by a great number of sugary options each day.

Most people consume more sugar each day than they are supposed to (four to five times the recommended maximum). Even if the sugar detox isn't permanent, it can train the body to survive without sugar and begin to ease sugar cravings. The health benefits of reducing sugar in one's body are numerous. By decreasing the amount of sugar in your diet, you are lowering your risk for medical conditions and improving your mental health. You will also experience several physical benefits by doing so. However, it can be quite difficult at first. We crave sugar and are surrounded by so many options with much-added sugar.

Sugar is quite addictive. It has been shown to affect the same parts of the brain that nicotine, cocaine, and morphine do. It makes us happy to eat it, and we look forward to it. Although this doesn't seem detrimental, this is not good when sugar affects the body negatively. The body also needs more sugar as time passes, as it becomes tolerant to the sugar and needs more of it to allow for the same effects to occur to the body. When one consumes sugar, they experience a rush of energy, which can feel good and uplifting. One that cuts out sugar, however, will not be getting the same rush, and their body will have intense cravings for sugar and the rush that comes with it.

With sugar, detoxes may calm the effects of sugar withdrawal. When this occurs, one may experience a number of side effects as a result of cutting out sugar from their diet. One may experience cravings, may have difficulty focusing, may have depression or anxiety, and may find it difficult to get proper sleep. One may also experience headaches, low energy, light-headedness, dizziness, nausea, tingling, and fatigue. This will make it difficult for the person undergoing detox at first. One may typically get past these feelings if they stick with it for ten days. However, most that attempt sugar detoxes don't realize this and think that their bodies still need sugar. This is not true. The body must simply go through an adjustment phase before being comfortable without sugar.

How to Sugar Detox

Before beginning a sugar detox, you should plan for it and determine how you will do it. Although you can try a sugar detox for a long period of time, such as thirty days, it is typical to detox for three to ten days. This will help you to go cold turkey and completely eliminate sugar for that period of time. This will give your body time to adjust, yet it won't seem like so long that it is unrealistic for you. For this period of time, you will completely cut out any added, refined, artificial, and natural sugars. It is highly beneficial to seek help from a medical professional while on a sugar detox. They may give you any advice based on your health. This advice can be personal, and you should seek the advice of a medical professional before beginning a detox in case of any health conditions that would prevent you from doing so. The professional will also ensure that your diet remains balanced while on the detox. Although you are cutting out sugar, you should still be well-fed and be getting all the proper vitamins and nutrients while you are on the detox.

You may also try easing into a sugar detox. You may decide to do this in a few ways. You may first decide to focus on one meal, such as improving your breakfast. Then, you can work at lunch. Then, you can improve your dinner. You may also work on cutting out sugary snacks and desserts. You may also ease into it by cutting out certain foods and cutting out more each week until you reach a level of sugar-free goodness. You may first work on beverages and then move to foods. Some people may benefit more from easing into a sugar detox. This can occur over a certain period, such as over four weeks. You may divide the detox into four stages to make it more realistic for you.

It's also important that you take care of the mental aspects of going on a sugar detox. You may want to journal to have a place to jot down your feelings. You should remind yourself why you are going on a sugar detox. It is important to remind yourself of the health benefits of going on a sugar detox to know that you are helping your body and mind by embarking on a sugar detox journey.

Benefits of Sugar Detoxes

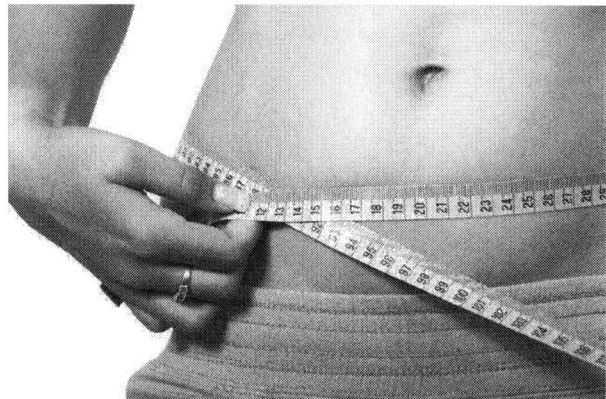

Sugar detoxes provide those who go on them with a number of benefits. Sugary foods tend not to have great nutritional value. Replacing those foods with more nourishing foods can really help the body to function better. The body's digestion, metabolism, and overall health will be improved. The body will be able to produce and use energy much more efficiently and effectively. Plus, the body won't experience crashes that it does when filled with sugar.

One will also enjoy the benefit of weight loss that comes with sugar detoxing. Cutting sugar is a great way to shed some pounds. Sugar helps the body to store more fat. By eliminating sugar, the body will decrease its stored fat. This will help you to have more energy and decrease your risk for health problems. Those who are overweight or obese have an increased risk of health issues, especially that of heart disease. Additionally, losing weight will help you to have more energy and be able to move more easily. You will also have higher self-confidence and self-esteem.

You will experience mental benefits by cutting sugar. You will regenerate the mind by detoxing. Instead of using glucose to fuel your brain, your mind will rely on more sustainable sources of fuel. Instead of crashing and becoming sluggish, you will be able to focus and concentrate better. Your mind won't be foggy from all of the extra sugar anymore. It will be easier for you to pay attention to what you love instead of being dragged down by sugar. Your cognitive function will be improved. Instead of being easily distracted, you will be able to think again. You will have more energy again. This will help with both thinking and moving. When consuming sugar, you may have a spike of energy that's quickly followed by a crash. When you crash, your body hits a low. You don't have any energy, and you are unable to concentrate. Eliminating sugar eliminates the crash that comes with it, allowing you to think better and have more energy.

You will see an improvement in your appearance. Your teeth and gums will be healthier after cutting out sugar. You will also improve the health of your skin, as acne can be caused by a surplus of sugar. Water retention will be reduced, so the appearance of bloating and swelling will improve. This can occur in the stomach, arms, legs, and fingers.

You will also decrease your risk of certain health problems. By decreasing the amount of sugar in your diet, you are decreasing your risk of developing heart disease. Your body will also be able to manage Type 2 Diabetes more efficiently and effectively. Reducing sugar will reduce your risk of non-alcoholic fatty liver disease, too. Your risk for Polycystic Ovarian Syndrome will also be reduced. You can really help your health by decreasing your sugar intake.

Detoxing Tips

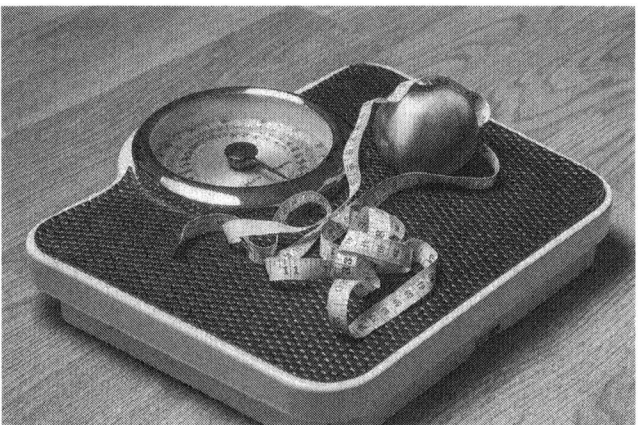

It can be difficult to go on a sugar detox. There are a few ways to make it a bit easier for yourself, though. There are several strategies for making your transition from your normal diet to going on a sugar detox. It can be a tough adjustment for your body, especially since your body will still crave sugar at first. You may seem depleted of energy, and your body will try to overcompensate for the decreased amount of sugar by giving you intense cravings, especially for sugary and high-carb foods.

One way to make detoxing easier for yourself is by quitting completely and quickly. Instead of trying to ease into a diet with less sugar, it is better to "shock" your body. Although you may experience more intense cravings and side effects, you won't experience these for as long. Your body will be forced to get used to it quickly, and your withdrawal symptoms will subside more quickly. It's like jumping into a cool pool instead of easing in. Your body will be forced to get used to it more quickly. Instead of feeling a little cool and going back on your decision, you will get used to it more quickly. This way, you'll be used to it before you even have the chance to second-guess yourself. It is best to simply cut out all sugary prepackaged foods, sweetened beverages, and white flour all at once. That way, you also won't be tempted to rely on one food for your sugar intake. For instance, if you only cut out sweetened beverages at first, you may be tempted to eat white flour and sugary foods to compensate for that. You may even justify worsening some habits as a result of improving others.

It is beneficial to increase your water, protein, and fiber intake. Protein will help your body to stay full for longer and keep your energy levels up. Fiber will help you to keep full for longer and regulate your blood sugar. This will help to decrease the likelihood of headaches, nausea, and cravings. You should drink more water as well. Staying hydrated will help you to avoid overeating. Since hunger and thirst feel similar, drinking water will help you not to mistake thirst for hunger. Staying hydrated will also help with digestion and will help minimize cravings.

It is best to avoid artificial sweeteners. Although it may seem beneficial to replace sugar with alternatives, it can impede your progress. These sweeteners will lead to sugar cravings and will leave your body dependent on sugar still. It gives the body false hope that sugary foods are still allowed.

It's also important to manage your overall health. There are aspects besides your diet that you must pay attention to. Managing your stress and dealing with your emotions in a healthy way is a great way to help with minimizing sugar cravings. It's also crucial to exercise. This can help assist with cravings, low energy levels, and fatigue. Ensuring that you are receiving a proper amount of sleep will also help with cognitive function, energy levels, and improved food choices.

Going on a sugar detox can be truly beneficial for your health. By cutting out processed foods, artificial sweeteners, sugary beverages, and grains for even just ten days, your body will get a chance to reset. You'll start off on a fresh slate; this will allow you to go in any direction with your diet. You will feel much better and experience great physical and mental health benefits from going on a sugar detox. It is important to understand what it is and why to do it before doing a detox.

Chapter 9: Taking Care of Your Mental Health

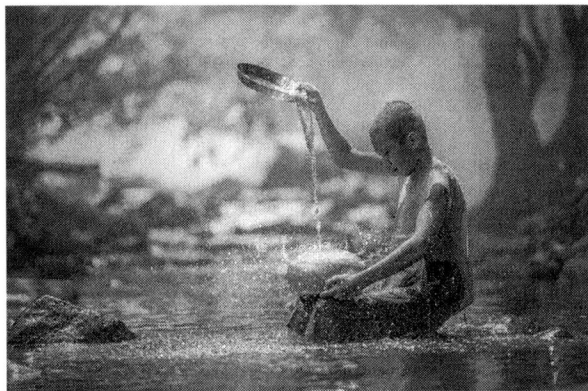

Taking care of your mental health is just as important as taking care of your physical health. Oftentimes, we neglect our mental health and only view "health" as physical health. However, your mental health can have a direct effect on your mental health. When you neglect your mental health, your physical health will suffer as a result. You must become more aware of your emotions, learn what makes you happy, stop negative body-talk, start practicing positive body-talk, practice self-care, love yourself, and learn how to practice self-respect and self-compassion. Doing these will really help you to improve your mental health.

Becoming More Aware of Your Emotions

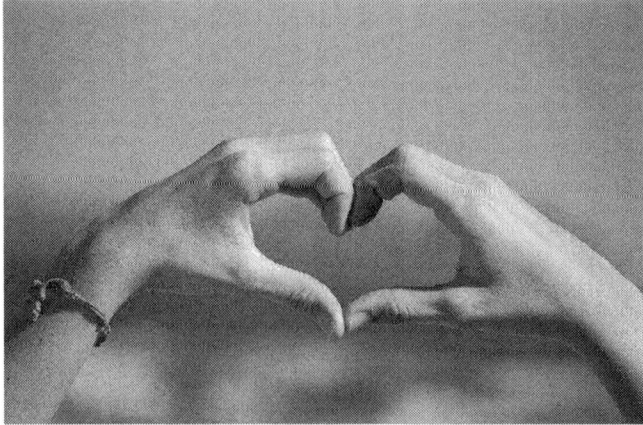

It's crucial to become more aware of your thoughts, feelings, and emotions so that you have a better grasp of how you're feeling. You will understand as well how you can handle yourself when you feel a certain type of way. You must be able to tune in to these thoughts and choose an appropriate way to respond to them. Your body may give you some more obvious hints that you feel a certain type of way. For instance, you may tear up when sad, yell when angry, and smile when happy. However, you can easily be sad and not cry. You don't have to yell to feel angry. It's important to develop an awareness of your emotions. It's best to control your emotions, not let your emotions control you. You can change your mindset and even direct your emotions.

One way to become more aware of your emotions is to look for patterns. Perhaps you feel similarly around a certain person, after performing a certain task, or after visiting a certain place. Jot down everything that makes you upset. There are probably patterns when it comes to this. Perhaps you feel the same stress each time you have a shift at work longer than nine hours. You should reflect on this and understand what triggers certain emotions.

Throughout the day, check-in with yourself. Understand what you are feeling and try to understand why you are feeling that way. It will help to realize what causes certain emotions. Learn how you handle certain emotions, too. When you feel angry, do you tend to take it out on others? When you're stressed, do you eat certain foods or eat more than usual? Notice the habits associated with your feelings so that you may gain a better understanding of your responses.

Try to have certain activities that you use as reflecting activities throughout the day. Perhaps you can reflect on your feelings while in the shower. Going on a walk is a great way to allow yourself some time to think. You spend all day paying attention to the needs of others and trying to read others' emotions. However, you must take some time to check in with yourself and understand how you are feeling. If it's hard for you to tap into your emotions, consider your behavior. Do certain people, places, or situations cause you to change your patterns? You may see an impact on your productivity, energy levels, or communications with others. These are great ways to identify how you are feeling.

It is necessary also to consider what helps with certain emotions. Perhaps you identify that you are feeling sad. Try to understand what helps you cope with certain emotions. When you're sad, you may find that talking to friends helps you every time. You must not only understand how you are feeling and what caused that feeling, but you must also understand how to cope with the different feelings that you experience throughout the day.

Learning What Makes You Happy

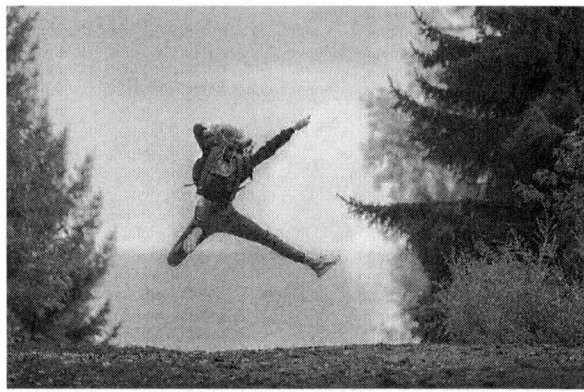

When you identify patterns in your emotions, you will be able to see who and what makes you happy, as well as where you are most happy. Happiness is evident when you are able to better communicate with others, your energy level is up, and your productivity is increased. You will be able to think more clearly. You will have a more positive outlook on life and will find more enjoyment in the activities you partake in. You may also find yourself living in the moment more, as opposed to dwelling on the past or worrying about the future.

You may already have some ideas in mind for what makes you happy. Identify places that you go that always leave you feeling happier. Understand which people in your life increase your happiness. It's also important to identify certain tasks, situations, and events that make you feel happier. You must key into your own emotions. It may be tempting to see others get happy over certain things, yet those may not make us truly happy. For instance, your aunt may adore cooking, but you may think of it as simply mediocre. Perhaps you really enjoy the experience of eating out at a restaurant. You must not base your happiness on other people, social media, advertisements, popular culture, or anything other than your own feelings.

You can start over with happiness and really take the time to understand how you feel about certain things. Jot down any time that you feel truly happy, worry-free, and energetic. You may make your list more specific to find out what you love. It's possible that you can't stand going to the gym alone, and it feels like a chore to you. However, going to the gym with your cousin may leave you feeling good about yourself and refreshed.

Once you have identified the places, people, and situations that make you happy, incorporate them into your life more. Take time every day to do at least one small thing that makes you very happy. Allocate at least one time each week to do a bigger thing that makes you happy. Perhaps you enjoy writing and take the time to journal every night before bed. You may also enjoy going to the beach, so you may plan a few hours every Saturday to do that and really make the most out of it. If you aren't doing what makes you happy in life, you won't be happy and enjoy life. It's that simple!

Improving Your Self-Talk

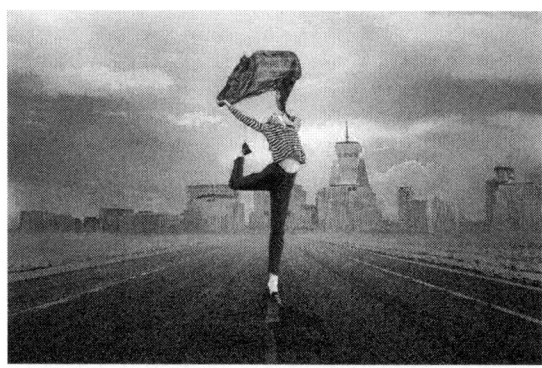

Your self-talk is your internal dialogue. It's what you tell yourself inside your head and the way you think about yourself. You may have positive self-talk, which is when you hype yourself up and have a pep talk with yourself. Negative self-talk is when you cut yourself down. You may think you're not good enough or that your body isn't the way you want it to be. You must increase your positive self-talk and decrease your negative self-talk to improve your mental health.

You must lower and stop your negative self-talk and negative body-talk. It is important to identify when you negative self-talk the most. Certain situations may increase your likelihood of having negative self-talk. It is important to identify this and stop it in its tracks. Otherwise, you can doubt yourself, lower your confidence, and feel unworthy. You may not feel good about yourself and judge yourself. However, you must not judge yourself. You must recognize all of the wonderful things about yourself and be proud of who you are. Aside from recognizing how you feel (and when), you should also begin to identify the patterns of your self-talk.

Eliminating negative self-talk is crucial. You can't blame yourself for everything. Everybody makes mistakes, and you must learn from mistakes to become a better person. A positive outlook on life is necessary. Focusing on the negative aspects of people, places, and situations is not okay. You can't let your worries or emotions get the best of you. Of course, not everything goes to plan. However, you can't always expect the worst in every situation. Life consists of many aspects, not just the negative aspects.

You must increase your positive self-talk. This is when you think positively about yourself. You are confident, positive, and motivated. This will help you to build positive thoughts. You will also improve your self-esteem by increasing the frequency of your positive self-talk. You will be more productive, be more satisfied with your life, improve your health, and feel less stressed. It's important to shift your internal dialogue from negative to positive.

It's important to check in with yourself to ensure that you are thinking positively. If you can catch yourself in the act, it will be easier to remind yourself that you are thinking irrationally. You may bring yourself back to where you need to be and switch your mindset. It is important to surround yourself with those who are positive so that you may be encouraged and inspired by them. When you surround yourself with negative people, you will be tempted to adopt the same mindset. They may also bring you down or criticize you, which may decrease your self-worth. Remind yourself how amazing you are, and remember that you can accomplish anything you set your mind to. Identify what makes you think more positively. Perhaps laughter and happiness can lead to positive self-talk. Spending time with a certain person may also help with this. Identify what works for you. You should spend more time doing these tasks and being with these people, especially when you find yourself having negative self-talk.

Practicing Self-Care

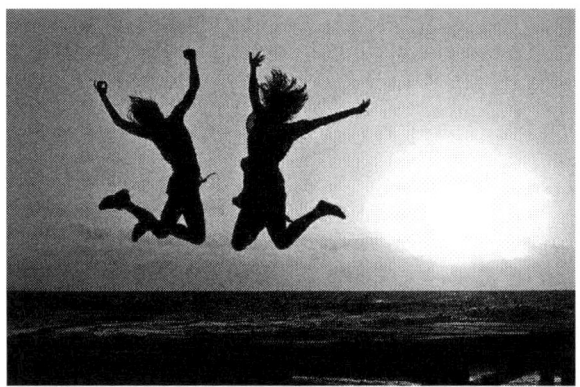

Of course, you probably care about yourself. You want to live and care about yourself. However, self-care is more than just caring about yourself. It's about going out of the way to do something for yourself to take care of your mental, emotional, or physical health. It's very important to practice self-care, yet it's typically not done as much as it should be. By practicing self-care, you will improve your health, your mood, and your relationship with yourself. You will also be able to care for others better.

Practicing self-care is doing something that will make you feel better and happier. Although it is about improving your health, it must also be something that you enjoy. It can't be forced. Running may be a great way to get exercise and improve your health. However, it is not self-care to force yourself to run when you don't genuinely enjoy running. When you practice self-care, you will feel better. It is necessary for you to practice self-care often to ensure that you are taking care of yourself.

Many people refuse to practice self-care. Although it is a wonderful trait to care about making others happy and to go out of your way to do so, you must take care of yourself. Some view self-care as a selfish act. It is quite the opposite. You must practice self-care so that you take care of yourself properly. When you practice it, you will feel much better, and your ability to care for others will improve. When you feel happy, you will be able to spread that happiness to others more easily. You can't love someone else if you don't love yourself first.

There are many ways to practice self-care. However, there is a proper way to do it and make it easier for yourself. Although you can go out and get a full spa treatment every week at your local spa, that can be quite costly. You don't have to make self-care expensive, time-consuming, or complicated. It should be able to fit into your routine easily. You must also make the active choice to plan out and set aside time for self-care. It must be thought of as self-care in order for you to truly enjoy it and all of the benefits it offers.

There are many activities and choices that you can make to practice self-care. One way is to cut out the things in your life that you don't enjoy. Don't talk to people who bring you down. Don't attend events that you don't like. Do what you love. Another way is to take care of your diet and exercise. You may get a proper amount of sleep. Exercising (the way that you like to) is a great way to practice self-care. Monitor your health with doctor visits, dentist visits, and therapy sessions (if desired). Take time to relax. This could be in whatever way you choose. Some enjoy at-home spa days; others enjoy meditating. You can try yoga, reading, writing, drawing, or whatever it is that brings you peace. You can also plan to spend time with friends and family. Overall, find activities that make you happy and actively plan for those activities.

Loving Yourself

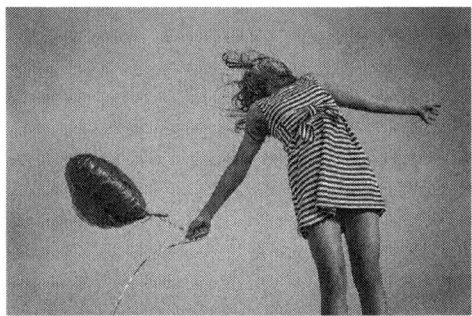

Loving yourself is crucial for your mental health. You must love and appreciate the person you are. This will help you to feel more confident and increase your positivity. It is important that you realize what a great person you are. You must not cut yourself down or think of yourself poorly. Your self-confidence and self-worth will increase when you love yourself more. You may find it easier to trust others, communicate with others, and form relationships with others. You will develop a better grasp of who you are and what you love in life. It will be easier to take care of yourself, and you will value your health more as a result of loving yourself more. You may also find it easier to work, as your productivity and ability to focus will improve.

There are several ways for you to practice improving your ability to love yourself. This will help you to feel better about yourself and gain independence. Instead of depending on others for love, the love for yourself will be internalized. You will develop a much deeper appreciation for life. You may also find that you learn more about yourself.

To love yourself more, you must enjoy spending time by yourself. Find a hobby or activity that allows you to be alone and enjoy yourself. This can improve your confidence and help you to try new things. Perhaps you commit to learning about a new subject. You may try learning how to bake on your own. Creative hobbies help you to express yourself while having some fun along the way. A great way to gain confidence is by going places by yourself. This will teach you that you don't need anybody else to have fun; you can be your own best friend. Traveling and exploring new places is another way to love yourself. You will also learn more about the world around you and what you really love in life. Practicing self-care is another great way to love yourself.

You must also shift your mindset. It's important to accept yourself for the whole person you are. There will always be aspects of yourself that you can work on improving. You must also accept that you will feel pain. You will make mistakes. Life happens. However, you can't blame yourself for everything that happens to you. You must, however, take responsibility for your actions. This means accepting your triumphs and mistakes. You must also care about your mental, physical, and emotional health. Loving yourself also means taking care of yourself. You must react appropriately to situations based on what you know about yourself. Treat your body and mind properly. It's important.

Practicing Self-Respect and Self-Compassion

It is also important that you practice both self-respect and self-compassion. You must respect your body and mind. Self-respect is having confidence in yourself and having grace, honor, and dignity. It is the respect that you have for yourself. You like yourself, regardless of your performance. Even if you have a bad day or make a mistake, you will still love and respect yourself. It creates a strong and healthy relationship with yourself, which can really help your mental health and will allow you to treat yourself well. You will respect yourself for all aspects of yourself, both your strengths and weaknesses. This will be evident to others, and they will respect you more as a result. You will also recognize your self-worth, and this will disallow others to put you down or use you. You will understand the amount of respect that you deserve, and you won't let yourself or others put you down as a result. You will know who you are, so you won't have to find yourself through other people. You won't need to only be around certain people to "feel yourself" because you'll already know who you are. You won't need to seek love, attention, and respect from others because you will be happy with the person you are. You won't need others to justify who you are. You will also want to treat yourself well and take care of yourself because you know that's what you deserve. You also won't tolerate those who don't treat you the way that you know you deserve to be treated.

Self-compassion is also crucial. It is similar to having compassion for others, yet you are having compassion for yourself. You will take care of yourself, especially when you sense that you are in pain. You will be understanding and kind to yourself. Warmth, care, and helpfulness to yourself will come naturally to you. It is also understood that you won't always be perfect. Suffering, pain, and failure are natural and happen to everyone. Those with self-compassion won't judge themselves for making mistakes. They will instead understand that everyone makes mistakes. When pain and suffering occur, it is important to care for yourself and help yourself to feel better. You will be able to value your health and happiness by being kind to yourself and not judging yourself for any imperfections. You will also recognize how to love yourself yet also allow yourself to love others and experience love from others.

Taking care of your mental health is crucial. It can have just as much of an effect on you as your physical health can, if not more. You must become more aware of your emotions to care about your emotional health. Learning what makes you happier can help you to make yourself happier. You must improve your self-talk. It's important to practice self-love, self-compassion, self-respect, and self-care. It is also crucial to learn to love yourself. These are all ways to improve your mental health and be a better person.

Chapter 10: Repairing Your Relationship with Food

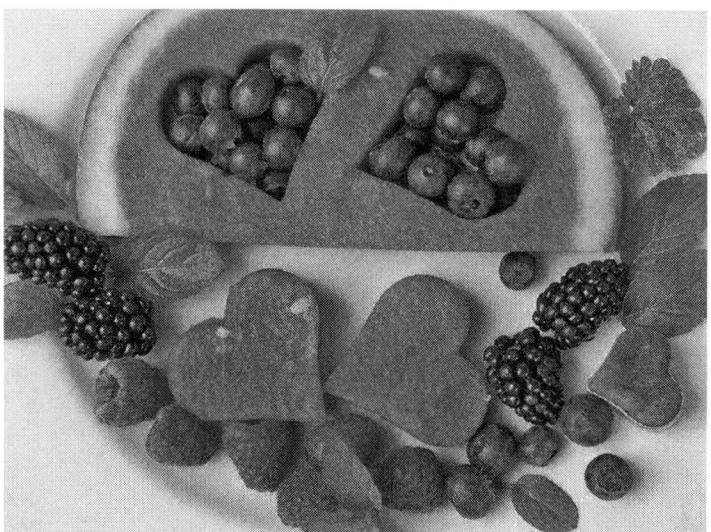

It is important to repair your relationship with food, especially if you have gotten off track with it. You must be able to recognize the signs of having an unhealthy relationship with food. If you identify that your relationship with food is unhealthy, you must be able to find a way to turn that around. It is also important to learn to love food without having to overeat. You must also learn how to value your health. You have one body, and you must treat it properly to have the best health that you possibly can. It's important to take care of yourself.

Signs of an Unhealthy Relationship with Food

You may realize that your relationship with food isn't the best. There are some obvious ways to tell that your relationship with food isn't healthy. Sometimes, it's more difficult to tell that your relationship with food is in need of improvement. There are several signs that you may need to improve your relationship with food.

If you try to hide your eating habits, you may have an unhealthy relationship with food. Perhaps you constantly snack at home and have frequent binging episodes. Around friends, family, and others, you may try to hide these tendencies or make different food choices. This is normal to an extent. Perhaps you feel more motivated to make different choices around different people. If you have a friend who is a vegetarian, you may choose more plant-based options around them. However, if you feel so guilty or ashamed about your eating habits that you feel the need to hide them or pretend that you eat differently, there may be an issue. You may "wear a mask" when it comes to food. You may pretend to eat a certain way while in public. As soon as you get home, you eat completely differently. This is due to the guilt that you feel.

If you exercise according to how much you eat, you may also have an unhealthy relationship with food. Perhaps you ate a 300-calorie donut and can only justify it if you run enough to burn 300 calories. You base your exercise off of how much you eat and try to burn off what you eat. Similarly, you may obsess over your weight. Each time you eat, you step on the scale. If you weigh yourself every day or even several times a day, there is a problem. Developing a fixation on your weight is unhealthy, both physically and mentally. You may end up exercising or starving yourself to get the weight that you desire. It will destroy your self-esteem.

If you are constantly trying new diets, paying for every plan, and trying every new trend, there may be a problem. You constantly try a diet, don't stick with it, and move on to the next one. You will never feel satisfied with your results and will only end up disappointed in yourself. This is a way to develop an obsession with dieting. You may view foods as "good" or "bad," especially when you develop the dieting mentality. This is unwise, as you will restrict yourself and end up craving the foods that you restrain yourself from eating, even more leading to binging episodes. When you constantly switch from diet to diet, you won't make any progress.

Building a Healthy Relationship with Food

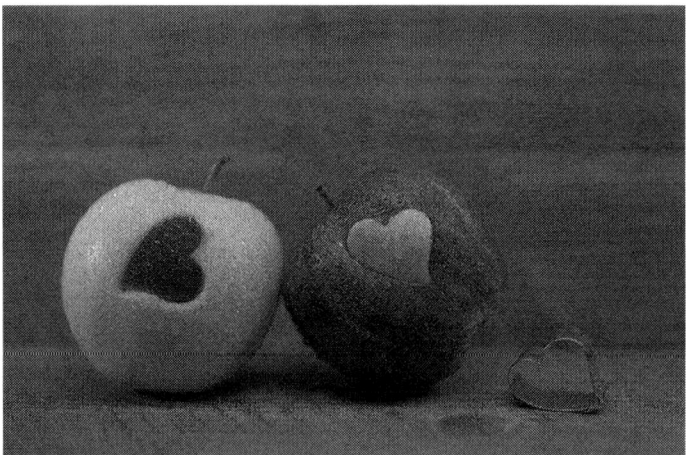

After recognizing that your relationship with food needs to improve, you must start rebuilding a healthier relationship with food. Food should not be a source of anxiety or guilt. It is not a coping mechanism. Food is necessary for feeding your body. It should also satisfy your soul. Those with a healthy food relationship will truly enjoy food and the whole eating experience that comes with it.

To begin building a healthy relationship with food, you must accept all types of foods. Although there are foods that have more nutritional value than others, you can't label which foods are "good" and which are "bad." This will only lead to guilt associated with certain foods.

It's all about how your body feels. When you begin labeling foods, food will begin to play mind games with you and make you feel bad. If you occasionally have foods with little nutritional value, that is okay. You won't gain ten pounds from a single meal that lacks nutritional value. It's important that you don't punish yourself for eating nutritionally-lacking foods.

To build a healthy relationship with food, surround yourself with good options. Eliminate foods from your home that can be tempting. If there is a certain food that you are trying to stay away from, keeping it in the pantry will certainly not help. Additionally, remind yourself that it's okay to say no. Perhaps your friend gave you some baked goods that they made. It's okay to have a bit and give the rest away. You don't have to eat something just because it's on your plate. If you've already eaten dinner and your family invites you to dinner, you don't have to eat again. Allow yourself to say no.

However, you don't have to say no to everything. You don't have to cut out all "junk food." Allow yourself to enjoy cookies, cake, French fries, and other such foods in moderation. As long as every meal doesn't turn into a cheeseburger and French fries, allow yourself to enjoy the foods you love. Having a salad for breakfast, lunch, and dinner is neither realistic or enjoyable. It isn't all or nothing. If you have an overall healthy day but slip in a little snack that isn't the greatest, that's okay. As long as the majority of what you're putting into your body makes you feel great, that's good.

Try tracking your foods. This doesn't mean that you have to count calories. In fact, it's better not to track calories, as it isn't an accurate measurement of nutritional value. However, it's important to jot down everything you eat (even for a short period of time, such as a week) so that you get an idea of what you really eat throughout the day. Perhaps you don't realize how much you eat or what you eat. This will help to put it in writing and allow you to see it. After doing this, you can analyze it. Are you happy with your eating habits? If so, great! If not, you can make adjustments until you are happy with your eating habits.

Loving Food Without Overeating

Just because you love food, you don't have to eat constantly. You can have an appreciation and love for food without constantly shoving food in your mouth or reaching for another snack. You must appreciate food as fuel for your body. It should be something that makes you feel good. There are several ways to stop yourself from overeating.

One way is by paying more attention to what you're eating. This can be done in several ways. One way to do so is to start keeping a log of what you eat. This will have you think more about what you eat since there will be a record of what you ate and how much of it you ate. You may also minimize distractions while eating. This way, your brain will truly register what you ate. Put away devices and other distractions while you are eating. You can truly appreciate your meal this way.

You may also allow yourself to eat the foods that you truly crave every so often. Instead of depriving yourself of French fries and eventually caving in, you can prevent this. When you deprive yourself of a certain food that you crave, you will most likely end up binging this food and overeating to compensate for the time without this. However, if you occasionally allow yourself to have some fries, you will satisfy your craving and prevent this from occurring.

Another important way to avoid overeating is by regulating your portions. Avoid eating from the container. If you eat chips from the family-size bag, you will likely overeat without realizing it. Eating from a container is an easy way to lose track of how much you've eaten. You may try meal prepping to portion your foods properly and avoid overeating later. It is much better to put no matter how much food you'd like onto a plate or into a bowl so that you avoid eating from the container. When eating out, don't feel obligated to eat the whole meal. Restaurant portions are typically larger than the recommended portion size. It's okay to take home some of your food.

Watch your emotions. By controlling your emotional and mental health, you will greatly reduce your likelihood of overeating. You won't feel the urge to overeat to cope with your stress or other negative emotions. It is also wise to come up with a list of healthy coping mechanisms to go to when you are feeling down. Instead of ordering an entire pizza for yourself, you may choose to go for a walk or talk to a friend. By taking care of your emotional and mental health, you will reduce these binging and overeating episodes and help improve your relationship with food.

Learning to Value Health

It's crucial to value your health. You have one body. It's important to treat your body well so that it can treat you well. When you care about your health, you take care of yourself better. When you take care of yourself properly, you will reduce your likelihood of developing a number of health problems. Taking care of your mental health can help improve your mental and physical health. Taking care of your physical health will improve both your physical and mental health. Additionally, you will feel much better about yourself. Your whole outlook on life will grow to be more positive.

Surround yourself with those who value their health. If you surround yourself with people who lounge all day long, neglect their mental health, and don't take care of themselves, you are likely to be negatively influenced by those people. Surround yourself with people who take care of themselves and encourage you to do the same. This can make a huge difference. You can share goals with those people. You can encourage each other and share your progress towards your goals together. It's great to have people that can push you to be the best person you can.

Make it a point to remind yourself to take care of your health. Each night, set your goals for the next day. Every morning, remind yourself why you are doing what you are doing. Remember why it's so crucial to fill your body with good foods. Before working out, think about why you are doing so. It is good for your body. Schedule time for a little self-care every day. Place a high value on health in your life. If you feel inspired by it, create a dream board, or surround yourself with inspirational quotes. On social media, follow accounts that encourage and inspire you. Make a list of all the benefits of health. When you are healthy, you will be more productive. You will be able to form better relationships and communicate better. You will be able to accomplish more. Your chance for health issues will decrease. You will be able to get more out of life. It'll be more common to experience genuinely happy moments. You will be able to move more easily. The list can go on forever. Remind yourself each day of at least some of these benefits. This will accentuate the importance of caring for your health and valuing it more in life.

It is important to take care of your health. You must understand if you have developed an unhealthy relationship with food. If you have, you must be able to build a healthy relationship with food so that you may enjoy the eating experience. As important as it is to love food, you must also ensure that you are not overeating. It's crucial that you learn to value your health. This way, you can treat your body well. You will be motivated to love your body and really pay attention to your health.

Chapter 11: Eating Disorders

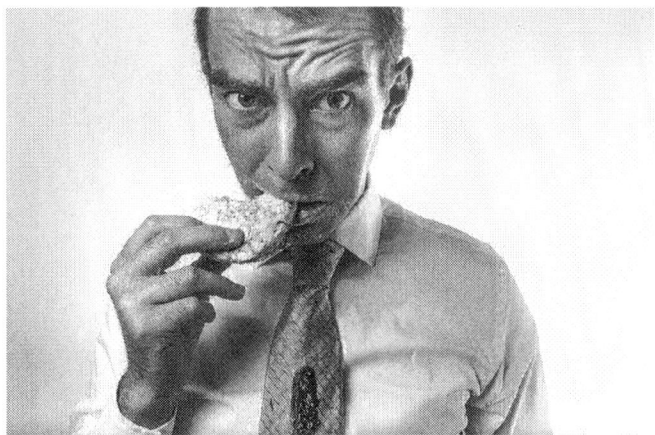

Eating disorders can be serious. They can have serious consequences for your health. It is important to understand the different types of eating disorders. You must also understand the causes of eating disorders to determine the mental aspect behind them. You should also familiarize yourself with the symptoms of eating disorders to identify if you may struggle with an eating disorder. You will also need to understand the proper ways to overcome eating disorders. They can be quite serious. Oftentimes, one won't even be aware that they have an eating disorder. Their actions are normal to them. It is important to educate yourself on eating disorders to prevent and/or overcome an eating disorder.

Types of Eating Disorders

There are several different types of eating disorders. These each has its own characteristics, symptoms, and effects on the body. Eating disorders can be serious, and attention must be given to them to ensure the health of the individual struggling with the eating disorder. One that struggles with an eating disorder will not be able to go on with their daily life due to a constant preoccupation with food. Their concerns about food, weight, and body image will interfere with their life and can result in serious health issues.

Anorexia Nervosa

Anorexia nervosa will result in weight loss (or for children the inability to gain weight). One will not be able to maintain a healthy weight. This is often accompanied by poor self-image. Those with anorexia will prevent weight gain in several ways. They may restrict their diets heavily and count calories. They may exercise compulsively (perhaps working off any "extra" calories). They may prevent themselves from eating certain types of foods. Weight loss may be hidden with loose clothes. They may also purge (either by vomiting or laxatives), and binge eat.

Bulimia Nervosa

When one does binge and purge, this is known as bulimia nervosa. One who struggles with this will be caught up in a constant cycle of bingeing and purging. They may try to hide their bingeing episodes from others and will "undo the damage" by purging it all afterward. A person who vomits after meals may struggle. One who uses diuretics or has evidence of much uneaten food may be struggling with bulimia. They may also drink excessive amounts of water or become seemingly obsessed with breath fresheners. There may be the development of dental issues and calluses on the hands as a result of self-induced vomiting.

Binge Eating Disorder

Binge eating disorder (BED) is characterized by frequent urges to binge-eat. They will not be able to control such episodes and may overstuff themselves to the point of discomfort. Afterward, they may feel guilt, shame, and anxiety as a result of the episode. Those with binge eating disorder will not try to "undo the damage." They will simply eat a large quantity of food in a short period of time. This binge will not be able to control themselves or stop themselves from eating more. They may try to hide food for the purpose of bingeing and will attempt to hide the actual action of bingeing.

Avoidant Restrictive Food Intake Disorder

Those with Avoidant Restrictive Food Intake Disorder (ARFID) will not maintain a proper and healthy weight. They may lose weight very quickly. They limit themselves to very specific foods. This is not due to a desire to lose weight or because of poor self-image, but because they are "picky." The selection of foods to eat is narrow and typically becomes even narrower over time.

They may even begin eating items that are typically not regarded as food and don't have significant nutritional value. When this occurs, it is known as pica. One may eat paper, hair, paint, ice, clay, or other substances. Those with pica may worry about choking or vomiting. They may also increase their risk of health problems as a result of an improper diet.

Rumination Disorder

Those with rumination disorder will regurgitate their food and re-chew or re-swallow their food. When regurgitating their food, the individual will not be upset, stressed, or disgusted. It may even seem natural for one to do so. They may also spit their food out after re-chewing their food up.

Unspecified Feeding or Eating Disorder

Unspecified feeding or eating disorder (USFED) is where one will be affected in their daily life by a disorder significantly. They may be impaired in their social life, occupation, or education (as well as in other areas of their life). They may not have the full symptoms of another eating disorder, yet the eating or feeding disorder will have a significant impact on their life and lead to distress. There may not be enough information to make a more specific diagnosis of the person. However, there will be symptoms of some type of eating disorder present. It may not be certain what type it is exactly, though.

Purging Disorder

Purging disorder occurs when one purges frequently. They will not, however, have the bingeing episodes before that are the key characteristic of bulimia. This will occur when one has a poor self-image or wishes to lose additional weight.

Night Eating Syndrome

Night eating syndrome (NES) is where the individual will eat a significant portion of their meals after their dinnertime meal. They may also wake up throughout the night so that they may eat. Those with night eating syndrome will eat at least a quarter of their daily consumption after their evening meal.

Other Specified Feeding and Eating Disorders

This is the classification for those who have symptoms of other eating disorders but don't quite match another eating disorder perfectly. They may have bingeing episodes followed by purging. They may also binge-eat. Those with OSFED may excessively diet, have poor self-esteem, and exercise excessively.

There are several different types of eating disorders. They all have different symptoms and can all have a serious impact on the individual's health. If left untreated, the individual can develop a number of health problems. It may even be fatal if left untreated for a long period of time. This will depend on the intensity of the eating disorder as well. However, it is important to recognize the symptoms of eating disorders to understand if one may have an eating disorder.

Causes of Eating Disorders

Eating disorders are complex. Each individual will have their own variation of an eating disorder if they have one. There are numerous causes, and the reasoning behind the development of an eating disorder will vary for everyone. However, there are some common causes of eating disorders that may be true for a great number of people. It's important to understand what causes eating disorders so that they may be prevented and understood more. The underlying cause may be helped if it is identified.

Genetics

One reason for the development of an eating disorder is due to genetics. The individual may have an increased risk of developing an eating disorder based on their genes. This is a heredity trait, which means this increased risk can be passed down to one's offspring. Those with a family member with an eating disorder are much more likely to develop one themselves.

Personality

One's personality may also be a contributing factor in the development of an eating disorder. One who frequently experiences obsessive thinking is more likely to develop an eating disorder. This is because the person is more likely to develop an unhealthy obsession with food, weight, body, exercise, and eating in general. An individual who is a perfectionist will want the perfect body and may do anything to achieve that. One who thrives off of rewards and punishments will also be more likely to develop an eating disorder. They will reward themselves when they lose weight or achieve their goal. This may be in the form of a binge or other unhealthy reward. Similarly, they may punish themselves. Perhaps they look in the mirror and don't like what they see. They may purge, starve themselves, or exercise obsessively to change their image. One who is impulsive and excessively persistent may also be more likely to develop an eating disorder.

Trauma

Those with trauma or with past events that had a great effect on them are also more likely to develop an eating disorder. They may feel ashamed of themselves or guilty about themselves and use the eating disorder as a way to express this. They may also wish to harm or punish themselves for the trauma. It may also be the result of their past. For instance, those who were bullied about being overweight may express that pain through an eating disorder. Eating disorders can be an expression of one's pain and emotions.

Coping Mechanism

Similarly, one may use the eating disorder as a coping mechanism. They may lack the ability or knowledge to utilize healthier ways to cope. It may be an outlet for their emotions. This is a way to express one's pain.

Outside Influences

One may also develop an eating disorder as a result of outside influences. Those with unrealistic bodies that are portrayed on television, in magazines, and on the Internet may cause one to believe that their body is not good enough. As a result, they will do whatever they can to change their bodies so that it matches this unrealistic ideal.

Overcoming Eating Disorders

Eating disorders can be dangerous. It's important to understand when you have one. When you identify what you may struggle with an eating disorder, it is important to take care of yourself and overcome the eating disorder that you have. It may not be easy. However, it's important to take the necessary steps to take care of yourself and watch out for your health. Otherwise, you are risking serious consequences. Eating disorders can take a toll on your health. The longer that they are left untreated, the worse that they will become. Your body will suffer if you don't work towards helping yourself.

Listening to Yourself

To overcome an eating disorder, you must listen to yourself. Listen to your thoughts and feelings. You must understand how you feel so that you can treat yourself accordingly. If you sense that you are unhappy, identify why that is and how you can help yourself cope in a healthy manner. You may also identify what triggers you. If you can learn how to stop yourself from reacting to certain situations in an unhealthy manner, you can really help yourself. You must also learn to listen to your body. Your body will send you signals on what it needs.

Learning to Love and Accept Yourself

You must also learn to love and accept yourself. It's important to be patient and understanding with yourself. You will make mistakes. You are not perfect. Your body will not look like others' bodies. You must love and accept yourself for who you are. If you punish yourself for your imperfections, your physical and mental health will seriously suffer. Train yourself to find aspects of yourself that you love. Learn to love your body and surround yourself with people who encourage you. Learn how to avoid comparing yourself to others. Everyone has their own strengths. Learn to appreciate your strengths.

Seeking Help

If you have tried to help yourself with your eating disorder and haven't had luck, it is crucial that you seek help. You can't be embarrassed or feel shameful asking for help. If you don't seek help, you will suffer. You may seek the help of someone close to you. Opening up with someone about your struggle may help you. They may be able to push you in the right direction. Choose someone that you are comfortable with so that you can really open up to them. You may also seek professional help. Seek out a medical professional that you can talk to and receive professional help from.

Understanding the Causes and Symptoms

Eating disorders are serious. There are several types of eating disorders, and it's important that you understand the causes and symptoms of both. You must also understand how you can overcome eating disorders. If you leave an eating disorder untreated, you can face serious consequences on your health. Understanding the symptoms of an eating disorder can help you to consider if you may struggle with an eating disorder. Understanding the causes can also help you understand how you may prevent an eating disorder from developing. Preventing and treating eating disorders is crucial.

Chapter 12: Tips and Tricks

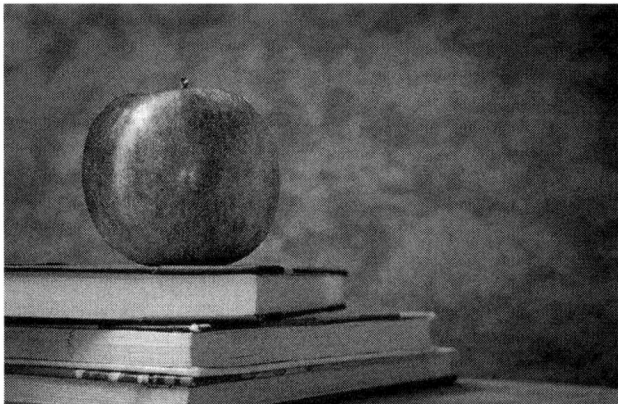

There are some additional tricks that you may learn. There are some simple ways to improve your health. These are simple tricks, yet they can have a great impact on your health. You may also learn how to implement healthier eating habits. By slightly changing your habits, you can really help your health. You may also learn to be happier and healthier overall, which will help you to get more out of life and experience genuine joy in your life. You will also learn some tips and tricks to learn how you can manage any poor eating habits that you may have.

Little Ways to Improve Your Health

There are many quick and simple tips to improve your health. Implementing these in your life can make a huge difference.

Drinking More Water

Make an effort to drink more water. Replacing the sugary beverages that you consume with water can make a huge difference. Even if it's only one drink a day to start off, you will be much better off. Make an effort to minimize or eliminate soda from your diet. Even fruit juice, tea, and lemonade can be loaded with sugar. Water is the best option, as it contains no sugar and hydrates your body. We need water to live, and it helps the body run more effectively and efficiently.

Exercising

Take some time to exercise. Only a little time is necessary. If going to the gym for an hour five days a week seems overwhelming to you, don't worry! You don't have to spend hours upon hours every week working out. In fact, five minutes a day is better than nothing. You can go for a short walk every evening to wind down after work. There are many videos online with short exercise routines that you can accomplish in under ten minutes. Even doing a few push-ups and sit-ups here and there is better than nothing. Carve out some time every day to dedicate to moving around. A great way to incorporate exercise into your routine is by scheduling classes to go to, especially with friends. This way, you can choose something that you like doing, and you will have to go. Your friend will count on you, and you will most likely have to pay.

Having Time for Yourself

You should also schedule a little bit of time each day to devote to yourself. This way, you can relax and unwind. It will give you time to collect your thoughts and focus on your goals. You may also enjoy some mental and emotional stability by doing so. This can reduce your stress, and you will feel more motivated to take care of yourself. Remind yourself of your goals during this time. You may also focus on what you would like to improve with your existing routine. You don't even need to spend a long time each day doing this. Even taking a minute to really relax and breathe can make a huge difference.

Tips for Healthier Eating Habits

Improving your eating habits can be as simple as slightly adjusting your routine. You may do this in a few ways. One way is to rid yourself of unnecessary snacks. Go through your refrigerator and pantry. Get rid of any snacks that you don't need in your life. If you aren't surrounded by unhealthy temptations, then you won't be as likely to reach for them. You may also choose to replace your snacks with healthier options. Start surrounding yourself with more fruits and vegetables. You may even plan out your snacks to ensure that what you are eating is right. Prepare proper portions of healthy options. One example of a potential snack is apple slices and peanut butter. If these are already prepared for you, the excuse of not having enough time to choose a healthier option will be invalid. Bring healthy snacks with you. Whether you put them in your car, in your bag, or bring them to work, it is good to have healthy options with you so that you aren't as tempted to grab a quick bite at a fast-food restaurant instead.

Eating More Fruits and Vegetables

One way to improve your eating is by incorporating more fruits and vegetables into your life. Instead of white rice, try cauliflower rice. When making pasta, shred some carrots into the sauce. Choose broccoli over French fries when eating out. Add some mushrooms to your grilled chicken. Replace chips with dried fruit. There are numerous ways to incorporate fruits and vegetables into your diet, and they can really boost your health and add some nutritional value to your diet. An easy way to boost your diet with fruits and veggies is to make smoothies. This is a great way to pack in your fruits and veggies. Plus, you can make them tasty! You can even make smoothie bowls. Salads are also a great way to load up on fruits and veggies.

Lessening Your Sugar and Salt Intake

Another way to boost your diet is to stop adding sugar and salt to your foods. Most food is already loaded with an excess of sugar and salt. While eating out, resist the urge to use the salt shaker. When cooking, reduce the amount of sugar and salt that you add to your foods.

Choosing Healthier Options

You may replace your foods for healthier options. Start swapping fried food for grilled food. Grilled chicken is a much better option than chicken fingers. Make the switch from refined grains to whole grains. Swap out any meat for leaner options. Reduce the amount of red meat and try to eat more turkey and chicken.

When shopping at the grocery store, make a list ahead of time. Plan out what exactly you need. This will reduce shopping for extra items. Make sure that you stick to your list. It can help you to eat before you go grocery shopping. That way, you won't be tempted to buy the entire store just because you're hungry. Planning ahead can help you to make better and healthier decisions. It may also help to come up with recipes for the meals you plan to make and buy according to that. This will help you be more motivated to cook those meals.

How to Be Happier Overall

Everyone likes to be happy. There are many small habits that you can incorporate into your life that can boost your happiness. When you do this, you are also helping to improve your mental health. When you are happier, you also experience negative emotions less. This will allow your emotional and mental health to improve. When you boost your emotional and mental health, you will be able to make better decisions regarding your health and can take care of yourself better.

Adjusting Your Sleep Schedule

Slightly changing your sleep schedule can make you happier. Simply waking up fifteen minutes earlier than usual can greatly impact your happiness. You can start your day off the right way and set the bar high. Waking up a bit early will allow you more time to enjoy your day. You can have more time to get ready instead of feeling rushed. Instead of waking up and immediately feeling stressed, you are starting the day off with a better mindset. You may take this time to ease into your day. You may also use it to go over your goals for the day and sort out your to-do list. It will change your whole attitude.

Cleaning Up Your House

Cleaning up a bit can make a huge difference. When your space is cluttered, you won't be able to think properly. If your workspace is cluttered, you will struggle to focus, as you will be distracted and overwhelmed by the mess. If your bedroom is a mess, you won't be able to sleep as well. When your kitchen is a mess, you won't make wise choices in what you eat. A cluttered pantry or refrigerator may seem overwhelming. This can be frustrating and lead to a preference for eating out, as you won't want to sift through the mess for food. When you are less stressed, you will be able to enjoy life more and will be happier.

Undergoing Social Media Detox

It is important to take a break from social media. Although social media can be a great way to communicate with others, it can easily become toxic if it is overused. People have a tendency to compare themselves to others, and social media is a prime example of this. You will find yourself comparing yourself to others, yet you must stay on your own path; everyone has different goals. Reduce the time you spend on social media, and you will find your happiness will increase. You may even consider a social media detox.

Expressing Gratitude

One way to be happier is by expressing gratitude. Think about all of the things that you are thankful for, as well as how grateful you are for yourself. At least once a day, remind yourself of one thing that you are grateful for (bonus points if it's something about yourself). By looking for the positives in life, you are shifting your mindset. You will start to see the good in life, and you will be much happier as a result. It's always possible to find joy in life.

Managing Poor Eating Habits

There are many simple tricks for combatting unhealthy habits. You can change your bad habits by slightly switching what you do. Just by making small switches, you can make big differences.

Listening to Your Body

Make sure that you take the time to listen to your body. Understand any emotions that may trigger certain eating habits and learn how you can handle these. Listen to your body to decide when you are hungry and when you are full. Don't keep eating if you're full, and make sure that you feed yourself when you're hungry. If you keep eating after you're already full, you are overeating. Starving yourself will most likely lead to a bingeing episode later. Watch out for yourself and prevent future issues before they even occur.

Reducing Your Food Stock

Reduce the amount of food in your house. Although you can clean your kitchen and make it appear decluttered, you must truly keep it clean. Don't buy what you already have; maintain your kitchen's cleanliness. When you only have the very best foods in your kitchen, you are more likely just to put the very best foods in your body. You should clean out your cupboards and drawers. Make sure the counter is also clean so that you may actually use it for cooking. Once you have gotten your kitchen to the point where all of your foods are of higher nutritional value, make sure that you don't bring back any of the foods that you wished to eliminate in the first place. Put the foods that you really want to eat where you can see them. You can put your "best" foods on display, and you will be more inclined to eat them.

Reducing Distractions While Eating

Remember to reduce distractions when you are eating. In addition to paying attention to your food by not watching any devices or such, you should also eliminate audible distractions. Although you may enjoy listening to music or podcasts, try to make meals special. Set aside that time for eating and eating only.

Regulating Your Portions

Regulate your portions. Choose smaller utensils, bowls, and plates. The smaller bowls and plates will allow you to think that you are consuming more. Smaller utensils will require more bites to eat the same amount of food. When you think that you are eating more, your brain will tell you that you are full sooner. You will be satisfied with less food. Even if the bowl is smaller, a full bowl of food still registers as a full bowl of food, regardless of whether or not it's a bit smaller. You may also consider switching to smaller glasses for beverages besides water.

Having an Eating Schedule

You may establish scheduled eating habits. When you follow the same daily schedule, your body will get used to eating at a certain time. This will also help you to keep track of your eating more easily. Instead of eating more than you should when you are bored, you will know when exactly it is time to eat. You may also have an eating ritual. Do the same task before you eat every time, and your body will be alerted that it is time to eat. You may even enjoy eating more when you have a ritual to look forward to.

There are many tips and tricks to help you out. Improving your health is quite simple. You can improve your health by adding small tasks to your daily routine. The same is true for improving your eating habits. Similarly, happiness may be increased in one's life by making slight switches. You can help make your poor eating habits into better habits by also utilizing some simple tips and tricks. Making improvements doesn't have to be difficult.

Conclusion

Thank you for making it through to the end of *Emotional Eating*! Let's hope it was informative and able to provide you with all of the tools you need to achieve your goals—whatever they may be.

The next step is to implement the habits that you learned. You can continue your research and continue starting healthy habits. After reading this book, you will understand how you can work to improve your eating habits and health overall.

These are key concepts that will help you to improve your health. When you eat better, your body will be happy. Treating your body better will make you feel better. You will experience the physical aspects of this, such as having more energy and being able to move better. You will experience the mental aspects of it. You will be more motivated to take care of yourself and your health. This will also allow you to be more productive and have a better ability to focus. You will also be in better control of your emotions, which will have a great impact on improving your emotional eating habits.

It is important to combat your bad habits once and for all and start implementing healthier eating habits. You need to discover the proper way to actually enjoy the food that you eat. You have to recognize the signs of an unhealthy relationship with food and know how to repair it. You will learn how to value your health.

It is important to work on your mental health. This will help you to control your emotions and get a grip on your emotional eating. Understand what mental health is and how you can work to improve your mental health. By improving your mental health, you will also be helping your physical health to improve. Understand the proper mindsets that you can work to adopt. Identify which mindset or mindsets that you wish to work on. You should learn how to plan and achieve goals, but just goals that are realistic and achievable and how to stay motivated despite obstacles.

Do you need a mental boost with achieving goals, staying motivated when issues arise, having a healthier body, overcoming addiction, or having a healthier mind? This is important to keep in mind. You may also work on mastering mindfulness and incorporating mindfulness techniques into your daily life. Identify why you wish to master mindfulness. Perhaps you have food cravings. Perhaps you struggle with compulsive overeating. You may wish to enjoy your food more. Mindfulness can help with all of these and in other areas.

Emotional eating is eating that is triggered by certain emotions_or_situations. It is important that you understand the causes and symptoms of overeating, as well as ways to help eliminate them. You need to learn how emotional eating is caused by more than your emotions. You must monitor all aspects of your health if you want to improve your eating habits. Healthier habits can result from taking care of both your physical and mental health. By learning how you can take care of both of those aspects, you can learn how to help with emotional eating. You can experience all of the wonderful benefits of living a healthier lifestyle as a result.

There are other areas of mental health to work on as well. Understand if you would like to become more aware of your emotions. Perhaps you need to focus more on what makes you happy. You may need to improve your self-talk and practice self-care. You may wish to love yourself more and practice self-care and self-compassion. Make a plan for repairing your relationship with food. If you have identified that you have an eating disorder, start working towards overcoming that.

There are several steps to improving your overall health. You must understand emotional eating. Identify if you are an emotional eater and take steps to improve your habits. You can also learn more about what physical health entails and how you may improve your habits. When you work to improve your physical health, your mental health will also get a boost. Understand if you have an addiction to sugar or to food, in general. Identify your plan for combatting that addiction. Consider going on a detox to get your body used to the idea of thriving without the foods that you are addicted to.

There are other ways that you may work on your emotional eating. It will really help to start a journal. This is a great way for you to write down your emotions. You can plan out your goals and anything else you need to do. You can also track your portions and the types of foods that you consume throughout the day. If you have tried to work on your health on your own but have seen no results, another way that you can improve your health is by seeking the help of a professional. A final way to help yourself is surrounding yourself with good influences on social media, with the people whom you surround yourself with, and in your refrigerator or pantry.

Autophagy

Heal, Detox, and Self-Cleanse Your Body; Speed Up Your Metabolism with Intermittent Fasting to Lose Weight Easily; Stay Healthy and Promote Longevity with an Anti-Inflammatory Keto Diet

by ALAN DIETER

© Copyright 2019 by Alan Dieter - All rights reserved.

The information contained in this book is not designed to replace or take the place of any form of medicine or professional medical advice. The information in this book has been provided for educational and entertainment purposes only. The information contained in this book has been compiled from sources deemed reliable, and it is accurate to the best of the Author's knowledge; however, the Author cannot guarantee its accuracy and validity and cannot be held liable for any errors or omissions. Changes are periodically made to this book. You must consult your doctor or get professional medical advice before using any of the suggested remedies, techniques, or information in this book. Upon using the information contained in this book, you agree to hold harmless the Author from and against any damages, costs, and expenses, including any legal fees potentially resulting from the application of any of the information provided by this guide. This disclaimer applies to any damages or injury caused by the use and application, whether directly or indirectly, of any advice or information presented, whether for breach of contract, tort, negligence, personal injury, criminal intent, or any other cause of action. You agree to accept all risks of using the information presented inside this book. You need to consult a professional medical practitioner to ensure you are both able and healthy enough to participate in this program. All rights reserved. No part of this publication may be reproduced, distributed, or transmitted in any form or by any means, including photocopying, recording, or other electronic or mechanical methods, without the prior written permission of the publisher, except in the case of brief quotations embodied in critical reviews and specific other noncommercial uses permitted by copyright law.

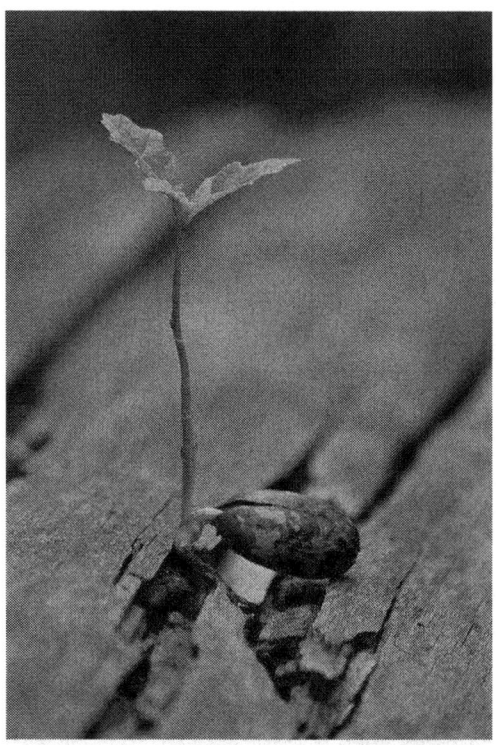

Table of Contents

Introduction **663**
Chapter One: **664**
What Is Autophagy? **664**
The Specific Functions of Autophagy 665
Autophagy Process in the Cells of Mammals 666
Major Types of Autophagy 667
Autophagosome Formation 667
The Self-Cleansing Process 668
Autophagy to Heal and Detox Your Body and Regenerate Your Mind 672
Three Ways to Boost the Symptoms of Autophagy 673
Feasting & Fasting: 675
Trying to Strike the Perfect Ancestral Balance 675
Weight Loss Through Autophagy 675
What Are Lipolysis and Lipophagy? 676
Autophagy and Ketogenesis 676
Autophagy and Insulin 677
Autophagy and Loose Skin After Weight Loss 677
Does Autophagy Enable You to Lose Fat? 678
Three Ways to Activate the Process of Weight Loss 679
Chapter Two: **680**
Fat-Burning Strategies **680**
Ways to Burn Fats 680
1. Begin Practicing Training of Strength 680
2. Follow a Diet High in Protein 681
3. Try to Sleep a Lot 681

4. The Diet Should Consist of Vinegar 681
5. The Consumption of Fats That Are Healthy 682
6. Drinking Beverages That Are Healthy 682
7. Increase Fiber Intake 683
8. Decrease the Intake of Carbohydrates That Have Been Refined 683
9. Raise the Cardio 684
10. Consume a Lot of Coffee 684
11. Practice the Sprint Interval Training 684
12. The Diet Consisting of Probiotics 685
13. Add the Consumption of Iron in the Diet 685
14. Start Fasting 686
Intermittent Fasting 687
Types of Intermittent Fasting 687
Effects of Intermittent Fasting 688
Insulin Resistance and Ketosis 691
The Resistance in Insulin 691
The Way It Works 692
More Fat, Less Sugar 694
Negative Effects of Sugar Consumption 695
Good Sugars (and Fats) 696
Advantages of Healthy Fats 696
The Not-So-Healthy Fats 697
Fat or Sugar? 697
Aerobic Training 698
Aerobic vs. Anaerobic Exercise 698
The Improvement of Endurance Through Aerobic Training 699
How Long Is the Training Period? 700
Health Benefits 701
Effects on Body Performance 701
Effects on the Brain 702
Disadvantages 702
Exercises That Are Like Aerobics 702
Take the First Step 703
Chapter Three: 704
Reducing Inflammation Through Autophagy 704
Effects of Autophagy on Other Inflammatory Pathways 706
Anti-Inflammatory Keto Diet 707
Using a Plant-Based Keto Diet to Reduce Inflammation 707
Inflammation Cut Down by Ketogenic Diet 707
How a Plant-Based Ketogenic Diet Can Help to Cut Down on
Inflammation Further 709
The Keto Diet (Introduction and Explanation of the Keto Diet and Its
Benefits in Relation to Autophagy) 711
Diet Changes That Can Boost Autophagy 712
Keto Diet and Inflammation 715
Anti-Inflammatory Foods 716
How Fasting Can Stimulate Autophagy 718
Best Foods/Drinks to Stimulate Autophagy Process 718
Green Tea 719
Coffee 719
Cinnamon 719
Coconut Oil 719
Chapter Four: 720
Longevity with Autophagy 720
Dietary Restriction/Reduced mTOR Signaling 721
Germline Removal 722
Reduced Mitochondrial Respiration 722
Forced Activation of Autophagy in the Extension of the Lifespan 722
Pharmacological Activation of Autophagy Contributing to Longevity ... 723

Spermidine 723
Resveratrol.. 723
Tomatidine 724
The Anti-Aging Process Through Ketosis State 725
Nutrition to Make Your Cells Younger.. 725
Circadian Rhythm and Autophagy... 726
Circadian Rhythm and the Modulation of Autophagy 727
Sleep Optimization 728
How Diets Affect Sleep 730
Does Intermittent Fasting Affect Sleep?... 734
Why Choose Sleep Optimization?.. 736
Conclusion 738

Introduction

Hey there! Thank you for purchasing *Autophagy*, a book that gives you all the necessary information to attaining excellent physical health and body metabolism. This varies from the definition of autophagy and types of autophagy to the detoxification process and how to lose weight in the most basic way. Are you looking to reduce weight? Are you having trouble with your metabolism? Are you trying to use anti-aging products that have not worked for some time now? Well, if your answer is yes, this book has the right natural procedures and mechanisms that will not only make you look more youthful but also increase your stay here on earth!

Chapter one starts by introducing autophagy, the significant types of autophagy, as well as the formation of this process. The second section deals with the self-cleansing, detoxification, and healing of the body. The third part involves a critical analysis of how individuals can lose weight through the activation of this autophagy process.

Chapter two focuses on how to burn fat in the body, which can be done through intermittent fasting, introducing the consumption of healthy fats and less sugar, as well as undertaking aerobics training.

Chapter three discusses the ways through which we can lower the risks of getting an inflammatory disease. It also talks about the ketogenic diet and gives you a variety of meals that can stimulate the process of autophagy.

Chapter four introduces longevity that can be achieved through the process of autophagy. It ranges from the specific topics that discuss the anti-aging process, types of nutrition that make your cell rejuvenated and younger, the circadian rhythm that can be achieved through the process of autophagy, and the optimization of sleep.

This book is going to interest whoever comes across it to find out more about what autophagy is, what it entails, as well as the procedure to go about it. It is that simple and clear. Get yourself one of these detailed guides to healing, detoxification process, anti-aging, and losing weight—and use it to your benefit.

There are plenty of books on this subject on the market—thank you again for choosing this one! Every effort was made to ensure it is full of as much useful information as possible. Please enjoy!

Chapter One: What Is Autophagy?

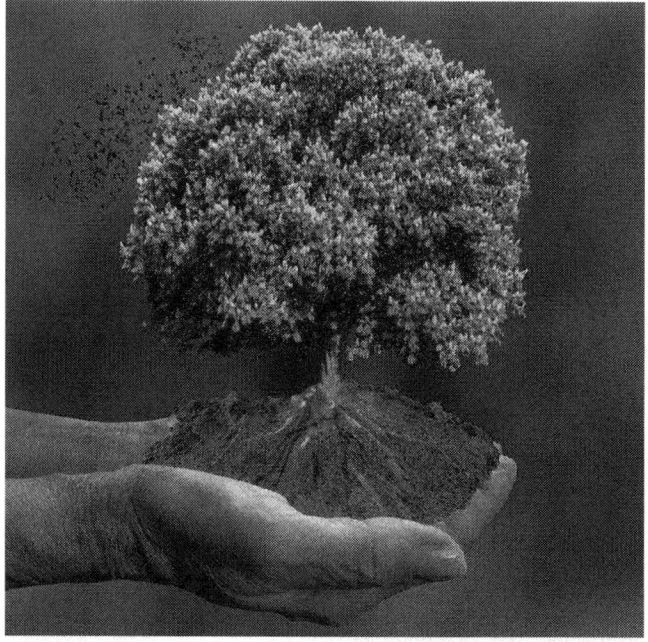

Living creatures—both plants and animals—have complex systems of behavior and physiological procedures to adapt to their ever-changing environment. There are uncountable stimuli that we are susceptible to on our day-to-day activities, and they all send a particular signal to the body. Consequently, this activates a chain response of events that ascertain how your metabolism, nervous system, and psychology react. Autophagy is part of this reaction, where the body of the organism is responding to specific changes or limitations in its environment

Autophagy engages in either an immediate or a deviant part of health. It's most uncomplicated—meaning that autophagy is usually an enormously compounded procedure that results in the change, excess, as well as the injured living macromolecules and the entire cell organs with the use of hydrolytic enzymes found within the lysosome. It is made up of consistent procedures of the autophagy enrolment, the emergence of the precursor autophagosome, its development, as well as its amalgamation with the lysosome, breaking down of the bulk contents, secretion carrying off the degraded outcome to the cytoplasm, and lysosome refinement. In this section, we will discuss the particular work done by autophagy and its underlying procedure.

The Specific Functions of Autophagy

Autophagy involves either an immediate or long-term effect on health and disease. In this section, we are going to look at its function in both health and disease. The tasks of autophagy in health are as follows:

- The control of the embryonic and primary postnatal growth
- Tissue homeostasis and the control of mitochondrial standard
- The protection of the cells against stress
- The response of tissue to nutrient deprivation for survival reasons
- The survival of cellular and physiological death of a cell during growth
- How a cell is involved in death during the treatment of radiotherapy or chemotherapy
- The remodeling of tissues during the evolution

The tasks played by autophagy in disease include:

- The energy supply, anti-aging, human malignancy, tumorigenesis, maintenance of the tumor, inflammation, ovarian cancer, colon cancer, and melanoma
- The storage of diseases in the lysosome
- Disorders to do with metabolism
- Cardiovascular diseases
- Cardiomyopathy of alcohol
- Myopathy of the skeletal muscles
- Atherosclerosis
- Diabetes
- Complications of being obese
- Degradation of lipid in the liver
- The diseases of the liver that are related to alcohol

- Pancreas diseases

- The management of cellular quality

- Genome protection

- The adaptive and innate responses by microbial pathogens to infection

- Defense of the body opposed to intracellular bacteria, parasites, and viral infections

- The intracellular pathogens' protection and the development of epileptic cells

Autophagy helps fight against infectious diseases. It does this by removing bane, which usually causes a defilement in the body, as well as by aiding to improve the way that the immune system of the body reacts to the banes. Intracellular bacteria and viruses can be removed by autophagy.

Autophagy betters the performance of muscles. By exercising, we usually put stress on the cells, resulting in energy raising; thus, the segments usually get tired quickly. Due to this, the process of autophagy aids in the elimination of damages and also maintains your energy levels.

What science can tell us today is that autophagy works to make your body function better. By cleaning up cellular junk, you will clear the way for cells to rebuild themselves with new parts. Sort of like that biological upgrade—giving an older car a more modern engine, so that it not only keeps running but "corners like it's on rails."

Autophagy Process in the Cells of Mammals

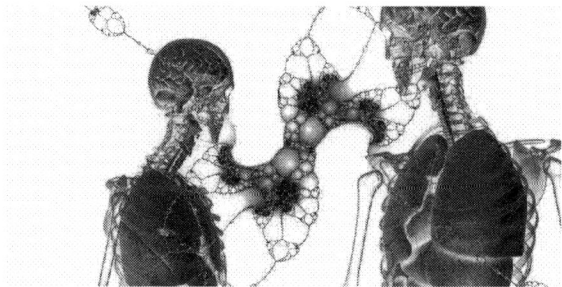

Even though the process moderates the adjustment of cells in various strain situations that involve starvation, this strain is seen as a problem—a multicellular organism cell can be able to solve consistently. The basal level of this process is seen in a lot of cells, hence being authorized to the suppositional detrimental clusters protein, which usually leads to a defective cellular. Consequently, the autophagy process in mammals is basically essential in aiding the cleaning of the intracellular of the injured proteins.

Therefore, the lack of a cleaning process would lead to the transformation of neoplastic. Mentioned earlier, lack of food is not so common in the cells of mammals on ordinary nutrition circumstances. As a result, it is necessary to find out the technique behind the regulation of autophagy under essential nutritional circumstances.

Major Types of Autophagy

There are three types of autophagy in the mammalian body.

I. Macro Autophagy - entire divisions of the cytosol whereby they are all secluded then transported for degeneration in lysosomes. These seclusions occur in the structure of autophagy. This process involves the innate authorized technique of cells that disposes of any defective or unwanted components in an organelle.

II. Micro Autophagy - is the immediate consumption of dispersible cellular components into the lysosome. It relocates the cytoplasmic material into the lysosome for the breakdown process through the direct division of the lysosome limiting membrane. As opposed to the other two, it is moderated in mammals by lysosomal activity, and in plants, it is reduced through vacuolar action (straight submersion of the cytoplasmic load. The cytoplasmic substance is confined in the lysosome by an arbitrary exercise of tissue introversion. In simple terms, microautophagy includes the direct introspection and amalgamation of lysosome/vacuole tissue under nutrient limitation.

III. The Chaperone Mediated Autophagy - is autophagy's conceptual manifestation that exists virtually in many kinds of tissues, including cells. It is distinguished in eukaryotes and not in yeast. For the reason of this specific feature, just the solvent proteins but not the entire organelle can be broken down through CMA. CMA is conditional on the inherent extracted heat shock cognate and recognizes the peptide series of the cytoplasmic parent material. Therefore, it is extra discerning than autophagy in its break down process. CMA performs duties for the stabilization of imbalanced energy and is best started up by metabolic or nutritious and oxidative tension.

Autophagosome Formation

Autophagy is an immensely compounded procedure that involves a series of steps of the inauguration of autophagy, the emergence of autophagosome predecessor, development of a phagosome, the amalgamation of an autophagosome and a lysosomal membrane, breakdown of cargo material, the deluge movement of the broken down content to be delivered to cytoplasm, as well as the refinement of the lysosome.

As for the cells of mammals, the process of autophagy development starts through the evolvement of a nucleus, in which the segregation membranes of diversified originations create phagophores, which then enlarge and merge to create a finished product that has two layers called an autophagosome. They are created at cytoplasm incidental places. After amalgamation with the lysosome, the cargo is broken down through hydrolases, followed by the renewal of lysosome virtually by the Golgi body. The segregation membranes could be produced from many origins—namely, outer mitochondria tissue, Golgi organ, Plasma tissues, and the Endoplasmic Reticulum. However, the Endoplasmic Reticulum origin is more attainable due to its protein synthesis aided by its ribosomes. The existence of a lot of autophagosome proteins near the endoplasmic reticulum also advocates that endoplasmic reticulum engages in a significant position in membrane source for the creation of autophagosomes.

Autophagy is implemented by the existing autophagy-related genes, which could also be connoted as Atg. Amino acid discerning in mammals and even indicators like growing and responsive oxygen breed control the undertaking of the protein kinases mechanistic target of rapamycin and the activated protein kinase. Both usually balance the process of autophagy by derailed addition of phosphoryl to the kinases unc-51-like kinase 1 and also unc-51-like kinase 2, as well as the initiation of autophagy outcome and the stimulation of the ULK kinases.

ULK is a section of the protein compound that contains autophagy-related protein 13, autophagy-related protein 101, and family-interacting protein 200. The unc-51-like kinase stimulates BECN1, which is the additional fragment of the protein network. The autophagy-practical Beclin-1 mixture carries the proteins protein 150—this unc-51-like kinase and the BECN1 multiplex position its location to where the formation of autophagy began.

The Self-Cleansing Process

In majority situations of our life, we have no self-cleaners. But other things demand quality of time and serious attention to get rid of dirt and waste that has piled up over a while. Come to think of it, what would happen if we dint regularly clean things or pieces of equipment? I know the expression you have on reading this is unpleasant. Our cars, desks, and kitchen would become toxic cesspools of dirt, and they would be sickening.

In the same way, this could occur to our bodies. If dirt and toxins are not thoroughly cleaned and thrown away, our cell productivity lowers, causing dull skin color, dark energy, fast aging, and weight loss. This is just what autophagy, your cellular self-cleaner, and talks about. Don't forget that in the literal sense, it means self-eating. This is because it takes up its own toxins and waste to produce younger and healthier cells.

This is how the process mainly works. Notably, our bodies are made up of different parts and organs that affect cellular functions. It is also made up of a lot of cells, each of which plays a significant role in the ways we function and live. A good example is the mitochondria, which is an organelle that gives rise to energy for a cell. Cells also carry proteins that are crucial for the working of a cell. These proteins provide structure to the cells and also carry out chemical reactions in the body. Besides, they act as messengers to relay a variety of information throughout the body.

Even though they're microscopic components, every cell chugs, and churns, manufacturing power, and elements that make your body carry out tasks the way they do, these cells play a role in how we think and feel. It provides the power to send signals, recall lyrics to a song, rational decisions, and even calculate rent payments and anything else you will do on your day-to-day lives. These cells are always operating. At many times they carry out a good job specifically at the early stage. Each item is usually new, and the networks function together in a consonance manner; therefore, everything continues functioning well without any problem. The work is done efficiently by all cells, and this usually results in the body being very healthy and fully energized.

That doesn't mean each cellular system works all the time correctly. Our standard cellular system becomes injured with use over some time through those unavoidable and speeds up Agers explained earlier. The majority of the people assume that wear and tear is a certainty of life and that no matter what we do, our bodies will break down because of aging. Surely, we cannot go against the natural arc of life and death, but we can definitely hinder the impacts of aging. At this point, we are going to see why.

Our cells degrade sections of themselves through segregating them into vacuoles and assimilating them. Consequently, they brought about waste material consisting of dead organelles, injured proteins, and oxidized pieces; this waste has to be eliminated. And not unless the waste is disposed of properly, that dirt stays and piles up in the body. That building up of trash is a critical influence in the rate of aging. The toxins get in the way and cause everything to malfunction. It could sound like jargon from a biology lesson, but in reality, it is when the toxins damage the system of our cells, it is a massive factor in the aging process. It makes your skin look older, your body becomes slow, your energy drops drastically, and the hormones scatter all over. Do you want that? Cause I also don't want that to happen to me.

This is the reason why autophagy is necessary for human health. It's the same as cellular garbage is being disposed of, taking the defective sections and destroying them, so that they wouldn't cause a distraction anywhere else. If it is functioning correctly, then it has undergone self-renewal degrading old useless structures to create space for new ones. The product is a brand new, more young, and energetic structure that would allow us to be more dynamic and look younger.

You can just imagine how that plays out in our day-to-day life. Increased youthful cells mean that you have healthier and softer skin, your body undergoes less fatigue, your metabolism rate being better, this will result in the cells to be able to generate energy all over the body from the muscles to your brain cells to your internal organs.

Many researchers term autophagy as a strategy or mechanism used for survival. In that, it speaks about how a cell would react to specific changes in the environment to ensure the health of a body. This makes sense because all living organisms are out there trying to survive to stay alive.

This knowledge has indeed resulted in the innovation of treatments for aging and finding natural cures for diseases like cancer, diseases like cancer, and infectious diseases. Major labs around the world saw the first known gene responsible for autophagy in mammals. They say the waste-removal function is what keeps us healthy.

Usually, autophagy hums along silently behind the scenes in the maintenance of the body's well-being mode. It suddenly kicks in the high gear during stressful times, acting as a protector to the body when there are limited amounts of food or water. The body stimulates the process of autophagy to slow down the aging of your body, reduce inflammation, and speed up the natural ability of your body to function. It also helps your body fight off disease-causing microorganisms to boost longevity. The human body can naturally activate the autophagy process.

There are a lot of natural ways through which you can increase the autophagy process of your body. To cleanse the cells and lower the rate of inflammation, and in general, retain your body functioning, you need these techniques discussed below. Remember that since autophagy is a response reaction to stressful conditions, you are required to trick your body into thinking it is under some amount of stress. This is how to go about it:

Eat High-Fat and Low-Carbohydrate Foods

I will be emphasizing on the significance of taking in fats to stimulate autophagy fats should be considered as a ruling macronutrient in our diets because it differs from protein. Where the protein could turn into carbohydrates and be sugar, but fats cannot do that. Particularly in the Keto diet, the intake of low carbohydrates and also the intake of high fat will offer your body an edge in as far as autography is concerned. The movement from a glucose burning to ketones that takes place in a Keto diet procedure impersonates the natural occurrence in a fasted state. This grows the chances of the autophagy process.

A lot of people have testified to the benefits of fats being in a replacement of high amounts of sugar for the activation of autophagy. They also argue that once the process began, it was a bit rough, but everything worked out along the way. You get used to the new diet within a week. You will be feeling much healthier

Try Out Protein Fasting

At least twice or thrice a week try to restrict the amount of protein intake to the utilization of 15 to 25 grams of protein every day. This limitation allows your body to be able to reuse proteins, which will lower the rate of inflammation and cleanse your cells without you struggling. Throughout this period of time, while autophagy becomes activated, your body cells are obligated to take up its own toxins and proteins to survive.

Try Out Intermittent Fasting

This usually refers to the habit of eating, whereby a person balances fasting and eating. It mainly focuses on which times you are supposed to eat, not really the types of foods to eat. There are many ways in which you can practice this kind of fasting. The simplest involves doing without breakfast, eating at noon, and the last meal before 8 pm. No food is permitted during the entire fasting period. You are only allowed to drink coffee, tea or water, and any other non-caloric beverages.

By doing this, you heighten your body's innate autophagy process. For example, protein fasting allows your body to close in on all those remaining toxins by cleansing your cells in the form of eating up these toxins to enable new ones to form. The proper disposal of these waste actually builds up a 16-to-28-hour fast. If the timings are irregular, it could cause hormonal imbalance in most women

This is because women are incredibly delicate to changes such as starvation or restriction of calories. So with that said, you can sidestep hiss problem by taking in a big diet breakfast and try to limit proteins and carbohydrates from your meal. While the fat tricks your body that it is not starving, you remain fasting. We are going to discuss intermittent fasting more broadly in the next section. Be sure to check it out.

Try Out Sprint Interval Training

This is another critical way to activate autophagy. Keep in mind that autophagy involves the body's reaction to stress, and in this case, high-intensity exercise puts you in stress spot. It stresses you sufficient enough to start up biochemical reactions. The right effects to make your muscles stronger without injuring your body. It also induces autophagy, which results in a boost in your longevity. Set a target to exercise approximately 20 to 30 minutes each.

Great emphasis is put on the less is more attitude toward exercise to activate autophagy in your body. Lifting weights and resistance training workouts for about 35 minutes each day is the most effective way to stimulate. It involves obtaining severe, temporary stress and allowing the body to take care of itself by disposing of waste substance through autophagy. You can try this out by taking intervals in training between low pace and brisk.

Get Restorative Sleep

You can garner the good of autophagy when you are sleeping too. Through sleep personality, which is also known as sleep Chronotype, helps you get knowledge of the benefits and effectiveness of sleep. An individual has a single of four sleep personalities that informs the way one functions throughout the night and during the day. Knowing your sleep personality allows you to set your body to stimulate the autophagy process with your circadian patterns or sleep cycle.

Autophagy to Heal and Detox Your Body and Regenerate Your Mind

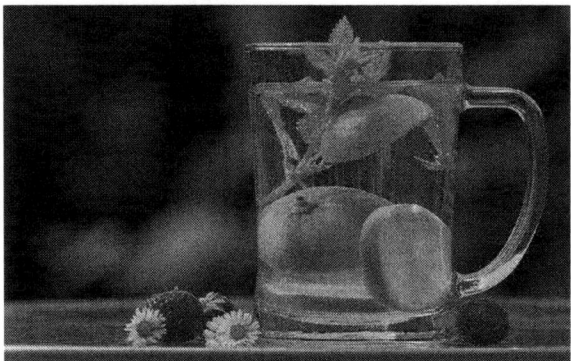

The term detox is undoubtedly the most misconstrued and misunderstood word in the health and nutrition sector—with the most significant wrongdoers being the vendors of 'detox smoothies.' The majority of the recipes of so-called detox smoothies carry more sugar than is needed in the body. The types of sugars in these mixtures are fructose that actually intoxicates the body.

Fructose metamorphosis is wholly distinct from that of glucose. While glucose is effortlessly metabolized and transformed into energy by almost all the cells in your body, fructose is at best handled in the liver. So a diet enriched with fructose is a day-to-day practice in the modern world. It deposits excessive amounts of injury to the main detoxifying organs.

Fructose is destructive to the liver as well as other toxic substances such as alcohol. And observing the rate of intake has grown to four hundred percent in the last five decades, it is not astonishing that fatty diseases of the liver have tripled during the same period of time. The majority of American adults suffer from fatty liver diseases that are non-alcoholic. So before you even think about getting smoothies for body cleansing, consider other options.

Your body is under the normal state of renewal. Every minute of the day, your body is degrading old, not useful cells to give space for the growth of new cells that will be reproduced. New proteins are created as others are used up. If a cell gets to the termination of its usefulness, it experiences a process known as apoptosis, famously known as cell death that has been programmed. This is a sequential procedure for the body to get rid of cells that have worn out. The cell is degraded into component sections and from there 'eaten up' by various immune cells when the necessity arises.

There are other times when it is only specific parts of a cell that need replacement, something close to the replenishment of energy battery in your TV remote control. It could not necessarily mean that an entire organelle needs to be replenished. Autophagy refers to the metabolic procedure where weak, broken or old cellular structures get renewed, repaired and reused through a self-cannibalization in the body

Let us see what autophagy does when it comes to detoxing and anti-aging.

This sequential metabolism utilizes structures that dispose of waste known as lysosomes. These organelles degrade and recycle cellular parts. The component sections are then turned into amino acids, which are proteins building blocks, and moved to other parts of the body where they are used to revitalize cells and get rid of waste materials. Now, this is what detoxcation truly means at the very profound level means

As this inner cleansing removes cellular clutter, aging is contrasted because what is old is made new again. And the satisfaction of autophagy goes well far and beyond looking and feeling more youthful.

This operation also helps to wipe out pathogens while creating newer and powerful immune cells. A more powerful immune system means excellent resistance to infectious diseases. Additionally, it improves monitoring against mutated cells and safeguards the wholeness of the cell's nucleus that prevent cancer cells from being created in the first place.

Research also reveals that autophagy helps in lowering inflammation, and resistance to insulin can enhance the symptoms and outward look for individuals suffering from an illness like Alzheimer's disease and even Parkinson's disease. Think about autophagy as your body's natural program for recycling. It makes us more sufficient in the ability to remove defective sections, prevent cancerous growths, and halt metabolic dysfunction such as diabetes and obesity.

In this other section, we will see how to make sure your body does not switch off these disease-fighting and detoxification process.

The primary diet that stops Cellular Detoxification includes high taking in of carbohydrates and, consequently, the release of insulin hormone in the body. This means that the fresh juices that are pressed, veggies smoothies that are mainly termed as detox beverages would switch off the autophagy (detox procedure) the same case applies to honey and sweetened desserts praised in the Paleo Blogs.

An individual should also watch out for excessive protein consumption. The majority of people do not know that a single protein can be easily transformed into glucose through a process known as gluconeogenesis. And researches have also conveyed that the amino acid called leucine completely halts the process of autophagy. This supposedly doesn't mean that an individual should limit consumption of protein to the extent that you may restrict carbohydrates intake, although it is vital to understand that diets rich in proteins could trigger powerful insulin reactions in some individuals and slows the healing process of organelles.

Three Ways to Boost the Symptoms of Autophagy

There are three significant ways to increase the activation of these internal detoxification, healing, and regeneration of mind. These vital factors include practicing fasting, the introduction of the Ketogenic diet, and body exercises.

Fasting

The most primary driver is fasting. Especially, intermittent fasting. The autophagy occurs in different degrees and a variety of organelles. Generally, if your blood sugars and level of insulin are low, they will automatically activate the autophagy process. How long exactly do you need to fast?

Following 16 hours of fasting and eating within 8 hours fasting plan on a daily basis can be essential in the stimulation of the autophagy process. The majority of individuals observe an eating window, which is even more compressed. They take in food within four hours and fast the other hours of the day that are left.

Extended fasting provides even more essential benefits to the body. Many scientists' advice on the introduction of quarterly water fast for at least five days is the best thing you could do to maintain the process of healing and detoxification to improve disease resistance process and longevity

Ketogenic Diet

The second process involves the ketogenic diet introduction to our day-to-day activities. When fasting is considered more valuable in the health sector, the majority of people prefer strictly sticking to a variety of diets that includes paleo and Keto diet. Let's take a look at the ketogenic diet.

Keto diet usually involves the consumption of foods or meals that have a high content of healthy fats, moderately low protein, and, last but not least, are low in carbohydrates. By observing the Keto diet, we can trick the body into thinking it is under siege. This way, it activates the lysosome to degrade old and defective proteins in an individual's body.

This diet also introduces ketone bodies. These bodies are not only useful in cleansing the body cells but also switch on the chaperone-mediated autophagy mechanism (CMA). This procedure selectively reuses cellular waste, and yet the only thing you needed to activate this process is to limit the consumption of carbohydrates. With the Keto diet, an individual gets the same metabolic changes and significance as fasting without actually fasting.

Exercise

Finally, there is a third most effective way to heighten the autophagy process. This involves exercise. In research on animals, scholars found that dreadful activity tends to switch on the autophagy process in the cardiac and skeletal muscles. It also consists of the stimulation of autophagy in the pancreas and liver by renewing and reusing significant metabolic tissues.

Some scholars would argue that autophagy is automatically activated after thirty minutes if acute exercises; however, it starts the process of breaking down and self-eating of toxins after about eighty minutes of vigorous exercise. This process substantiates the fact that a shorter duration but high-intensity activity is of high significance compared to the long term and less intensity cardio.

Feasting & Fasting:

Trying to Strike the Perfect Ancestral Balance

Even in real life, there is a saying that says that too much of everything is poisonous. While autophagy is beneficial to the human body, too much or too little of it could be harmful to your body. Therefore, this calls for the ability to balance between both so that you can avoid killing yourself while trying to undergo these severe changes in your day-to-day activities.

Nonetheless, there's substantial evidence that the severity of the autophagy process is something we can adjust to; it is an evolutionary process of reaction to either feasting or famine during stress periods. If not dealt with naturally, these toxins could kill us, so the best outcomes would be seen after getting used to these techniques over a while.

To obtain optimal health and reap the benefits of the nearest thing we have to natural healing and detoxification of the body, we should incorporate the natural lifestyle of our ancestors of feasting and fasting to enable cellular growth when eating and cellular cleansing when we are fasting.

Weight Loss Through Autophagy

The majority of individuals who are practicing fasting are either doing it to reduce diseases causing microorganisms, or to lose weight. Especially people with signs and symptoms of obesity use this mechanism to lose excessive fats. More specifically, to increase longevity and become more energetic.

Intermittent fasting researches have not established an essential benefit over consecutive energy limitation diets. It only works if a person can adhere to it consistently. Unfortunately, most research on IF is poorly constructed and doesn't consider the differences between fasting routines.

However, losing weight isn't the same as fat loss, and it doesn't mean you're getting healthier or activating autophagy. Conventional calorie restriction diets don't guarantee autophagy and may block it completely.

Most of the longevity benefits of fasting are mediated by autophagy. Deficient autophagy promotes aging and disease. Furthermore, autophagy regulates lipid metabolism through lipophagy.

What Are Lipolysis and Lipophagy?

To lose body fat, you have to first "release" it from the adipose stores. This process is called lipolysis. It is the degradation of fatty acids, triglycerides, and cholesterol by autophagy. It contributes to lipid droplet degradation in many cell types.

Lipophagy uses 'acid' lipolysis in lysosomes to degrade cellular triacylglycerols, which store free fatty acids. Lipid stores are metabolized by lipophagy to fuel mitochondrial beta-oxidation and regulated to maintain energy homeostasis. Impaired lipophagy promotes fatty liver and dysregulates body mass.

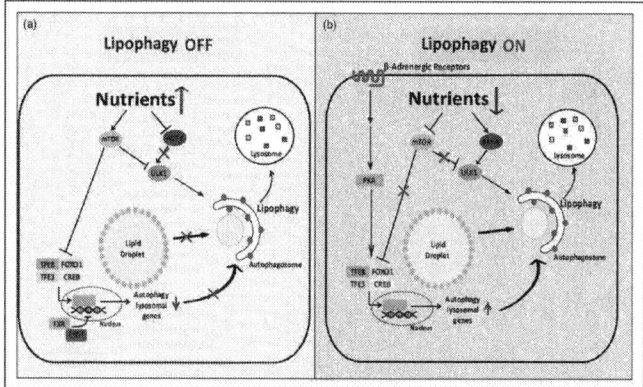

How many lipids get degraded by lipophagy depends on the supply of extracellular nutrients and overall caloric balance. The cells adjust the amount of lipophagy based on their nutritional status.

Autophagy and Ketogenesis

Another pathway related to lipolysis and fat loss is ketosis. It's a metabolic state characterized by elevated ketone bodies, which are energy molecules created from beta-oxidation.

You can be in ketosis without autophagy, and you can have autophagy without ketosis. It's just that, usually, you'd see them together because they follow similar principles.

Autophagy is essential for the synthesis of ketone bodies. Autophagy deficient mice have decreased the production of ketones by the liver.

While inadequate renal autophagy does not impair Ketogenesis, mice with deficient autophagy in both liver and kidneys have lower blood ketones and physical activity under starvation than those who lack autophagy in just the liver. You need autophagy to induce proper Ketogenesis.

If you're on a calorie-restrictive diet, but you don't have autophagy, you'll inhibit Ketogenesis, which lowers the amount of available energy your body has access to it. Body fat is fuel, and you shouldn't feel tired of hungry even when you have sub 10% body fat.

With enough autophagy, you'll enable Ketogenesis to kick in, which raises ketones in your blood and gives more energy to the brain. Most people find it easier to diet and fast when they're in ketosis.

Autophagy and Insulin

Conventional weight-loss diets are anti-autophagic and anti-ketogenic because they promote eating low fat, high protein, high carb at a high eating frequency. This will inevitably interfere with both Ketogenesis and autophagy. If you eat very often throughout the day, then you're preventing the formation of autophagosomes by raising insulin.

The autophagy of the impaired macrophages usually causes the resistance of insulin when it comes to the condition of obesity because the inflammatory adipocytes produce too many reactive oxygen species, which autophagy would frequently clear out. Being obese promotes inflammation, which makes you even more provocative and obese while not being able to heal that inflammation because of suppressed autophagy.

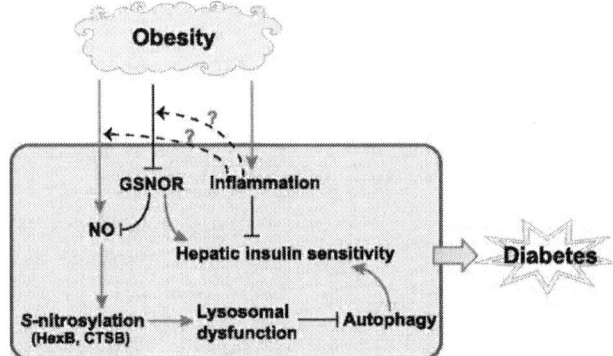

Mice deficient in autophagy show larger adipocytes in the visceral tissues, which are fat, increased liver fat, reduced tolerance to glucose, as well as being resistant to insulin.

So, not only are a ketogenic diet and fasting great for lowering insulin and thus activate autophagy, but they also help to protect against developing insulin resistance.

Autophagy and Loose Skin After Weight Loss

It's said that autophagy can eat up loose skin and tighten it up after you've lost a bunch of weight. However, that's only true to a certain extent.

A 2014 study in Japan found that aging fibroblasts have decreased autophagy. Fibroblasts create collagen in the skin, which causes wrinkles and loose skin.

Another 2018 study from Korea found that aging fibroblasts experience an increase in the production of unwanted materials, which results in skin aging. The researchers said that the role of autophagy is very important, as it aids the counteracting aging process to the skin by keeping the fibroblasts healthy.

Autophagy may help with slowing down the aging of the skin, but it's not eating up wrinkles and loose skin. It only supports the processes that keep the skin more elastic and able to tighten up faster.

In cases of extreme weight loss, fasting and autophagy can help with preventing excess loose skin. You will inevitably have some loose skin after losing a bunch of weight. However, if you lose weight with fasting, you'll have more autophagy, which can help your skin adapt to the new weight quicker.

Calorie restrictive diets without autophagy will probably create much more loose skin because, as we've seen in studies, autophagy is central to at least keeping the fibroblasts and collagen production active.

Does Autophagy Enable You to Lose Fat?

The number of adipocytes is a significant determinant in how much fat mass a person has. Unfortunately, it's said that the total count of the cells that are fat usually remains the same when one becomes an adult or following a loss of weight. About ten percent of the cells that are fat are usually developed every year at all the ages of adults and also the total mass of the body indexes. Autophagy is the process of cellular turnover that increases the rate of cell renewal. Theoretically, increased basal autophagy and specific degradation of adipocytes may enhance this because you'll be breaking down things more effectively.

You're not going to lose fat unless you're at a caloric deficit, even if you have a lot of autophagy. Fasting for three days and then over-eating will still make you gain weight if you consume excess calories.

Autophagy does not make you lose fat directly because your overall energy balance determines it. It's just that autophagy promotes the metabolism of lipid droplets and fatty acids through lipophagy and ketosis.

If you want to know how to start intermittent fasting for autophagy, longevity, anti-aging, and improved body composition, then check out my book.

Three Ways to Activate the Process of Weight Loss

While autophagy occurs throughout the body regularly, there are three primary ways to speed up the process and encourage the body to take its stance against unwanted fat cells. The following three triggers play a key role in weight loss, to begin with, but when used to stimulate autophagy, they take on an entirely new level of efficiency.

Exercise – Exercise stresses the body and can cause small tears in muscle tissue. These micro-tears aren't necessarily harmful, but they take a toll on the body and can increase your risk of injury if not given ample time to heal. This is where autophagy comes in. By helping to clear away the broken and damaged bits of cells associated with the micro-tears, they make way for new cells to form that help to regenerate the muscle tissue.

Autophagy Fasting – Like exercise, fasting creates stress on the body. Intermittent fasting, or going for a few hours a day without eating, may help to control diabetes and minimize a person's risk of developing heart disease. Fasting also works in the brain as well and may help fight neurodegenerative disorders. By eliminating deteriorating brain cells, some studies state that cognitive function may improve when a person uses intermittent fasting. Some people fast for 12 to 18 hours, while others prolong the fast for as long as 36 hours, depending on the results that they hope to achieve.

Decreasing the number of carbs that you consume will also trigger autophagy processes. For this trigger to be active, you would need to fast for up to 18 hours or longer. This forces the body into a state of ketosis. During the other six hours, the use of carbohydrates is minimal, forcing the body to feed on itself for the fuel it needs to function. However, cutting out whole grains to reduce carbs is a risky proposition, with the recent studies connecting low overall grain consumption to cancer (particularly colon cancer).

Chapter Two: Fat-Burning Strategies

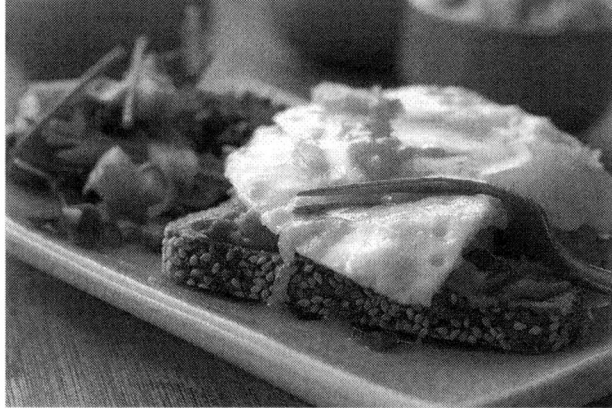

Fat burning refers to the innate utilization of stored fat by the body during certain conditions. It could be either activated or induced in many ways or can naturally happen without us knowing. The burning of fat can be the body's way of surviving in low-energy conditions.

Ways to Burn Fats

Whether you are considering the enhancement of your health, in general, or you want to attain that summer body for a new bikini, the process of burning fats is quite a task. Specific techniques can help an individual to increase the fat burning process on their body. The best ways to burn fat in your body involve:

1. Begin Practicing Training of Strength

This exercise involves a training activity that demands the shrinking of the muscles with another person. It helps to create the mass of muscles and grows your power to be able to pursue work that needs toughness. Nearly all the training of the strength usually consists of weight lifting exercise so as to be able to acquire more muscles. Through the various researches, we are able to understand that strength training produces multiple health benefits like a fat burn and gaining muscles.

Resistance exercise could also assist in the preservation of masses that are free from fat, hence the increase in the level of calories in the body, which usually burns when you are resting. Performing bodyweight training, lifting weights, and using gym resources is one of the simplest ways to begin strength exercise for burning excessive fats.

2. Follow a Diet High in Protein

Inclusive of meals which have a lot of protein is the efficient method which lowers the food appetite while burning a lot of fat. The consumption of increased protein quality is linked to a reduced risk in belly fat. Increasing your protein intake may also heighten your ability to feel full in your stomach because proteins take time to digest in the stomach, thereby reducing appetite and reduction in calorie consumption to help lose weight. The good examples are eggs, seafood dairy products, meat, and legumes, which consist of a lot of proteins.

3. Try to Sleep a Lot

Sleeping at an early time will help you prolong the burning of fats in the body and also the increase of a lot of weight. Several types of research have discovered a link between having a quality sleep period and losing weight. A research conducted on females indicated that the women who were having a sleep period of about five hours in a single night were at the risk of adding more weight compared to the women who had quality sleep of about 8 hours in a single night. A lot of studies found out that deprivation of sleep usually leads to various changes in the hormones of hunger, which will also lead to the appetite of a person to increase and also a person being at risk of having the problem of obesity. Even though every person is different when it comes to the duration of sleep they usually have, a lot of researchers have found out that getting quality sleep of about 7 to 8 hours of sleep period in a single night is very essential, as it will result to losing weight and other benefits which are associated with the health of the body.

A person should be having a single sleeping period pattern something they do every single day, they should decrease the amount of caffeine that is taken just before going to bed and also decrease the level of electronic usage during the time to sleep so as to have a sleeping pattern which is healthier than the ones experienced before. Therefore, one should know that when you get a quality sleep pattern will result in the low chances of increasing your weight.

4. The Diet Should Consist of Vinegar

This is usually because the vinegar is widely proven to contain substances that help increase the health of a person. To add on that, it usually beneficial when it comes to the health of the heart and also the control of the blood sugar levels, and therefore by increasing the level of consumption of vinegar will aid in increasing the burning of fats process, which has been proven by various researchers. Consuming about one to two spoons of the vinegar every day will eventually aid in decreasing the weight of a person. Through the consumption of the vinegar, a person will be able to experience an appetite reduction.

5. The Consumption of Fats That Are Healthy

Through the increase in the consumption of a lot of fats that are healthy will eventually result in weight loss, even though it is viewed as impossible. This is usually because the fats tend to take time to digest and hence aid in the process of stomach emptying in a slow manner, thus causing the reduction of hunger feelings and also the reduction of having an appetite. Various researches indicate that constant following of a diet that consists a lot of fats that are usually healthier which have been extracted from nuts and also olive will result to the weight management of the body whereby a person will have less risk in gaining weight as compared to someone who does not practice this. Many studies have proven that loss of weight can be achieved through the use of vinegar, and therefore, just by taking a spoon of olive oil or even the oil from coconut will eventually be able to lose the weight. Therefore, this process will be very beneficial to a person who is having a diet so as to be able to lose weight.

You should always know that the fats that healthy also contain more calories; therefore, you should be able to balance the consumption level of these fats even though they are healthy. This can be achieved by changing the consumption of taking all fats in general and change to consuming the fats that are healthier. Because fats usually take time to digest; therefore, consuming it will aid in the reduction of your appetite. Thus, its consumption will be beneficial in losing weight in the whole body.

6. Drinking Beverages That Are Healthy

Changing from the consumption of the drinks that are usually high in the levels of sugar to the dinks that are so low on sugar levels will result in the increase of the process of burning of the fats. Therefore, one should avoid drinks the intake of beverages that contain a lot of sugar, for instance, soda, which contains a lot of calories, which usually gives the body a little benefit but a lot of damages. The alcoholic drinks usually consist of a lot of calories, which will also cause the inhibitions in the body to reduce; hence, the person under the influence will be at risk of overreacting to things. Therefore, the consumption of the drinks that usually contain a lot of sugar together with alcoholic drinks will eventually result in gaining a lot of fats around the belly of a person. The limitation of these drinks will be very beneficial, whereby there will be a decrease in the consumption of calories, thus keeping them away from developing the belly fats. You should, therefore, change to drinks which do not contain calories that will help with your health—for example, the drinking of water. Drinking a lot of water every day and more specific around meal times will result in loss of weight. The consumption of green tea is also a good way to help improve your health, whereby it contains caffeine and contains a lot of antioxidants, which will help in the process of burning fats and also increase the rate of metabolism.

7. Increase Fiber Intake

The dissolved fibers usually suck up water and shift through the track of digestion hence aiding a person to feel satisfied for a long period. Therefore, increasing the consumption to consist of a lot of fiber will be very beneficial, as it will guard the body against gaining weight and also the concurrence of fats. Research indicates that the consumption of every ten grams of dissolved fiber will lead to weight loss in between 4 to 5 years, even without following any diet or being involved in any exercise. The consumption of fruits or vegetables will help in the process of burning fats in the body. Therefore, the increase in consumption of a lot of fiber is highly linked to the loss of fats, low consumption of calories, and a general loss of weight.

8. Decrease the Intake of Carbohydrates That Have Been Refined

You should decrease the consumption of the carbohydrates that have been refined hence being able to lose the fats in the body, and this is high because the carbohydrates that are usually refined lose their nutrients in that process hence containing a low level of nutrients and also fiber. Usually, the carbohydrates that have undergone the process of refining have high levels of the glycemic count, resulting in crashes and spikes in the sugar levels of the blood, which will eventually cause high hunger levels. Many types of research indicate that a meal that contains a lot of the carbohydrates that have been refined usually results in the development of fats around the belly. Therefore, the consumption of the carbohydrates that have not been refined will help in the weight loss process in the whole body and, more specifically, around the belly. Many researchers argue that the people who usually consume refined carbohydrates were at risk of getting health problems like the fats around the belly, while the people who consumed the carbohydrates that were not refined were at a lower amount the development of such problems. To be able to do away with such problem you should lower the level of consuming the carbohydrates that have undergone the process of being refined and increase the consumption of the carbohydrates that have not been refined as they contain a lot of nutrients and also have a lot of fiber and reduce the level of hunger in the system and be better health-wise.

9. Raise the Cardio

The exercise of aerobics is a famous type of exercise that is used to train and also exercise the organs of the body, specifically the heart and the lungs. Through doing this will result from increasing the burning of the fats in the body, as it is an operative way of achieving this. Therefore, the increase in aerobics resulted in the burning of a lot of fats, which is around the belly, which can be seen in many types of research. The aerobics can be able to add the mass of the muscles while decreasing the fats around the belly and also the weight loss in the general body. Many professionals have argued that it is important to have aerobics exercises of about 150 to 300 minutes every week. This can be achieved through running and also swimming, including other types of aerobics, which are beneficial to the health of the body. This will also result in lower the total circumference of the waist of the body and also aid in burning off the excess fats in the body, even having a positive effect on the mass of the muscles of the body.

10. Consume a Lot of Coffee

Drinking coffee helps in the burning of fats because caffeine is a very important component that usually speeds up the process of burning the fats in the body. The caffeine, which is included in coffee deeds as the main stimulant, which usually affects the rate of metabolism positively and also encourages the degradation of the acids that are fat in the body. Many research shows that a person can be able to boost energy and even improve the metabolism process through drinking coffee, which contains a lot of caffeine. The high consumption of caffeine is usually linked to the slow gaining of weight. Through drinking coffee, you will be able to benefit a lot, as it also helps in maintaining weight loss in a person. To be able to get the benefits fully through drinking coffee, one should eliminate the sugar and also the cream and, therefore, just drink the coffee in black or add a little milk so as to be able to keep away from the consumption of more calories.

11. Practice the Sprint Interval Training

This is usually a form of practice that joins the first intense of activities which have a small period of recovery so as to be able to increase the rate of the heart. This can be beneficial, as it aids the burning process of fats, as well as it has a positive effect on losing weight. Therefore, through this, you can be able to lose weight in just a week by just practicing it for just 25 minutes a day, and you will be able to see some remarkable changes in your weight. Changes will be vivid, even without altering your lifestyle or what consist of your diet. Through this, one will be able to reduce the fats, which usually accumulate around the belly and even decrease the total circumference of the waist. Through this process, you are also able to burn a lot of calories in just a short period as compared to the others. This process will help you in the burning process of the calories of up to 35 percent, hence being more efficient than the other forms. For the best way to start with the sprint interval training, you should start by balancing between the process of walking and also the action of running slowly for a period of about one minute. You can even choose to balance the exercises—for example, doing a few push-ups and then doing some squats—which will be very beneficial to the person. Therefore, this process is proven to be able to help in the burning of a lot of calories within a small period of time.

12. The Diet Consisting of Probiotics

This is usually a form of bacteria that is usually beneficial to the body of a mammal, and it is located in the digestive tract, and it has been proven to be able to benefit the health of a person. These bacteria, which are in the gut, have been indicated to help big time in many things—for example, the immunity of the body and also the health of the person's mind. Therefore, through the increase in the consumption of probiotics by taking meals that consist of the product, which will benefit the body in so many ways, including the burning process of the fats and also the management of a person's weight. Many types of research have been conducted, and the results are the same whereby the individuals who consumed the probiotics were able to lose weight and more specifically in the reduction of the total percentage of fats in the body but the others they still had a lot of fats and were able to gain a lot of weight. Many types of research indicate that the consumption of the probiotic eke out aided many people who had a diet that consisted of a lot of fats and also a lot of calories, and they were able to the accumulation of fats in the body and also maintained the general weight of the entire body.

13. Add the Consumption of Iron in the Diet

Everyone knows that iron is a very important mineral, as it comprises a lot of functions in the body. The lack of iron mineral in the body will affect the body negatively, whereby it will affect the thyroid gland, which is located on the neck and usually produces the hormones that usually help stimulate the metabolism process in the body. Many types of research indicate that having a diet that is low in iron will result in the thyroid being less effective in performing its duties, as well as the thyroid hormones production will be interrupted. The famous indicators of hypothyroidism, which is viewed as the ineffectiveness of the thyroid will consist of experiencing some form of visibility in the body, some exhaustion of the body, running out of breath, as well as the addition of the bodies weight. Treating the insufficiency of iron in the body will ensure the body functions well and also that the function of the thyroid glands to be more effective; hence, the body will be able to prevent issues like running out of breath and even encourage the activities levels. Research has also discovered that the people who usually get treated for the insufficiency of the iron mineral in the body enjoyed the high level of weight loss. People should start including the right amount of the iron minerals in their diet so as to experience the benefits it comes with. A person should be ready and eager to include the iron mineral in the meals so as to be able to reach the levels of iron that the body really requires so as to be able to maintain the energy levels of the body. This is easy, as you can find iron in dairy products—for example, meat. The insufficient iron in the body will lead to the thyroid not functioning well hence affecting the body negatively in so many ways.

14. Start Fasting

This is usually a diet program that involves the balancing of periods to eat and the periods that you should fast. A lot of researches usually indicates that intermittent fasting aids in the reduction of weight and also being able to lose the fats in the body. Some of the various results of the fasting usually involve the propositional fasting in a day, which is a type of fasting that consists of the alternation of the fasting days and the days of frequently eating. The research I found out that the day alternation fasting of about 3 to 12 weeks resulted in a weight loss of about seven percent and also helped in lowering the level of the fats in the body. Therefore, by eating in between 8 hours of the day also helps to lower the percentage of fats in the body and also maintains the mass of muscles. There exist a lot of methods of fasting, which usually consist of different patterns of eating and also of abstaining from taking any meal. Therefore, you should look for a method that will fit with your schedule and routine to be able to see which of the methods work best. This is because there exist a lot of many methods to aid in the weight reduction process and even improve one's health. The introduction of a new lifestyle that is healthy will be very beneficial.

Intermittent Fasting

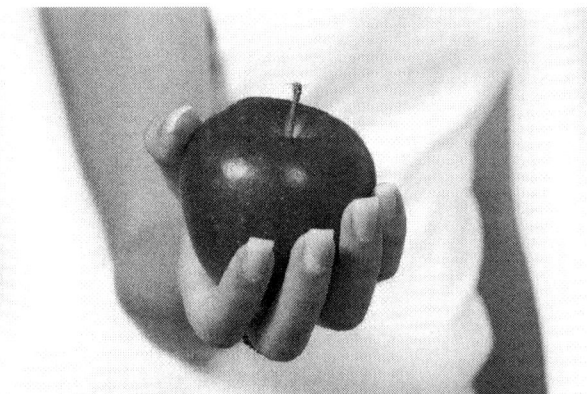

It usually refers to the various sequences of eating that surrounds the time that a person eats and fasts. It usually does not portray the food that a person should consume but talks of *when* to consume the food. Therefore, it is not a diet but a guide in giving the direction of when to eat the food. The recognized fasting method usually consists of a person being able to abstain from food in a period of 16 hours and should be practiced within two times a week. Many humans have been practicing fasting since the Ancient Times. The people during these times were not equipped with shops or sophisticated technology. All they had were crude weapons, which helped them survive—but at times, they went to sleep or stayed hungry the entire day. Through this, the humans were enabled to stay for long periods without eating, hence being able to fast over time. Many people have been practicing fasting for religious reasons—for example, the Muslims who usually have a month of fasting. The same case applies to Christians. Though a lot of people usually practice fasting for religious purposes, it is very important to health, as it helps solve a lot of health issues—for example, being obese. There exist various methods of practicing fasting, which usually consists of being able to balance the days of fasting and the days of eating. Therefore, to be able to achieve this, you should eat a small quantity of food or abstain from eating during the days you are fasting. Through this, you will be able to improve your health.

Types of Intermittent Fasting

The following consist of various methods of intermittent fasting:

16:8

The most common one is the fasting of between sixteen hours and being able to eat within eight hours. This method usually consists of missing breakfast and also restricting the consumption habits to a fewer number of hours—for example, 2 to 10 pm—then, abstain from consuming food for almost sixteen hours straight. This will have an impact on your health.

Eat, Stop, Eat

The second method is eating and then stopping and then eating again. This method usually consists of practicing fasting for a full day, which is twenty-four hours in a single week. You should be able to do so one time or repeat the fasting in the same week. This will also have a positive impact on the health of the body.

5:2

The next method is known as the five to ratio two. This method usually consists of the consumption of only five hundred to 600 calories in any given two days in a week, but there is no limit of the remaining days of the week.

Calorie Reduction

The fourth method usually consists of the decreasing consumption of calories, which usually has a positive impact on losing the weight of the body. A lot of people usually suggest that the first method is the simplest and that it is more sustainable, and a person can be able to follow. This method is the most famous type, as many people know about it as compared to the rest, as it is viewed as an easy way to achieve the benefits of fasting.

Effects of Intermittent Fasting

When a person abstains from the consumption of food, a lot of effects are experienced in the entire body. This will be able to change the levels of the hormones so as to be able to access the fats that have been stored. This will also result in the cells stimulating the important process of repairing and also alter the gene-to-protein process. The following are some alterations that usually happen in the body when a person is fasting:

The Hormone Responsible for Growth in Humans

These type of hormones usually increases, and it has many benefits to the body of a person—for example, it usually helps in the fighting the increase of fats in the body and even results to the gaining of the total mass of the muscles. This will be very beneficial to the body, as it makes the body much healthier and being energetic and strong. Therefore, the fasting process usually helps the improvement of the body's health.

Insulin

There are improvements in the sensitivity of the insulin in the body, as well as, the levels of insulin will lower very quickly, thus enabling the body to use the fats that were stored. Therefore, this will improve the accessibility of the stored fats to be reached and used hence promoting the health of the entire body.

The Repair of the Cellular

When a person is fasting, the cells usually stimulate the process of repairing the cellular, which usually consists of the process of autophagy, wherein the cells will be able to undergo the alimentary process and eliminate the proteins which are not functioning and the old ones which usually accumulate in the cells.

The Expression of Genes

These are usually the alterations that usually occur in the duties or roles of the genes which are linked to longevity and guarding the body against getting any diseases. The alterations in the level of hormones, the role of the cells, as well as the expression of genes, are the result of the benefits from fasting, which improves the health of the body. Therefore, when you fast, the hormones which are responsible for growth in humans will increase in number while the levels of the insulin will shift downwards. Due to fasting the cells of the body will alter the expression of the genes and then stimulate the process of repairing the cellular.

Weight Loss

Losing weight is very important, and many people share this, as it has become an issue in society, hence becoming a mutual cause for the individuals to try and fast. Therefore, consuming fewer foods, the process fasting usually leads to a direct lowering of calorie consumption. The fasting process also alters the number of the hormone hence being able to increase the loss of weight in the body. This will also aid in dropping the levels of insulin and boost the levels of the hormones that are responsible for growth in humans and also boosts the discharge of hormones that are responsible for the burning of fats in the body. Due to these alterations in the hormones, hence fasting over a short time period will boost the rate of metabolism in the body. Through the consumption of less and burning calories, the process of fasting usually results in losing weight and thus improves the health of the entire body. Many types of research indicate that the process of fasting can be a beneficial way to lose weight hence being viewed as the best tool for losing weight.

Many types of research prove that through fasting, a person will be able to lose weight, and therefore, the eating sequences can be able to result in a weight loss of about three to eight percent with a given period of about three to twenty-four weeks.

Researches also indicate that people who practiced fasting experience a drop in the total circumference of their waste of about four to seven percent and also illustrated a decrease of the fats around the belly which usually accumulate around the organs of the body and result to diseases which are very harmful to the body. To be able to achieve these, you should be able to consume fewer calories in general. You are advised that when not fasting, you should not consume a lot of calories, as it will hinder the achievement of these benefits. The process of intermittent fasting will help in the addition of metabolism at the same time, aiding the person to eat fewer calories so as to promote the benefits associated with fasting. Therefore, this method is very useful in helping a person to lose weight and also decrease the fats around the belly.

The Health of the Heart

Through fasting, you will be able to lower the bad low-density lipoprotein cholesterol, which affects the heart.

Cancer Prevention

Through fasting, you can be able to prevent the development of such ailment, which is dangerous for the body.

The Health of the Brain

Through fasting, you will be able to add the level of the brain hormone, which is the brain-derived neurotrophic factor and will enable the growth of cells of the nerve that are new.

Fight Against Aging

Through fasting, you can be able to add on the lifespan as researched on some rats, which enabled them to live longer. Through fasting, you can be able to experience a lot of benefits that are associated with the brain and also the body. This can result in the loss of weight of an individual and also lowers the rate at which a person is at risk of getting type two diabetes and other diseases. This will also play a major role in longevity. People usually view healthy consumption as way too easy, but it usually requires a lot of effort to be able to maintain and make it a daily routine of your life.

If an individual is below a normal weight bracket or has ever experienced disorders when it comes to consuming meals, the person should seek the advice from a professional like a doctor so as to be able to start fasting.

As a result of fasting, a person will experience a lot of hunger and be weak, resulting in the brain not being sharp compared to the normal days that an individual is not fasting. This will take some time for the body to get used to the new lifestyle, which involves abstinence from eating meals for a given period of time. To be able to practice fasting, one should not be included in the categories below:

- People who have any type of diabetes

- People who have a problem with the regulation of sugar in the blood
- People who have decreased blood pressure
- People who are under any medication
- People who are under the general normal weight
- People who are pregnant

Insulin Resistance and Ketosis

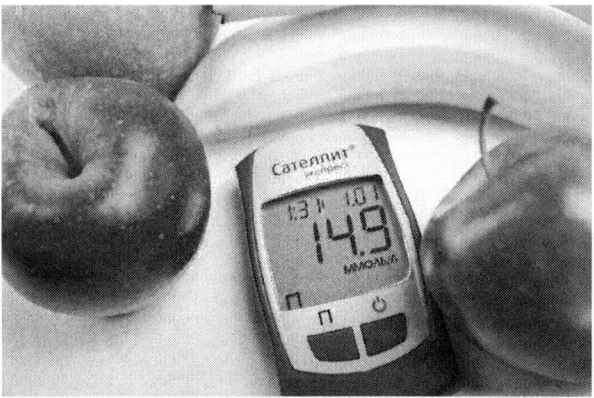

The Keto diet usually consists of the consumption of fewer carbohydrates and more fats, and it really helps in weight loss. This is possible, as it alters the metabolism in the body—stimulating the use of fats as energy in lieu of sugar. This will help in promoting the good health of the body.

The Resistance in Insulin

The insulin hormone plays a major role in the body, as it aids the body to be able to control the sugar levels of the blood. If the sugar levels in the blood are above constantly for a long period, it will result in some dangerous health problems through a condition referred to as hyperglycemia. This will increase the risk of getting diabetes. In type one of diabetes, hyperglycemia usually generates due to the lack of insulin production by the pancreas. In type two diabetes, the organs and also the tissues of the body tend to drop their capability, which helps in responding to the insulin produced in the body. The pancreas usually attempts to make it up through the production of even more insulin, but it never enough hence resulting in the occurrence of hyperglycemia.

The general level of sugar in the blood which is usually viewed as the normal level but many researchers have proven it wrong while arguing that what people think is the normal sugar level in the blood is not, as it is more than that hence being higher than what is viewed as the healthy level.

They exist a lot of ways that insulin usually aids in the control of the sugar levels in the blood. This can be achieved through the sending of signals to the liver to cut down on the manufacture of the glucose, and the other is through the absorption of the glucose and then being converted to energy. The resistance of insulin is a complicated disorder that usually has no single source. This will result in the liver becoming resistant to insulin, specifically during the time or period it neglects to lower the manufacture of glucose in the body in reply to insulin. The cells can also resist insulin when they are in need of more quantity of hormones so as to aid them in using glucose. But the major cause in the decrease tolerance of glucose in the Keto diet was high because of the resistance in the liver of the insulin. Many researchers have investigated what causes the resistance of insulin and also type two diabetes, which is not known. The act of the body resisting insulin is the worst news one could get from a doctor, but this can be controlled by the Keto diet, as it aids in altering the way the body usually functions. If an individual observes the symptoms which are associated with the resistance, the best advice so as to be able to fight it is usually the Keto diet, which will help improve the situation whereby the body will be functioning well without any issues.

The Way It Works

The liver usually contains cells, fats, and muscles—and when they fail to help in the absorption of the glucose, which is in the blood, and since the sugar in the blood has nowhere else to go, it results in the blood containing a lot of unnecessary sugar. This will result in the pancreas boosting the production of insulin so as to able to balance the sugar levels in the blood. To be able to moderate the amount of the sugar in the body's blood, the pancreas is responsible for that and also helps in the dealing with the extra sugars but not all the time as the organ gets worn out and fails to give a standard amount of the insulin so as to be able to manage the raised levels of glucose in the body. This will result in the damaging of the architecture of the cells of the body with time, and therefore it fails to take control of the little levels of glucose in the body.

With time, it fails completely, resulting in diseases like diabetes. Due to this, the excess glucose in the body just comes around in the blood with no specific place to go hence resulting in the levels of sugar in the blood to continue to raise, which is dangerous to the health of the body. All of these will result in the body having high levels of sugar in the body's blood and also the increase in the levels of insulin in the body. They are therefore leading to diabetes hence requiring medicine so as to be able to balance the levels of insulin and the glucose levels in the body. In many examples, people usually get to know they are experiencing the resistance of insulin condition very late hence being at the late stages. This will help the person to be checking the levels of sugar and also insulin in the body on a daily basis. If you are found to have these problems, you will require to start the treatment immediately so as to be able to manage the levels of sugar in the body so as to enable the body to function well.

The resistance to insulin is referred to as the condition of diabetes, as this will result in the diabetes disease due to the levels of insulin and also sugar levels in the body. If an individual does not change their lifestyle which comprises of the diet one usually follows, will not help in the management of sugar levels of the body hence resulting to the type two diabetes which is highly associated with having a lot of sugar in the blood and it is resistant to the insulin and also results to various problems which are associated with the issue usually include experiencing stroke or even cancer of any type. These medical problems that are associated with the high levels of the sugars in the blood have resulted in the loss of many lives in the world, and the remaining individuals are also at risk due to the verse lifestyle we usually have. To be able to prevent this, the world should start considering following a diet so as to be able to manage the levels of sugar in the body.

Many types of research indicate that a lot of people in the world usually have the condition of the resistant insulin in the body, but they do not know it yet but will soon learn about it. This is usually because a lot of people in the world do not visit the hospitals for check-ups more often but rather visit the hospitals when they are sick or feeling unwell. Through the consumption of a lot of carbohydrates and also a diet that usually consists of a lot of sugars due to the lifestyle one is used to. Other reasons include a lifestyle that is usually stationary, which also raises the body's glucose levels because the cells in the body are usually inactive to be able to use the body sugars. This can be dealt with through some exercises so as to be able to use the present glucose in the body.

Below are some factors that are responsible for the stimulation of the resistance of insulin in the body:

1. Age - the resistance of insulin can be able to affect individuals of all given ages, but it usually worsens when growing older

2. Race - many people with the American roots and also the Asian Americas, are usually at high risk of getting this condition

3. When a person has high blood pressure

4. Experiencing inflammation

Therefore, people should visit the hospital more often to have checkups so as to be able to know the functioning of their bodies. This will lower the chance of it worsening because it was detected late. Therefore, if it is known earlier, you will be put on medication early enough, which will help you more.

Because the body usually attempts to balance the levels of insulin and also the sugar levels in the blood through its own mechanisms hence taking a long time to be able to get the resistant of the insulin. Therefore, a lot of people usually recognize the symptoms when it is at its peak.

More Fat, Less Sugar

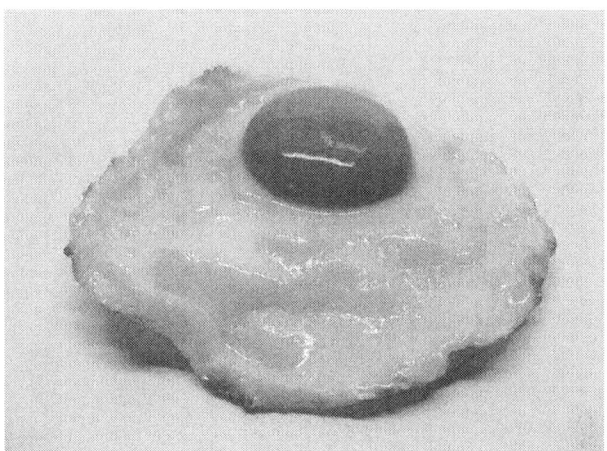

For many decades, the nutrition industries have an emphasis on the war against the consumption of fat, making consumers convinced that lowering fats in your diet is vital to losing weight. However, it is advisable to know the contrast between good and bad fats and the effects of sugar consumption on the body.

If you walk down the supermarket aisle, you will discover an endless variety of 'healthy' foods. They may have been branded the fat-free tag or termed as reduced fatty foods. However, these foods could do more damage than good to the body. What the dietary industry does not reveal to a consumer is that these foods are inflated with extra sugars, chemical additives, and preservatives that are used to increase flavor and taste.

Added sugars are more harmful than fats in as far as your weight is concerned, it can also begin to damage about every other aspect of your health. By lowering your fat intake, you could be removing a variety of potential health benefits provided by healthy fats. Many consumers are left in a dilemma asking themselves is it fat or sugar.

Negative Effects of Sugar Consumption

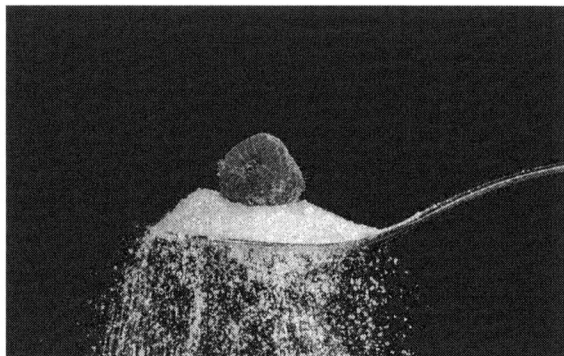

Sugar has been seen to activate the rate of inflammation, which could actually be the root cause of most disease-causing organism survival. Sustenance of high inflammation levels, in the long run, has been connected to an increase in the risks of suffering from conditions such as diabetes, heart diseases, and immune disorders. Recent studies argue that loading up on added sugars may even cause cancer. There's a direct connection between the two, mostly since obesity increases your likelihood to get a variety of cancer types

As you may already know, intake of sugar has also been linked with higher chances of obesity, insulin resistance, and metabolic syndrome, all of which can cause chronic disease.

Additionally, sugar is very addictive and can activate the release of dopamine, which is a neurotransmitter that controls the pleasure and reward centers in the brain — consequently leading to symptoms of sugar withdrawal when you halt the consumption of sugar. Remember that the disadvantageous effects limited mostly to added sugars found in manufactured and processed foods. A good example is soft drinks and sugary sweets.

Good Sugars (and Fats)

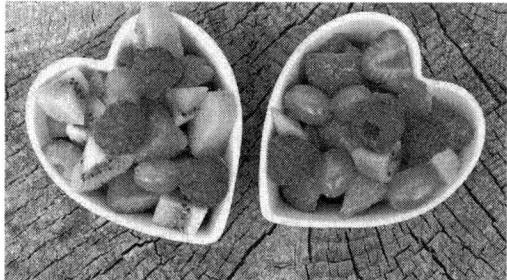

There are a lot of healthy foods—for example, fruits carry natural sugars—but they also store a variety of vital nutrients together with fiber lowers the sugar absorption as well as nullify any possible harmful impacts on health. While added sugar is believed to be unhealthy globally, fat is regarded as an essential part of the diet, which has a lot of health benefits.

Advantages of Healthy Fats

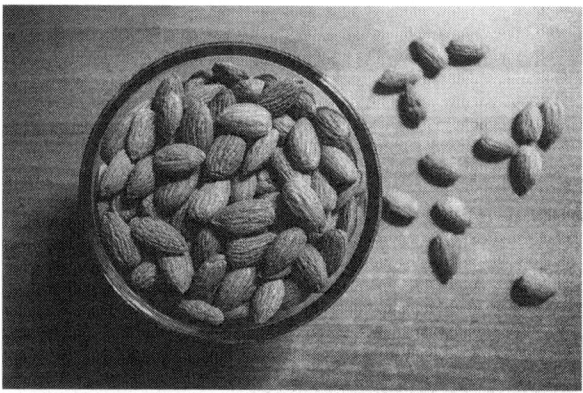

Unsaturated fatty acids found in foods like avocados, olive oil, and almonds can actually boost heart health, lower cholesterol levels, and alleviate inflammation. Particular saturated fatty acids, such as coconut oil, may also have health benefits and have been linked to better brain function and increased fat burning (if eaten according to a planned calorie intake). It may be viewed as contrary, the addition of the fats that are healthy will influence the emptying of the gastric thus maintaining your health through making the body feel full for a long period to cut down on having cravings and boost the loosing of weight, however, not all fats are created equal.

The Not-So-Healthy Fats

While fats found in whole, unprocessed foods such as nuts, seeds, and oils are jam-packed with benefits, the fats found in highly processed foods are not at all good for your health. Trans fats, for example, are found primarily in processed foods and hydrogenated vegetable oils that are linked to various ranges of the unfavorable conditions of the health—for example, heart diseases, including diabetes. Steer clear to stick to healthier sources of fats instead to help optimize your health.

Fat or Sugar?

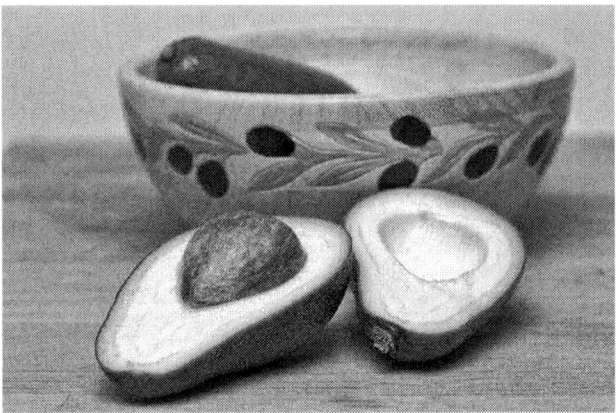

The healthiest and most sustainable way to improve your health is to make minor changes for healthier choices. Sugar is highly addictive and has been associated with some adverse effects on health. Healthy fats, on the other hand, are an essential part of the diet and may actually aid in weight loss, improve heart health, and reduce inflammation. For this reason, it's best to swap the sugar out of your diet and fill up on healthy fats instead.

Please keep in mind that Even if some fats are considered healthy, it's best to eat them in moderation so as to be able to shed weight. Adjusting the calorie consumption crucial for weight loss, and fats, even the healthy ones, have a lot of calories.

If you want to become your healthiest self, opt for the meals which include the oil extracted from the coconut, some fruits like avocados, fatty fish, nutrient-rich nuts and seeds

I also suggest skipping the sugar from processed foods, sugar-sweetened juices, energy drinks or sodas, and other unhealthy sources.

If you need to add a hint of sweetness to your favorite baked goods or beverages, do select natural sweeteners like raw honey, stevia, and dates.

Not only can these components provide a bit of extra flavor, but they also carry vitamins, minerals, and antioxidants that make them a much better preference to plain, white, processed sugar.

Aerobic Training

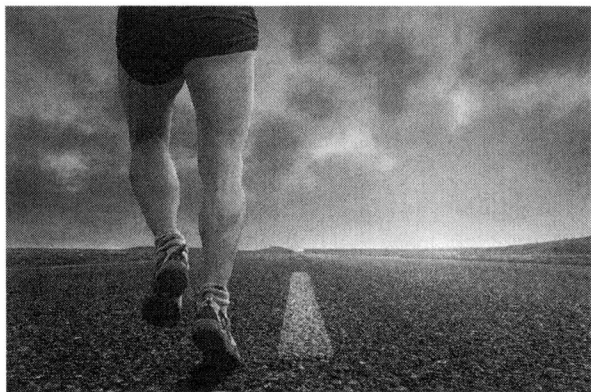

Aerobic training is a process that strengthens your lungs, heart, and your body, in general. It improves the performance of your skeletal muscles. The main aim of aerobics training is to increase sports functions and enhance training response. This specific type of training involves activities that an individual does participate in that raises their heart rate and makes breathing much tricky. The activities must be constant and consecutive.

These activities may be done either indoors or outdoors. Which usually includes print activities which include exercises of walking or even swimming activities and many more. Many exercises are considered to be aerobic when they are done more often in—for example, the sport of tennis. The exercises of the aerobics usually include the forms that are not able to count. Therefore, it is usually done at a level that is balanced over a great duration of time. Therefore, many activities are viewed as aerobic, which helps boost the working of the body physically since, through this, the body will be fit hence ensuring the perfect working of the body. The muscles of the leg are usually involved when it comes to the exercises of aerobics, which usually have a positive effect on the body.

Aerobic vs. Anaerobic Exercise

There are a lot of differences between the aerobic exercise and the exercise that is usually anaerobic, which is highly due to the strength of the training activities and also running short distances. Which will be beneficial to the body. These types of exercises usually differ when it comes to the long period of the exercise and also the shrinking of the muscles and its production of energy inside the muscles. Many types of research have been done on the performance of the endocrine about its role in the shrinking of muscles, and therefore, these exercises are usually practiced so as to be able to boost the transportation of the myokines and also aid in the development of tissues in the body and even have an effect on the reparation of the injured or damaged ones. This also aids in the reduction of inflammation in the body. This is very beneficial since it aids in the prevention of developing various diseases that are infectious. The production of the myokine usually relies on the total quantity of the muscles that have shrieked. Many types of research have found out that both the two exercises usually aid in the secretion of the benefits, which are associated with the endocrine benefits. In a lot of situations, the exercise of the anaerobic is, at times, accompanied by aerobic exercises because the productive anaerobic metabolic process should encourage the aerobic structure highly, as there is a high need for energy, which usually surpasses the capacity of the aerobic structure.

The Improvement of Endurance Through Aerobic Training

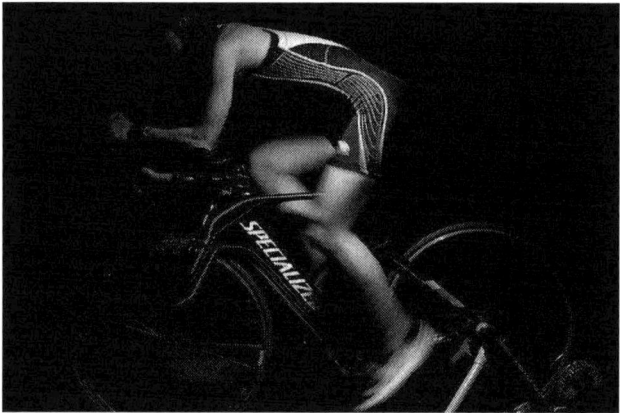

The aerobic exercises usually boost the quantity of the oxygen which has been breathed and its transportation from the lungs and also the heart of the body into the blood so as to be used by the muscles of the body. A person who is fit in the aerobic exercises can be able to train for a long period and is wide because the person's body has gotten used to the long hours of training and also the hardship that usually comes with the training. When such an individual does train, their heart rate is usually low, with short rates of breathing, as well as a decrease in the fatigue experienced by the muscles of the body and even increased levels of energy. After the exercise, the recovery period is usually short. The fitness in aerobic can be gauged in the lab through the use of a treadmill and also the use of cycling of the bicycle.

How Long Is the Training Period?

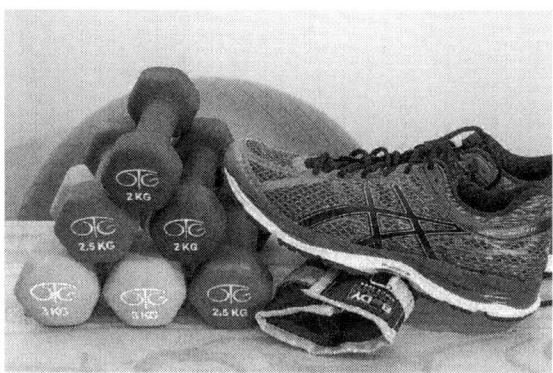

To be able to achieve the benefits that are associated with training of aerobics, a person should have an exercising time for about three to five times in a week, which should be of about twenty to sixty minutes per session of training. To be able to be fit and also increase that fitness, one can achieve it by adding a little time in between the exercises so as to enable the body to get used to the long periods of exercising. This will also enable the person to lose a lot of weight and also the fats which are around the belly. The people who are not yet fit should start with shorter exercising periods so as to also enable their bodies to get used to the training slowly and continue increasing the time span of the exercises over time so as also to enable the improvement of their fitness capabilities. By adding little time in the training plan over time, a person is usually able to prevent many injuries. Through cross-training, a person is able to lower the various risks to a lot of injuries. Through balancing the various exercises of the training will help to prevent these injuries. Therefore, a person should balance the training of activities that are usually vigorous and require a lot of energy with activities which do not require a lot of energy and are less vigorous—for example, walking or even jogging.

A person will be able to increase their persistence in the training by moderating the training levels to be enough. The intensity level of training is usually fun, and it will not lead to various injuries as compared to the training that involves high intensity. The training schedules of aerobics should be planned to be able to fit every person since people are different in terms of their levels of fitness. When training, people should be able to communicate comfortably without experiencing breathing problems. A person should be able to say some words without having any stress and then pause a little bit to breathe and then continue talking without any problem. If a person fails to do this, it shows that they have not trained well. The heart rate also plays a major role in understanding the fitness levels of the individual. The heart rate of an individual should be beating at an average of about 60 to 90 percent.

Through aerobics, a person is able to enjoy a lot of benefits, which is usually associated with the training of aerobics. By doing the aerobics exercises, a person is able to have health advantages, which usually involves the addition in the capability to be able to circulate a lot of air in less time.

Health Benefits

The known benefits that one enjoys by doing aerobics include:

- It aids in making the muscles that are involved in the process of respiration to be strong so as to enable the transportation of air from and to the lungs.

- It helps enlarge the muscles of the heart so as to improve the process of pumping blood.

- It also aids in boosting blood circulation.

- It usually lowers the risk of getting diabetes.

- It helps in adding the number of red blood cells.

- It usually helps in the promotion of mental health.

- It usually helps lower the risk of dying because of the problem linked to cardiovascular.

- It aids in the stimulation of growth of the bones and also lowers the risk of getting osteoporosis.

Effects on Body Performance

The following are the benefits which are associated with the body performance due to aerobic exercise:

- It aids in raising the storage capacity of the molecules of the energy in the body, which usually include a lot of fats and also carbohydrates.

- It also aids in the formation of new blood vessels, which enable the transportation of blood in the muscles.

- It even positively affects the activation of aerobic metabolism in the muscles.

- It also enables the muscles to be able to use fats as energy when a person is exercising.

- It usually boosts the rate the muscles will take to recover from the exercises.

Effects on the Brain

- It aids in boosting the architecture links of the brains.
- It also adds the density of the gray matter in the brain.
- It also boosts the growth of the neurons.
- It also helps the brain to be sharp in terms of memory.
- It also boosts the general health of the brain.

Disadvantages

- It is not the best practical way to develop the muscles of the body.
- It usually leads to a lot of injuries highly due to repetitiveness in the exercises.
- It is not the best way to burn fats in the body except when done more often.

The benefits, which are associated with both the health and even the performance, usually need the interval—and the rate of the exercises should be greater than the minimum time. Many researchers indicate that allocating an average of about 20 minutes and performed three to four times in a week will be very beneficial.

Exercises That Are Like Aerobics

The raised intensity of exercises usually adds on the resting rate of the metabolism in just twenty-four hours and helps in the process of burning a lot of calories as compared to the exercises that usually contain exercises that are low in terms of intensity. The exercises with a low intensity usually burn a lot of calories during the exercising periods, and this is high because of the time span added. During the period of training, you move large muscles over and over in your legs, hips, and arms. You will observe quick reactions in your body.

Your breathing pattern increases and becomes more profound. This expands the amount of oxygen getting into your blood. This means that your heartbeat rate increases, which consequently heightens the blood flow from your lungs to your muscles and back to your lungs.

In your body, the small blood vessels will widen to ensure the transportation of more oxygen to the muscles is efficient. They deliver back waste products from the tissues such as lactic acid and deoxygenated blood (highly concentrated with carbon dioxide). Your body also generates an enzyme known as endorphins, which act as natural pain relievers which enhance your wellbeing in general.

Take the First Step

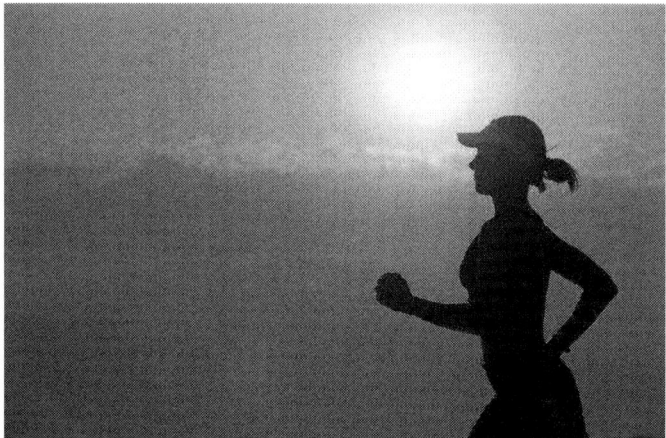

Are you ready to get your body energetic in activities? If the answer is yes, then here's a way to get you started on this great journey!

An important strategy in getting started is to start with small steps until your body has adjusted to the rhythm of your exercise—especially if you have been inactive for a long time or have a chronic health condition, you need to start slow. It is also advisable to get your doctor's guidance before you even consider starting this training.

Once you are set to get started, begin with slow walks for about five minutes both in the morning hours and in the evening hours. A preferred activity that consists of the body is usually viewed as beneficial—for example, bicycle riding or swimming. These equally allow you to not only burn calories but also involve your skeletal muscles in healthy exercise.

From there, make sure to add in extra few minutes to each session of the walk, bicycle ride, or swimming. This enables your body to adapt to the physical exercise slowly but surely. Picking up your pace bit by bit consecutively also helps your body fall into the exercise rhythm. Soon enough, you will be comfortable walking or doing vigorous exercise for longer minutes and will notice all the advantages of regular aerobics training. You could reap even more fruits if you do more and more training regularly.

Another potential aerobic exercise could include jogging, dancing, or skiing. Even if you are suffering from conditions that limit you from taking part in full aerobics exercise, you could talk to your doctor for alternative activities that could benefit your general health without harming your muscles or joints.

Chapter Three: Reducing Inflammation Through Autophagy

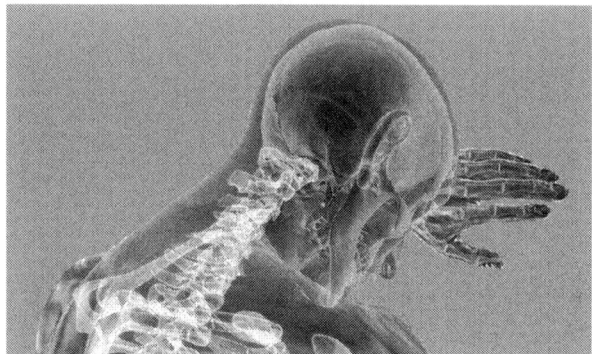

Autophagy is the homeostatic process that is involved in the scrapping of the organelles that are damaged, pathogens that have invaded, as well as the proteins that are denatured. The role played by autophagy in both adaptive and innate immunity is very important, as it influences the pathogens that cause inflammatory diseases. The discovery of autophagy mechanisms usually facilitates autophagy measurement, which is during the periods of pathophysiological and physiological procedures. Autophagy often plays a significant role in inflammation (which is through affecting development), the homeostasis, and the inflammatory cells' survival (which also includes the macrophages and the lymphocytes).

The mechanisms that usually depend on autophagy have been responsible for many inflammatory diseases. Inflammation often plays either a protective or destructive role in an injury. This can be caused by the physical, chemical, as well as biological agents and also include mechanical trauma, exposure to sunlight, through the x-ray and the radioactive materials, the extreme heat or cold levels, bacterial infections, viruses, as well as the corrosive chemicals. The inflammation pathogens include the changes of hemodynamic, leukocytes exudation, chemical mediators' releases, and even the hormonal response. Autophagy usually plays a significant role in the formation and also the pathogenesis of immunity response and inflammation. The process of autophagy interfaces with many cellular responses for stress pathways and also consists of direct interaction between the proteins of autophagy and even the molecules of immune signaling. This is highly brought out that the influenza virus usually triggers the Threonine kinase two, which is used to activate serine, which enhances the autophagy and also controls the activation of the inflammasome.

The critical role played by autophagy in the secretion of interleukin one beta can be seen in the primary human cells, whereby autophagy inhibition leads to an increase in the interleukin one beta production. In humans, the creation of the human tumor necrosis decreased by the inhibition of autophagy, thus suggesting a varying effect of autophagy on cytokines production. When it comes to the impact on autophagy there are essential differences between the humans and mice on the creation of interleukin 1 beta, whereby in mice the result is attributed to the activation or inhibition of inflammasome which is by autophagy while in humans the interleukin 1 beta mRNA transcription is increased when there is an inhibition of autophagy, but there are no effects that are seen on the activation of caspase 1.

Effects of Autophagy on Other Inflammatory Pathways

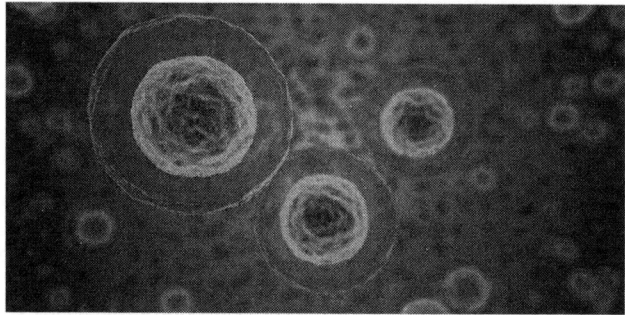

Autophagy usually has inhibitory effects on the activation of the inflammasome but also affects the inflammatory mediators that are independent of the activation of caspase 1. The autophagy restrains the activation of caspase 1, which results in the production of the ROS. Autophagy usually reduces the activation of the nuclear factor kappa B by selective degradation of the B-cell lymphoma complexes. The process is mediated directly through the cofactor of NSFL1C, which is a negative adjustment of the IKBKB, thus acting through the NFKB modulator that has been polyubiquitinated. Therefore, autophagy and inflammation are processes that are intertwined during the defense of the host. The process between the two plays a significant role in the pathogenesis and the treatment of many diseases.

Therefore, autophagy influences many significant components of the responses of immune hence helps in the inflammatory response regulation. Many people have suggested that autophagy developed as a primordial defense mechanism of eukaryote for the host. As this developed, the autophagy has been able to interact with other components of defense for the host like inflammatory reaction.

Anti-Inflammatory Keto Diet

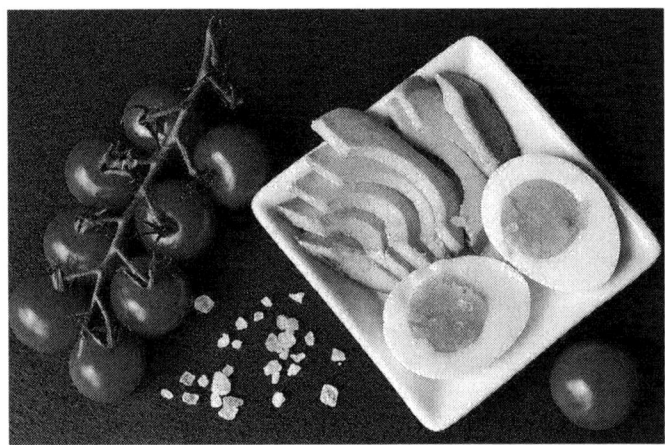

Using a Plant-Based Keto Diet to Reduce Inflammation

If you have been on the food that is ketogenic because of health issues or because you want to lose weight, it might seem to be a little extreme, but it works because many of our health problems usually are caused by inflammation. Therefore, we will feel well if we can reduce inflammation. If one is struggling to shed some weight, experiencing some acne, changes in the hormones, or experiencing chronic pain in the body—but it is not related to any injury—one should know that they have chronic inflammation in their body. When you have injured the direct body fluids to the damaged part of the body to try and heal it.

However, if your diet is causing chronic inflammation in the body, then this means that the body is fighting in opposition to the foods that it is not familiar with. Sadly, several foods that have been seemingly thought to have been healthy, which are modified genetically, have experienced pesticide spraying—or even the animal products that have been improved in an unnatural way can be seen as not being healthy.

Inflammation Cut Down by Ketogenic Diet

The ketogenic diet can achieve inflammation reduction by suggesting that one's fat intake should be 70 to 80 percent, while the protein intake should be between 15 and 20 percent, and the carbohydrate intake should be 5 to 10 percent. Something important to remember is that for every gram of the carbohydrates we take, the body claps about four grams of water. This is because a lot of the carbohydrates we take in are usually over-processed, which has negatively affected their nutritional profile. It is, therefore, essential to remember that even carbohydrate that is healthy and is found in their organic set up like oats, the wild rice, the quinoa, the sweet potatoes, the apples, and the bananas usually cause the body to hold a lot of excess fluids. Oftentimes, the people who are on a Keto diet typically remove the foods with high carbohydrates from the menu to be able to have control over the present inflammation in their bodies.

The diets that are against inflammation suggest that one should eat the foods that are high in antioxidants, which will help in fighting the oxidative stress in the body, which is responsible for getting a person fat, tired, or sick. This diet suggests that one should keep away from taking sugars and several other foods that have been processed, which the body was not made to take in. When the body fails to handle the several carbohydrates that a person is eating will result in the carbohydrates being converted into glucose. The glucose will build up in the bloodstream hence causing inflammation and also being kept as fat. If a person takes in a lot of protein, the body will convert the protein that is excessive into glucose through the process known as gluconeogenesis.

Through the intake of a lot of fats instead of carbohydrates, the body can convert the fats into energy instead of converting glucose to power, and the process is known as nutritional ketosis. This process usually occurs when the masses are not getting enough glucose to turn to strength, and this results in the kidney, making a lot of ketones, which is used for fuel. When the body uses fats as fuel instead of the use of glucose as fuel, one will be able to know they are in the ketosis process, and this also helps in promoting loss of weight. Through this one will be able to decrease some a lot of water weight which is extra and also one will be able to adapt to fat. When one is suited to fat, they are getting energy from the use of ketones instead of the use of glucose. Therefore, a person will not need carbohydrates the same way they once did. This will enable a person to be more in control of their appetite since they are not experiencing spikes of blood sugar the entire day since they consume glucose.

By decreasing the number of carbohydrates in the body, the Keto diet will do away with the extra fluids in the body, and hence, ketone Beta-Hydroxybutyrate will increase its levels in the body. The ketone can deactivate the chemicals which cause pain and inflammation in the body, and it does so without hindering the immune functions of the various cells, and this allows the healing process of the body to continue. The Beta-Hydroxybutyrate also positively affects the purposes of the mitochondrial, which usually makes a person healthy at the level of cells. Since the mitochondria are the power center of cells, so when the mitochondria are healthy will result in the whole body being healthy from both the inside and outside. This is because they can resist infections and the various inflammation causes. By the reduction of inflammation, you will be decreasing the chances of getting chronic diseases, as well as you will be able to control and manage the conditions that you already have. The sugar we use is very inflammatory, and in our daily lives, sugar is used in almost everything starting from breakfast. Sad diet usually consists of a lot of sugar, and therefore, when we eat carbohydrates, they will be converted into glucose by the body.

The ketogenic diet was initially formed to help in the treatment of children who had epilepsy, and it has been helpful, as it has enabled the children to function with the illness. Some physicians in the world have started to include the ketogenic diet into the treatment programs for the patients who have cancer, and through this, they have achieved remarkable results. The patients who are suffering from diabetes have been enabled to decrease the number of illness markers through the use of the ketogenic diet, which has helped control their disease.

How a Plant-Based Ketogenic Diet Can Help to Cut Down on Inflammation Further

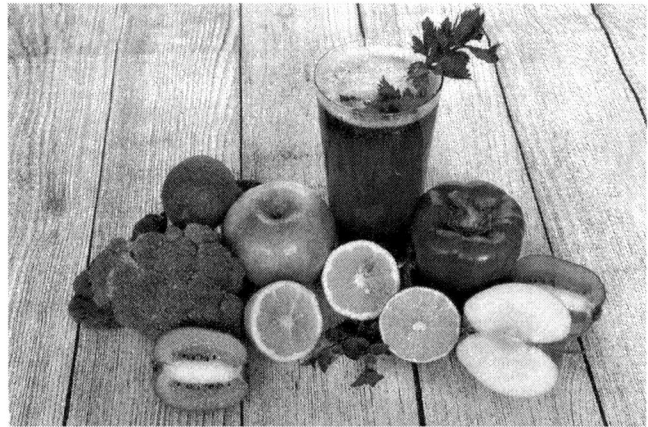

Many studies suggest that a diet that is based on a plant is usually anti-inflammatory independently. The Keto diet process takes away the fear people generally have from eating dairy products that are full of fats, which is a good habit. This is because our bodies need fats to be able to absorb the vitamins and also minerals and even to be satisfied after the meals. The Keto diet usually encourages the intake of dairy products that are full of fat, as well as it promotes the consumption of dairy products, which are very low in carbohydrates. If after going through the Keto diet for a while and you do not see any changes in the weight loss or you are experiencing health issues that are unexplained chances are that you may have an intolerance on the dairy products which you have not recognized. Many people tend to choose dairy, which grass-fed, and this is because they are healthy. But if your gut lining is being irritated by the dairy, you are advised to remove it from the diet for sometimes hence allowing the healing process of your gut. If you can feel well after eliminating the dairy from your daily diet, you may be able to include it back into the food. The meat, which is usually conventionally raised, is very inflammatory, and this is due to what the animals are eating as they are not eating what will promote their health; hence, the phrase we are what we eat.

If you are taking in too many proteins on your Keto diet, your body will be able to detect it and hence change the proteins to glucose through a process known as gluconeogenesis. Therefore, you may not be reducing inflammation due to the extra stress on your body. You should also make sure that you are furthermore eating foods that are rich in fiber with antioxidants to aid the body in fighting stress. If you are not a vegan and you want to try out a plant-based Keto diet, the following are some suggestions that will aid in the transition. You can be able to eat tempeh, a lot of beans, as well as eggs for proteins. Avocado oil, which too good, the MCT oil, some coconut oil or olive oils, some nuts seeds are also good plant-based sources of fat. The intake of olives, some sprouted beans, the avocados, and non-starchy vegetables will not be dense on the digestive system. Through this, you can save money because they are cheap compared to dairy and meat, which are always expensive. Through this, we can be able to save some cash by taking in a plant-based Keto diet

The expansion of your palate can be achieved through eating a portion of food that is plant-based, and this will help you be satisfied with the many varieties of plants that exist. Since the body usually processes the nutrients, you should eat a variety of some colored foods, and through eating a plant-based diet, this can be achieved. Even though the body does not need a lot of proteins as opposed to what we believe. There is a high possibility that it will increase gut inflammation from just eating a lot of beans than what you are used to on a plant-based keto diet. But by taking in the sprouted seeds, you will be able to limit the degree of inflammation, and you can be able to experience.

If you avoid fish while on a Keto diet, which is plant-based, you will end up having a low amount of fatty acids, which is classified as omega-3, and this is because they are usually found in fish. A fish oil supplement, you should always remember that the nutrients will always be better when absorbed through the foods.

The method of eating in the diet is usually restrictive, and sometimes it can be tough to maintain over a long time. You can be able to eliminate the ingredients from the menu which you suspect are the cause of inflammation for a short period and then you can add one by one after a while to be able to find out if they are the cause of inflammation or they are not. If you are worried that the Greek yogurt, which is usually full of fat or any other dairy products, may probably be causing inflammation, your body will let you know how it feels after abstaining from the consumption of dairy for a short period. The agency will also let you know if you should add the dairy products back into the diet or not.

If you are interested in trying out the Keto diet for vegans for some ethical reasons or some healing, it can be a good option, as well as it is doable. This is because most of the vegan diets are usually consist of a lot of carbohydrates, and the animals typically store fats while the plants do not store fats hence making it a little bit challenging to continue with the Keto diet of a vegan, but it is not impossible. A fully Keto diet for a vegan will limit the various foods that you can consume. This will result in difficulty in consuming the 15 to 20 percent calories from the proteins that are usually suggested on the Keto diet. Most of the protein sources for the vegans generally consist of carbohydrates, which will make it challenging to maintain the intake of carbohydrates levels between 5 to 10 percent of the total calories taken in a day a little confusing. The vegans usually prefer to use the pea proteins or other various vegan powder to be able to supplement their diet and precisely while limiting the intake of carbohydrates.

Beans, at times, have a negative inflammatory effect on the lining of the intestines—more importantly, if the grains are not sprouted. If you add the sprouted nuts and also seeds to your diet, you will increase the nutritional levels and also decrease the effects on the area of the gut. If you have been doing a Keto diet for some time, you will be able to add more carbohydrates in your diet from sources of plants and at the same stay in ketosis. You can also be able to modify random fasting when you feel worried about being in ketosis, which will aid the body in burning its fats rather than looking for glucose to convert it to energy.

The Keto Diet (Introduction and Explanation of the Keto Diet and Its Benefits in Relation to Autophagy)

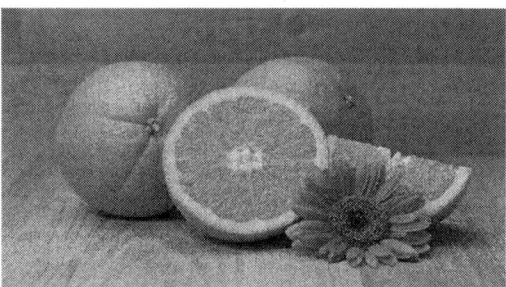

The Keto diet usually consists of a high quantity of fats, with a sufficient amount of proteins, as well as a low amount of carbohydrates—and it is usually used to treat and manage the negative issues brought by the struggle to be able to control the epilepsy disease in the young people. This is achieved highly because the Keto diet usually forces the body to burn and convert the fats to be used as energy instead of converting the carbohydrates. While usually, the sugars which are found in food are usually changed into glucose, which will be moved across the entire body, and it correctly plays a significant part in fueling the functions of the brain. But if the carbohydrates remain behind, the liver changes the fats into the fatty acids and also ketone bodies. The bodies of ketones usually go in the brain and replace glucose as an energy source. Therefore, an increase in the level of bodies of ketone in the blood, which is referred to as ketosis, usually leads to a reduction in the frequencies of epileptic seizures.

Half of the total of the children and the young people with the problem of epilepsy that has tried this diet has been positive, as it has helped in decreasing by almost half and has been effective even after stopping the diet practices. Many evidence shows that adults who have epilepsy will benefit more from the Keto diet and that the less strict regimes, such as the modified diet of Atkins, which are also similarly effective. The possible effects of this usually include constipation, an increase in cholesterol, slow growth, and even kidney stones.

The original diet used in therapy, which is for pediatric epilepsy, usually provides enough amount of proteins, which aids in the growth and repair of the body and also offers calories, which are sufficient in the maintenance of the correct weight and even height. The therapeutic ketogenic diet was initially formed to help in the treatment of pediatric epilepsy in 1920, and it was widely used in the following decade. The old ketogenic diet usually consists of a 4:1 ratio, which is by weight of the fat to the merged carbohydrates and the proteins.

This can be achieved through eliminating foods with high carbohydrates like the starchy fruits and also vegetables, the bread, some grains, and even sugar, but on the other hand, increase the intake of foods that have high levels of fat—for example, nuts, dairy cream, and even butter. Most of the fats in a diet are usually made of molecules, which are known as long-chain triglycerides. But the medium-chain triglycerides, which are formed by the fatty acids which have shorter carbon chains as compared to the quicker car from long-chain triglycerides, which are usually more ketogenic. A variation of the model diet, which is known as the medium-chain triglycerides ketogenic diet, often uses a type of coconut oil, which generally contains a lot of the medium-chain triglycerides hence help in providing half of the calories. A less amount of fats is required in this form of diet whereby a large number of carbohydrates and also the proteins can be consumed hence allowing a massive way of the food choices.

The plausible therapeutic use for the diet of ketogenic has been researched for several added neurological disorders in which some include the disease of Alzheimer's, the amyotrophic lateral sclerosis, the autism, brain cancer, experiencing headache pain, brain injury, the Parkinson's disease, as well as sleep disorders. The diet of ketogenic is a therapeutic mainstream diet that was created to bring out the success and also eliminate the limitations which are of the non-mainstream through the use of fasting to be able to treat epilepsy sickness. The physicians of ancient Greece were able to treat epilepsy and other diseases by changing the diets of their patients.

During the period of the 1960s, the medium-chain triglycerides were discovered to produce a lot of ketones bodies, which was per unit of energy than the usual dietary fats. The medium-chain triglycerides are usually absorbed more efficiently and are also moved to the liver through the hepatic portal system instead of the lymphatic system. The restriction of carbohydrates of the old ketogenic diet made it a little bit difficult for the parents to be able to make portable foods that the children will be able to tolerate. A physician in 1971 came up with the ketogenic diet whereby about 60 percent of calories usually came from the medium-chain triglycerides oil hence allowing a lot of proteins and also increased the number of carbohydrates by three times the old ketogenic diet. The oil used in the menu was usually combined with skimmed milk, then cooled and then drunk during the meal periods or was mixed with food. The medium-chain triglycerides diet later took over from the old ketogenic diet in several hospitals even though a lot of the implemented diets were the combination of both. By the year 2007, the food of ketogenic was famous and was found around the world, and it consisted of minor restrictive variants—for example, the adults were using the improved Atkins diet.

Diet Changes That Can Boost Autophagy

Autophagy usually means self-eating; therefore, it is understandable that the intermittent fasting and also the ketogenic diets are well known for triggering autophagy. The act of fasting is the best effective way, which is a trusted source that triggers autophagy. The ketosis is a diet that consists of a lot of fats and little carbohydrates, which usually bring out the same advantages of the practice of fasting without fasting, which is seen as a shortcut to implicate the same metabolic changes. This is the best, as it does not overwhelm the body with many external loads, but it usually allows the body a break to be able to focus on its health and also the repair of the body.

In the Keto diet, you will be able to have almost 75% of the total calories you take daily from the fats and also 5–10% of the calories from the carbohydrates. The shift in the sources of calories usually causes the body to move its metabolic pathways. It will start to utilize fat as fuel instead of glucose, which is often gotten from carbohydrates. Due to this restriction, the body will start to produce ketone bodies, which typically have a lot of protective effects. Many studies have suggested that ketosis may also result in starvation, which induces autophagy, which consists of various neuroprotective functions. The low levels of glucose usually occur in the two diets and always associated with low levels of insulin and also high glucagon. And the glucagon level usually affects autophagy.

Through fasting or ketosis, the body usually lows on sugar, which will result in having the positive stress that often wakes up the mode of survival repair. Even through exercises, one can be able to induce autophagy, which is achieved through a non-diet function. According to several studies, physical activities usually induce autophagy in the organs, which are parts of the metabolic regulation procedure. This will include the muscles, the liver, the pancreas, as well as the adipose tissue. If you are interested in the stimulation of autophagy in the body, you should include fasting and also incorporating various exercises into your daily routine. If you are on any medication, you should first consult the doctors for more information. Even if you are pregnant, or if you are breastfeeding, having plans to be pregnant, experiencing some chronic conditions—for example, diabetes—you should not fast without consulting your doctor or without professional advice.

Through the following steps, one will be able to increase the process of autophagy in the body:

By Eating a High-Fat and Low-Carbohydrate Diet

It is imperative to be eating fats to activate the process of autophagy. This is because the fats usually need to be the macronutrient that is dominant in the diet, as it is not similar to proteins. This is because the proteins can be able to turn into carbohydrates and then change to be sugar, but the fat cannot be ready. Especially a Keto diet, which consists of a high level of fat and also a low level of carbohydrate food plan, usually gives you a positive outcome when it comes to the process of autophagy. This process occurs from burning the glucose to ketones, which happens in the Keto diet, usually imitate what usually occurs innately in a fasted mode hence increasing autophagy.

By Abstaining from Proteins

You should be to limit the intake of protein once or even twice a week. This will give the body the entire day to be able to recycle the proteins, thus helping to cut down on inflammation and also aid in cleansing the cells without losing any muscles. At this time, when the process of autophagy is triggered, the body will be forced to absorb its own toxins and also its proteins.

By Practicing Intermittent Fasting

By not having breakfast and arranging to have all your foods within 8 hours, you will be able to increase the process of the essential autophagy of the body. Like fasting on the proteins, the intermittent fasting usually allows your body to be able to reach the lingering toxins through the process of cleaning up. You can be able to eliminate the toxins which typically build up within 16 to 28 hours fast. But if this is not done correctly, the intermittent fasting will be able to affect the women, whereby they cause hormone imbalances negatively. This is because women are usually more sensitive to the signs of starvation or the restriction of calories. Through eliminating the carbohydrates and also the proteins out of the meal, you will be able to remain in a fasting mode hence the body will believe that you are not starving

By Exercising Using High-Intensity Interval Training

Another way to be able to stimulate autophagy is usually through high-intensity interval training, which is very advantageous. You should always know that the process of autophagy is a bodily response to the stress; therefore, the exercise of high intensity usually places the body in excellent tension, and this is because it can stress the person to a point where it results in the change of biochemical. This will result in the body getting impact load, which aids in making stronger muscles is hence inducing autophagy without doing any harm. You can also be able to induce autophagy through lifting weights each day.

By Getting Restorative Sleep

You can also enjoy the benefits that come from autophagy while you are just sleeping. How you function during the day is determined by how you sleep as sleep play a significant role. A person usually possesses one of the four sleep personalities, and therefore, when a person knows which of the sleeping character they have, they will be able to plan themselves to have autophagy between the sleep and wake cycles.

Keto Diet and Inflammation

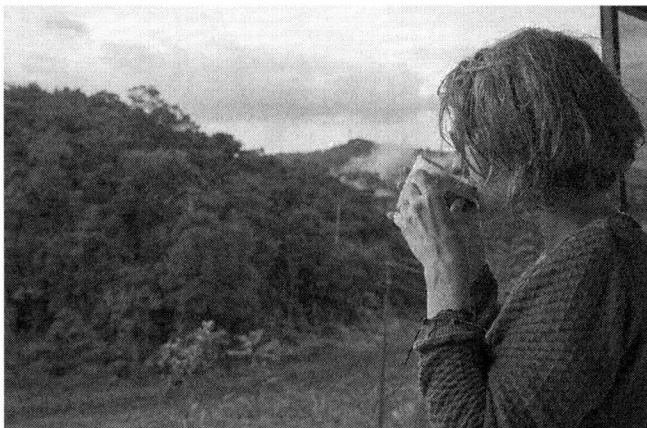

Most people have been using the Keto diet to aid them in reducing inflammation. Even though the Keto diet is not put up as a diet to fight inflammation, it usually consists of various foods that are anti-inflammatory and less inflammatory foods. The Keto diet often restricts inflammatory foods—for example, the foods that are processed, packed, or refined—as well as highly glycemic foods. The Keto diet usually pays more attention to the foods that are anti-inflammatory—for example, eggs, avocados, coconut oil, as well as low-carbohydrate foods like spinach. The Keto diet will let the body to experience ketosis for a prolonged time frame.

Even though the Keto diet will let a person in the reduction of inflammation through the process of limiting the intake of omega-6s, foods with high glycemic and also the highly processed foods which usually promote inflammation process and encouraging the consumption of omega-3s, various vitamins, absorption of minerals and also the antioxidants which usually calm inflammation hence the levels of inflammation will decrease and the body will begin producing a lot ketones which will aid in the reduction of inflammation. With inflammation described as a number one threat to our health, it can be best defeated through a healthy diet. There exist differences between the acute inflammation and also the chronic inflammation whereby the acute inflammation is usually the swelling and the redness that typically occur after having an injury while the chronic inflammation is the type of inflammation which often destroy the immune system of the body hence increasing its vulnerability to various health conditions. The chronic inflammation is generally associated with multiple diseases, which include the epidemic of cardiovascular, suffering from obesity, have high blood pressure, and many others.

Through the choice of your diet, you can control the levels of inflammation. The cells in the body are usually made of what you always eat. Certain foods can be able to trigger responses of inflammation that typically stress the body, thus weakening your immune system hence preventing the body from functioning normally. The best diet which will eliminate chronic inflammation is a diet that consists of low carbohydrates. The ketogenic diet usually contains substantial anti-inflammatory benefits. The best way to achieve this, you are supposed to remove the refined grains, sugar, as well as other food additives from your diet and replace them with healthy foods, which will reduce inflammation.

Anti-Inflammatory Foods

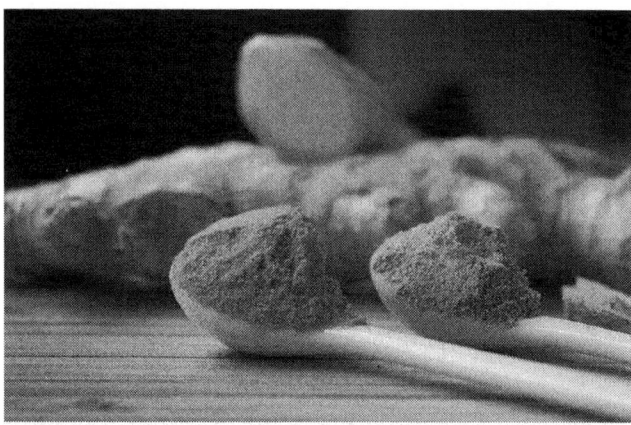

Turmeric

The turmeric is viewed as an anti-inflammatory product whereby turmeric curcumin has been found to consist of a lot of benefits, which aids in reducing inflammatory. The curry is delicious and also a functional food. The curcumin is usually 154 percent even more effective when it is mixed with the black pepper. When curcumin and the piperine are combined, it will help reduce inflammation very fast, and the curcumin remains in your blood hence giving protection against inflammation. Therefore, you should make the intake of turmeric a daily routine in your life to be able to maximize the benefits of health. Through this, you will be able to achieve the elimination of inflammation as turmeric is one of the best foods which are anti-inflammatory.

Ginger Roots

This type of root is best known to help calm a stomach, which is upset, but at the same time, it contains essential anti-inflammatory properties. The extract from the ginger usually inhibits the induction of the genes which are associated with the inflammatory response. Thus, ginger can regulate the biochemical pathways which are activated in chronic inflammation. Therefore, you should include more ginger to your meals, which will spice the food and also lessen indigestion and even lower inflammation.

Salmon

The salmon usually contain a lot of fat, whereby 3 ounces of salmon often include 1921 milligrams of the anti-inflammation omega-three fatty acids. Therefore, through the salmon, the body will be able to fight inflammation.

Macadamia Nuts

These nuts are the healthiest because of a lot of reasons, and more important is because they are the fattiest nuts. Macadamia nuts usually contain 75 percent of fat, and the fats included are healthy for the body and also help in reducing the inflammatory effects. Macadamia nuts also contain some magnesium, which aids in turning off the pain signals and also reduces the blood sugar, which are the positive impacts on the effects of inflammation. The magnesium deficiency may result in chronic and reduce inflammation; hence, it is beneficial to be including it in your meals.

Walnuts

The walnuts are usually high in carbohydrates, but as long as you remember to check your consumption, it will be very beneficial. The intake of magnesium is always necessary to prevent chronic inflammation and also lower the pains.

Healthy Fats

A lot of the vegetable oils which are found on the shelves of the groceries—for example, canola oil is sour and also pro-inflammatory. You should eliminate such oils and choose the ones that are healthier like coconut, use of organic ghee, which is obtained from the grass-fed cows and also olive oil.

Green Leafy Vegetables

The green leafy vegetables like kale and spinach are usually rich in anti-inflammatory polyphenols. These green leafy vegetables also contain a lot of antioxidants that regularly repair and also takes care of the damages. They also provide a lot of magnesium, which generally helps fight chronic inflammation. The green leafy vegetables usually contain a lot of nutrients, which helps lower the rate of swelling.

How Fasting Can Stimulate Autophagy

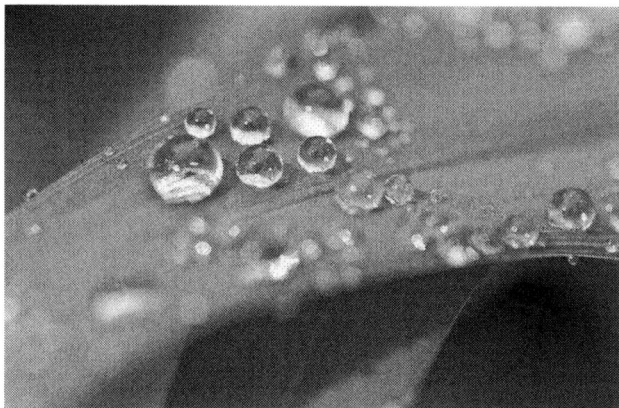

One of the best ways to promote autophagy is by practicing intermittent fasting. Through this method, digestion will be able to provide the nutrients to be able to maintain vital cellular functions, which happen during fasting and even eliminates the cells of organs that are damaged. Many types of research indicate that having an intermittent fast of about 16 hours will result in the autophagy being triggered. This usually consists of the alternations in between the periods of less protein intake and also the periods of moderating to the healthy protein intake. When you are fasting, the levels of insulin and glucose are usually low. Therefore, reducing the level of insulin often triggers the additional glucagon; hence, the body will naturally produce the hormones which will help in the stabilization of the levels of blood sugar.

The link to protein and also the added advantages of protein cycling is that even lowering the levels of protein will also promote the production of glucagon since there is neither both glucose or protein which the body can use as a source of energy. Therefore, as a result, the levels of glucagon will increase hence the increase of autophagy. Without the consumption of the proteins, the body will react by reusing its proteins to be able to extract the amino acids that are usable in the formation of proteins in the future.

Best Foods/Drinks to Stimulate Autophagy Process

Through the use of medium-chain triglyceride in the diet, one will be able to induce autophagy. This is the most abundant natural source of medium-chain fatty acids, which is healthy, and it usually changes into ketone bodies, which is a clean fuel for the brain and also the body. This results in the oil aiding in relieving hunger and also aids in the stimulation of autophagy through the increase of the level of ketone, especially when there are no carbohydrates.

Green Tea

You should try stimulating the pathway of autophagy through the use of polyphenols—for example, the epigallocatechin gallate, which is usually found in the green tea. Therefore, you should try and drink a given amount in a day or otherwise add a teaspoon of the matcha powder in your smoothie in the morning.

Coffee

Even coffee also contains polyphenols, which usually induce autophagy, which is also independent of caffeine. Due to this, several cups of coffee in a day is very beneficial to health and also have low risks even though it has a high amount of caffeine.

Cinnamon

Cinnamon usually contains a lot of antioxidants and is best known for its action in lowering blood sugar hence increasing autophagy. You should find the Ceylon cinnamon since it is regarded as the best quality of cinnamon.

Coconut Oil

Coconut oil is referred to as the best natural source of getting medium-chain fatty acids, which are healthy. It usually aids in reducing hunger and also stimulates autophagy through increasing the levels of ketone, especially when the carbohydrates are absent.

Chapter Four: Longevity with Autophagy

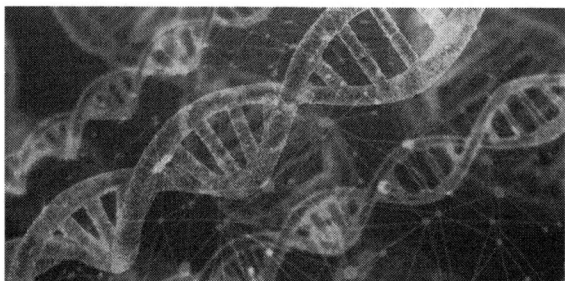

A lot of longevity-enhancement interventions usually work through the autophagy upregulation. A lot of the existing enhancement interventions for longevity, which have been tested regarding their effects, often suggest an addition in autophagy's cellular maintenance process. The focus point of this research community is the issue of aging.

The cells of the body usually react when there is a lack of nutrients, experiencing extreme heat through maintaining efforts over a long time. If the stress is very severe, it will result in a lot of benefits. The sad thing is that this approach does not have a lot of effects on the increase of the life span. To be able to live a long and healthier life, then you should look at strategies like the rejuvenation biotechnologies, which usually mend the damaged cells and tissues generally responsible for aging.

Through much advancement in the world, the aging molecular signature has been able to be discovered. The extraordinary conservation of the signaling pathways of the cells has been ready to be shown over many of the vertebrates and also the invertebrate species. Autophagy is usually the process of the cellular that came up as a nexus whereby the various pathways can converge. The activities of autophagy have been unveiled to be decreasing with the age of a person. Likewise, Caenorhabditis elegans have been revealed to cause an overall decrease in the activities in a lot of tissues consisting of the intestines and also the neurons. A similar reduction in the functions has also been noticed in many mammals, such as the electron microscopy investigation of the livers of the old mouse.

Many parties have recognized the critical role of autophagy in the effects of longevity, often enhancing mediating. The autophagy inhibiting in a mutant that has lived long usually nullifies the promotion effects of the mutation in survival.

To be able to demonstrate a natural connection between longevity and autophagy, a lot of groups have assessed the various effects of overexpressing the genes of autophagy. A good relationship between the activities of autophagy and the lifespan was shown in Drosophila. The overexpression of the autophagy-related 8a gene by the specific neuron usually results in the increase in the lifespan and also the reduction in the accumulation of the toxic protein aggregates.

Aging usually shows the organism's functional deterioration. The efforts to be able to find the downstream mechanisms in each of the longevity pathways, which often reveal that there are numerous but sets of different factors in each of the longevity pathways even though some of the elements typically work the same way. Recent findings recommend that the process of autophagy is one of the various connecting downstream mechanisms of all the paradigms of longevity. The autophagy activity is usually raised in long-lived, living things, and therefore, it is required for their increased durability.

Dietary Restriction/Reduced mTOR Signaling

The limitation of the diet is the best way that has been proved to aid in slowing the aging process and extend the lifespan in many species. Several molecular mechanisms are said to mediate the various effects of the restrictions of diets on longevity, which include the target of rapamycin also insulin. Through the use of amino acid, you can be able to induce restriction on your diet, which usually increases the autophagy process and even increases the CLS.

The nutrient sensor mammalian target of rapamycin inhibition often raises the CLS, and autophagy and the genes of autophagy are traditionally crucial for the rapamycin in the extension of the lifespan. In the aging of yeast, the role of autophagy is generally complicated. The elimination of autophagy 15, but not including the other autophagy genes which have been tested regularly, disrupts the extension of the RLS, which is always activated by the limitation of glucose, thus another way of restriction of the diet in yeast.

Many ways of restriction of the diet exist like the eat-2 mutants, which usually consist of the receptor of acetylcholine mutation that generally negatively affects the pumping of pharyngeal and also reduces the intake of food. The eat-2 mutants indicate a ban increased level of the green fluorescent protein - immunoglobulin G in the seam cells of the hypodermal. The eat-2 mutants' longevity is usually eliminated when the several genes of the autophagy are usually inactivated. In the eat-2 animals, some of the genes of autophagy are often transcriptionally activated by the several factors of transcription. Some research has shown that the autophagy of the intestines is very significant in the extension of the lifespan during the restriction of the diet. How the existing factors of transcription result to the autophagy and also longevity activation in the spatial and also temporal modes should be outlined.

The use of the TOR mediates the same as yeast the extension of the lifespan, which is activated by the restriction of the diet sometimes, and this is high because the TOR usually inhibits the eat-2 mutant; hence, it does not increase lifespan. The same as this, which is the same as the restricted diet worms, which help in the inhibition of TOR, usually aids in the lifespan extension in the factors of transcription. In the treatment of rapamycin in drosophila often results to a moderate expansion of the lifespan and this also process requires the gene of autophagy hence suggesting that the lowering of the TOR often extends the lifespan in the Drosophila at most through the process of autophagy which is similar to the yeast and also worms the treatments of rapamycin have been revealed to increase thought to the maximum and even the median lifespan of both the male and heterogeneous female mice. Many researchers have illustrated the various positive effects of rapamycin regarding the lifespan in mice through the use of different genetic histories. However, the positive impact of the autophagy process in these mice is not clear.

Germline Removal

The reproduction is usually correlated negatively with longevity in a lot of species. Therefore, the removal of the stem cells of the germline through the use of genetic mutation or by the use of microsurgery usually increases the lifespan in the drosophila. In worms, the mutants that are sensitive to temperature, which generally encodes the notch receptor elegant, indicate the lowering of the stem cells of the germline and also the extension of lifespan. It has been illustrated that the count of the green fluorescent protein-immunoglobulin G puncta is deficient in the germline; hence, the genes of the autophagy and the animals are important for their longevity. In the animal germline insufficient, a lot of the factors of transcription have been illustrated to induce the genes of autophagy. Surprisingly, the specific knockdown of the intestines of the genes of autophagy usually eliminates the longevity of the GLP-1, but it is different in the case of the mutants of daf-2, which shows the contrasts of the regulation of the autophagy in the individual tissues, which are between the conserved paradigms of longevity. The animals of glp-1 usually live long, as they have high lipase activity. Also, the same applies to animals of lipl-4, which aids the animals to live long. The overexpression of the lipl-4 often increases the process of autophagy and the lifespan; thus, the animals require the gene of autophagy to increase longevity. Therefore, the turnover of lipids by the process of autophagy is significant for the promotion of survival.

Reduced Mitochondrial Respiration

The free radical theory suggests that the process of aging is usually the product of damages of the cells through the oxidative process, which is generally over time. The injuries on the molecules are typically caused by the reactive species of oxygen, which created primarily from the respiration of the mitochondrial. Even though the damages caused by oxidation often heightens with age is still not clear if this process has effects on the aging of organisms. By reducing the respiration of the mitochondrial, you will be able to increase the lifespan of various bodies like mice and yeast. For example, in worms, electron reduction usually, transport chain components, which generally extends the lifespan of microorganisms during the larva stage, when they are inhibited. Several mutants of mitochondria, including the ubiquinone synthase mutants, often show longevity. The inhibition of the larva of the gene of autophagy genes often reduces the lifespan of the CLK-1 and also isp-1 mutants. These mutants show generally heighten in the numbers of the green fluorescent protein-immunoglobulin G-1 puncta in the cells of hypodermal during the larval period.

Forced Activation of Autophagy in the Extension of the Lifespan

The loss of the activities of autophagy has been shown to result in premature aging in a lot of species. The process of gene screening, which is involved in the yeast chronological lifespan, usually indicates mutants that have lived shortly, which experienced their mutation in the genes of the macroautophagy. The lifespan decrease in the elegant ATGL can be observed. The same results can be seen in drosophila. Even though the whole body knockouts of the genes of the ATG in mice usually leads to postnatal death and also the conditional knockout of tissue-specific of the ATG7 indicate several phenomena which are associated with age which include the aggregation of the inclusion bodies in the neurons, the lysosomes accumulation which consists of lipofuscin pigments, the disorganized mitochondria, the increased levels of oxidation of the proteins and also lower the mass of the muscles. Through the correlation between autophagy and the process of aging, it is beneficial to test if the forced stimulation of the process of autophagy aids the extension of the lifespan in animals. The same as this, the treatment of the TFEB agonists can help in the expansion of the lifespan in worms and also reduce the metabolic syndromes in the mice. The overexpression of the ATG5 in mice usually extends the lifespan in both the female and male mice. And also, the overexpression of the neuronal of the ATG8 is often enough to aid in the extensions of the lifespan in drosophila.

Pharmacological Activation of Autophagy Contributing to Longevity

Spermidine

The administration of the polyamine (spermidine, in particular), usually provides a lot of benefits for the health in a lot of species and also helps in the extensions of the lifespan of the yeast and other organisms like the mice. The survival of the cultured mammalian cell is usually increased through the treatment by spermidine, which is also included with epigenetic hypoacetylation of the histone through the inhibition of the activities of histone acetyltransferase. This will result in the correlates with transcriptional upregulation of various genes related to autophagy.

Resveratrol

The polyphenolic is usually a naturally occurring resveratrol, which is a compound found in the grapes and also stimulates the NAD-dependent histone deacetylase sirtuin. The administration of the resveratrol can aid in the extension of the lifespan of many organisms and, specifically, the lifespan of any microorganisms. This is specifically for the lifespan of the elegans, which usually depends on autophagy because the resveratrol does not extend the lifespan of the bec-1 of the treated animals. Resveratrol often increases the levels of DsRed-LGG-1 in wild-type animals. The above observations go in line with the findings of the mammalian cells whereby the pharmacological stimulation of the SIRT1 by the resveratrol treatment, which activates autophagy.

Tomatidine

Unripe tomatoes usually contain a natural compound known as cimetidine, which inhibits the age-related skeletal muscle atrophy in the mice. The tomatidine often extends the lifespan and also the health of the elegans. Through the use of the tomatine, many C. elegans behaviors are related to the span and also the health of muscles, consisting of the increase in the pumping of pharyngeal—and even the reduced levels of muscle cells that have been damaged are improved. The imaging of the microarray and the behavioral analyses show that the tomatidine usually maintains mitochondrial homeostasis through modulating the mitochondrial biogenesis process and also PINK-1, which is a dependent mitophagy. Research shows that tomatidine often stimulates the mitochondrial hormesis through inducing the production of ROS, which will activate the pathway of SKN-1 and also the paths of other cellular antioxidant responses hence the increase of mitophagy.

Through all this, we can see how the activation of autophagy plays a significant role in the process of longevity. The neuron-specific knockdown of autophagy after the reproductive period has been seen to be able to extend the lifespan in worms. Therefore, it is essential to understand the spatial and also the temporal regulations of autophagy and even their physiological importance to aging. It is also necessary to determine the process of autophagy contributes to the extension of lifespan and also which of the cargo of the autophagy is essential for aging and even longevity. The clearance of lipophagy and even the mitochondria are related to the aging of the C. Elegans. It is also important to test which of the autophagy stimulators are practical and are even applicable to humans.

Autophagy is the process of cleaning, which aids in fighting stress damages, which are usually created in the cells when they make energy. The protein aggregates often accumulate with effects that are toxic on the cells, which eventually leads to the death of the cells if the damage is not repaired. Therefore, these proteins should be eliminated to be safe, which is through the process of autophagy, which protects the cells against death. Through aiding the removal of oxidative damages, parts of the cells which are responsible for the operation of aging at the cellular level hence increasing the lifespan. Autophagy plays a significant role in the prevention of neurodegenerative diseases, which plays a role in the destruction of the aggregates of proteins that are responsible for these diseases.

The process of autophagy and aging are connected somehow whereby when the genes causing the process of autophagy are inhibited in the mammalian cells, there is degeneration, which looks like the degeneration we observe in the aging process. The aging itself usually comes with reduced autophagy; therefore, when one stimulates the autophagy process, we are mitigating aging. The many strategies used to slow the aging process in model organisms also result in the occurrence of the process of autophagy. When there is inhibition of the autophagy process during some extension of the lifespan—for example, the restriction of calories—it usually erodes the effect of anti-aging. The autophagy shows promise as a fundamental mechanism for maintenance and repair specifically in the process of aging

The Anti-Aging Process Through Ketosis State

Ketogenic diets can slow down aging according to many types of research. Through the intake of low carbohydrates and high consumption of a lot of fats usually prevents the conditions related to age—for example, diseases of the heart and others. During the time of carbohydrates starvation, the body regularly releases a chemical, which is known as the β-hydroxybutyrate, which plays the role of protecting them from the internal stress. The stress is generally connected to the genetic damages in the cells, which causes aging. The Keto diet often forces the body to burn fats instead of carbohydrates for energy, which starves the body of carbohydrates but not the calories.

Through following the intake of fewer carbs and the consumption of high-fat foods, you will be able to prevent conditions related to aging. The restriction of calories usually slows down the process of aging and increase longevity. High concentrations of the bodies of ketone are generally considered to be toxic, and an example is the diabetes of type one, which happens because of an increase in the number of ketone bodies, and this can also be a cause of some life-threatening medical emergencies.

The low level of the collections of the ketone is very beneficial, as it aids in the protection of cells from the oxidation stress, which is a factor contributing to aging. Research indicates that the restriction of calories diet will be able to slow the aging process and also increase longevity. B-hydroxybutyrate is a significant source of energy which is used by the body during periods of fasting, exercises, and even starving.

The B-hydroxybutyrate will block specific enzymes that will promote oxidative stress in the body, which end up contributing to the aging process. The test of the ketogenic diet in mice usually shows an increase in the B-hydroxybutyrate, which blocks the effects of the histone deacetylases enzyme, which generally works by inhibiting the action of two genes.

Nutrition to Make Your Cells Younger

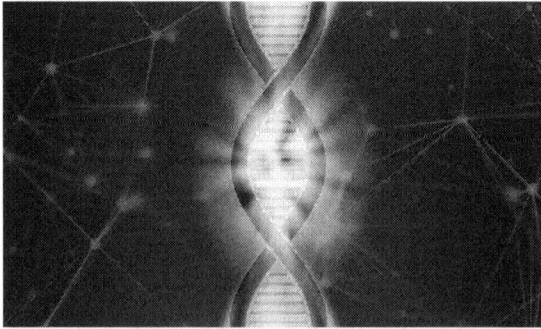

While we typically measure the age in years, the marking of biological aging is cellular aging. Therefore, the DNA of the cells can be able to tell us how much the bodies have aged. The telomeres are structures that are made up of the strands of DNA and proteins. Therefore, every time there is a division of the cells, the telomeres usually shorten until the cells are senescent and finally dies.

Consequently, the length of the telomeres is often the best indicator to show how old a battery is. While the process of shortening the telomere is often a natural process, the accumulated damages in the cells will speed up the process and result in the premature death of the cells. The damaged cells and also the shorter length of the telomere have been linked to chronic diseases and even cancer.

The factors which are associated with damaging the cells are environmental and modifiable. Therefore, you can be able to do something about them. These usually include the diet, the exposure to ultraviolet rays, a lot of alcohol consumption, and the lifestyle; hence, more stress can generally speed up cellular aging, while the practice of exercise keeps the cells young. Overall, researches find a significant association or rather a link between high adherence to any of these diets and longer telomere length.

Circadian Rhythm and Autophagy

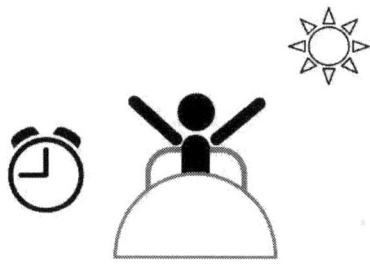

The mammalian circadian clock and the connection to the genes of the clock are being discovered and understood as a very important component in various anatomical disease processes that go over the production of hormones, the thermal arrangement, as well as the cycles of sleeping and waking up. A lot of researches indicates that the disruption which is associated with the clinical patterns, which usually consist of the long patterns of the job and even the travel of space, will affect the circadian pattern negatively, which will lead to diseases that will affect the entire systems.

This mammalian circadian clock is usually located at the suprachiasmatic nucleus, which generally lies on the optic chiasm to be able to attain the light through the help of the cells of the photosensitive ganglion, which are located on the eyes. The usually depends highly on the SCN is over gland of the pineal, the nuclei of the hypothalamus also the vasoactive peptide of the intestines to be able to manage various procedures which usually happens like the production of cortisol hormone and also the melatonin hormone, the response stress of the process of oxidative, and even the management of the temperature of the body which is linked to the cycle of the circadian.

The clock of the circadian usually supported by the cellular indications; also, the light got so as to be able to arrange itself with the time of the solar and also being able to period of 24 hours. Circadian Rhythm in Degenerative Disease and Cancer

The disease of the neurodegenerative and the lessen lifespan have been associated with the functions of the various circadian mammalian clock. In the study, the lifespan of the drosophila has been lessened into three choppy mutants consisting of the caladium articulatum, the cyco, and the timo. Specifically, the caladium articulatum mutants included important age-related shortages of locomotor. Through the restoring process, functions were able to help the Drosophila from the shortcomings of locomotor. The rising levels in the oxidative stress were discovered with the phenotype mutants, but the shortages also were seen to be able to agree well with loosing of the neurons of the dopaminergic.

Circadian Rhythm and the Modulation of Autophagy

Autophagy is the process that usually recycles the components of the cytoplasm in the cells for the remodeling of the tissue and also in the elimination of the organelles that do not function. The term macroautophagy usually refers to the classification of autophagy that has the role of recycling the organelles and also consists of the sequestration of the cytoplasmic proteins and the organelles into autophagosomes. These autophagosomes will combine with the lysosomes for the degradation and even recycling process. The microautophagy outlines the invagination of the membrane of lysosomal, which aids in the sequestration and digestion of the cytoplasmic components. The chaperone-mediated autophagy usually uses the cytosolic chaperones to be able to transport the cytoplasmic components across the membranes of the lysosomal.

Therefore, the process of autophagy can be the root cause of a lot of degenerative disorders like the disease of Alzheimer's, Parkinson's disease, Huntington's disease, and diabetes mellitus. The process of autophagy can also have effects on the decline of the cognitive and even the aging processes.

The circadian rhythm dysfunction during the loss of the cognitive and the aging process has been tied to the stimulation of autophagy. The chronic sleep fragmentation can influence the autophagy proteins in the brain, which will alter the recollection ability and also the perception. In addition to this, the autophagy process in the brain is usually not functioning when there are no PER1 circadian clock proteins, which often worsens the pathology of cerebral ischemia.

The loss of a wonderful circadian rhythm will eventually cause an increased risk for having nasopharyngeal carcinoma, cancer of the breast, as well as cancer, which is associated with the metastatic colorectal. The disruption of the clinic behavior, which consists of extended work shifts and even space travel, will negatively impact the circadian rhythm. At the level of the cellular, the management of the autophagy pathways, which usually consists of the wingless related integration site, is usually very crucial due to reasonable anatomical adjustment of the circadian pattern of the body.

Sleep Optimization

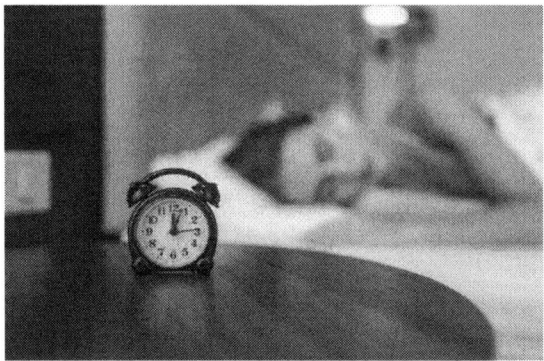

Sleep is usually a part that makes us human as we need it. You can argue that as a society, we are getting worse at sleep activity. Many people in the world today usually suffer from a sleep disorder, and only a few people typically get good sleep regularly. This is a very worrying trend that has a lot of negative consequences. Rest is a very important requirement of life; therefore, the quality and the quantity of sleep usually have a direct effect on the health regarding both the physical part and the mental. Deprivation of sleeping over a long period is generally connected to severe health issues like diabetes, suffering a stroke, diseases of the kidney, as well as the heart. Poor quality sleep has also been associated with obesity and also the experience of depression. In some researches show that having a proper sleep can promote longevity. Not only is sleeping necessary to maintain a healthy mind and also body, but it can also be actively used to improve each. Instead of viewing sleep as the inevitable activity of every day, we should be able to optimize it to be able to get the best benefits out of the rest.

When it comes to the health of the body, we usually push sleep aside and then focus on other contributors such as the nutrition and practice of exercise. This is understood as the impact on health is often more apparent. But sleep should be included in all the health plans. We should all know that sleep usually affects the out productivity and also focus. When you have been deprived of sleep, it is challenging to be able to do anything of advantage. Thus, it usually affects the function of cognitive. The ability to be able to solve a problem s, to be able to learn, as well as to be able to think and be more creative is usually affected by the quality of our sleep one typically has. The optimization of sleep is generally not complicated, as it requires some pure self-analysis and also some trials and errors. Our bodies usually respond to the routine of sleeping; therefore, by falling into one, the body will be able to discover when to sleep.

Consequently, this usually means you will be able to sleep comfortably and also have a higher quantity of sleep. The optimization of sleep can be robust. It can also have a positive effect on health and also productivity, and even has the power to be able to change the life. To be able to find the best ideal sleep program might take time, but it usually starts with awareness and practical action-taking.

A diet that usually consists of low fiber and has a high level of saturated fats will result in taking a change in the shutting of the eyes through lowering the quantity of heavy and also the slow sleep, which one can achieve at night. By consuming a lot of sugary staff will cause a lack of sleep, thus leading in the midnight wake-ups. A healthy diet, on the other hand, will help in the fast drifting off, as this kind of diet promotes quality sleep.

Any person with gastroesophageal reflux usually understands how bad it is to be able to go to bed with heartburn. Usually, the individual who is suffering from heartburn does experience sleep problems and other disorders—for example, insomnia, sleep apnea, restless legs syndrome, as well as daytime sleepiness. Through using the best diet, you will be able to create some deviation in the sleep patterns. Then, steer clear of a lot of fried foods or those with a lot of fat, spicy foods, alcoholic drinks, and even carbonated drinks when just about to sleep. For the best sleep at night, you should be able to eat a diet that is balanced which usually emphasizes on the intake of the fresh fruits, some vegetable, the whole grains and also proteins that are low in fat but are rich with vitamins, like fish, meat, poultry, and even the dairy. The B vitamins usually help in the regulation of the melatonin, which is a hormone that generally regulates the sleep cycles.

Through eating well, one can be able to lose weight, which usually helps a person to be able to sleep well, whereby they are able to get quality sleep. The lowering of the excess fats in the body, specifically among the middle parts, usually results in the optimization of rest a little bit easy; hence, there is no struggling to be able to get some sleep.

Nutrition usually has an important part in the health of the organisms, which has been proven through much research. You become what you eat acknowledges the importance of nutrition for the well-being of the body. This concept is usually talking about the addition of the dimension as the research demonstrates the various impacts of diet on optimization of sleep.

Researchers studying both the public health issues have a powerful connection between sleep and disease of obesity, hence there is a strong reason to know and always remember that improving the diet will also improve sleep.

The food and also nutrition usually have a profound effect on sleep. A healthy diet practice and also healthy eating habits typically lead to the promotion of both the higher quality sleep and even more total sleep time.

Researches have long discovered that there are links that exist between poor sleep and poor diet. The people with various types of sleep disturbances usually tend also to have inconsistent or consist of foods that are generally unhealthy. In many of the researches, it is to tell the direction of causality. As it turns out in the investigations, likely, sleep usually affects nutrition, and diet usually affects sleep.

How the body usually processes the food and also the nutrients often depends on what, or when, and how much you eat. Eating at a regular interval stimulates a sequence of reactions in the body, as well as the nature of these reactions, which will influence the ability to be able to fall asleep as well as the architecture of sleep. At the same time, when you get inadequate sleep, you will be able to be at risk of diseases like obesity due to poor diet choices.

The way that people usually respond to food is variable, and it can depend on the person's genetics, the environment, the stress, the activities, the gut microbiome, and other various factors. Researchers have started to deepen their understanding of the compound and also the interrelated network. As a result of this, it might be a little challenging to be able to state exactly how the diet or the food will affect the specific person, but at an overall level, therefore it is vivid that how we eat will directly affect how we usually sleep. This will enable an individual to be

How Diets Affect Sleep

Everyone usually has a diet that refers to what you eat or what your meals typically contain. But when the people are "on a diet" or follow up on a specific diet, it usually means that they follow or have a particular routine of a specific set of rules about what foods to eat and what not to eat. The food intake and how the body usually processes the food will affect the schedule of the sleep. Therefore, the consumption and how the body digests the food will affect the sleep patterns; hence, the different variety of diets that usually restrict some types of foods, or the nutrients will have different impacts on the sleep. In this section, we will outline several popular diets and their possible effects on the sleep pattern. However, you should keep in mind that many systems of the body are usually associated with regulating metabolism and meal processing. Since everyone is not alike, therefore people typically react differently to the same food or the same diet. A nutritionist or the doctor is usually in the best position to be able to give personal advice about the various diet for any individual who is willing to try the foods.

Vegan

The diet of a vegan usually avoids any product which is derived from the animals, which consists of the meats and also dairy products such as cheese, milk, and eggs. And because of the existing considerable restriction which are involved in the diet of a vegan, and it is common for the vegans to plan their meals or what they eat systematically, and this will help in avoiding some of the various negative impacts to the sleep patterns that usually come from overeating or the act of splurging on the extremely fatty or the sugary dishes.

There is no detailed study that has been able to document the effects of the diet of a vegan, but a lot of the vegan diets usually include complex carbohydrates, nuts, as well as fruits that also contain tryptophan and the melatonin which aid in promoting good sleep. A vegan diet regularly avoids some foods which usually disrupt the sleep pattern, such as the heavy meat-based dishes.

Transitioning into a vegan diet is, at times, reported to be able to cause sleep problems or instead disrupt sleeping patterns. This will be part of an adjustment period or will result in a change in the intake of nutrients like the drop in protein or the overall calories, which may make it a little hard to stimulate sleep.

Vegetarian

Vegetarians will not eat the meat products of any type, but they still consume other dairy products—for example, eggs and dairy—which are gotten from the animals. The same as the vegans, the additional planning which will be required to be able to eat a vegetarian diet will aid in adding consistency to a person's menu, which will make it easier for the body to process food without any disruption. The diets of the vegetarian usually include foods that are similar to the foods of the vegans' diet, which will promote sleep, which consists of the almonds, the fruits, and even whole grains. Just like the vegans, vegetarians usually avoid foods like meat consumption, which generally result from the sleeping problem.

Pescatarian

The pescatarian diet usually excludes all the meat products except for fish and other kinds of seafood. The pescatarians can eat other animal products like eggs and also dairy but always rely on fish due to the bulk of their protein. A lot of fish usually have omega-3 fatty acids and also contain vitamin D that will help in the regulation of serotonin and also the promotion of sleep. Even though the researches are still limited, there is some indication that through eating fish you will be able to gain the positive benefits which aid in promoting quality sleep

By avoiding the red meats, a lot of the pescatarians prefer vegetarians, usually include items like yogurt, nuts, and fruits, which will offer useful nutrients hence having a quality sleep.

Keto

The ketogenic diet is based around the reduction of the body's net carbohydrate intake to be able to put the body into ketosis process. Ketosis is a state whereby the body uses the stored fat instead of the carbohydrates to be used as energy. Ketogenic diets have recently developed in popularity, but they still require considerable research to figure out their advantages and risks fully. Some people usually describe the "Keto insomnia" or experiencing difficulty sleeping when they first begin this diet. This is typically related to the body's general process of adapting to being in ketosis. Keto diets are usually heavy in the consumption of meat, which, as discussed above, typically results in having several negative impacts on the patterns of sleep. However, a researcher in his finding argued that the study of the ketogenic diet in obese patients did not find any effects on sleep quality. The Keto diet is not the only type of food that consists of low carbohydrates. Many other diets, like the Atkins diet, usually promote the restriction of carbohydrates. There is a link between the diet one chooses and the sleep patterns. The practice of foods with high sugars often supports falling asleep very fast, but at the same, they may reduce the sleep quality or even alter the pattern of sleep; this usually relies on the type of carbohydrates and the period it is consumed.

Paleo

The caveman is also restricted to the types of foods that usually would have been readily available to the early human beings whose food was gotten through the process of hunting of animals and gathering of fruits and roots. This diet profoundly excludes refined sugars, dairy, the agricultural products such as wheat, and other foods that have been processed.

Several people who are on the Paleo diet indicate that their sleep improves while other people have insomnia, specifically at the beginning. The research found out that many people reported the experience of sleeping problems on the Paleo diet. The diet usually consists of nuts and fruits that include melatonin but commonly involves a lot of meat, which will have harmful effects on the patterns of sleep.

The Diet Consisting of Raw Foods

This type of diet usually includes the intake or rather the consumption of predominantly uncooked foods—specifically fruits, vegetables, as well as nuts. There is no substantial data from the controlled research studies about the raw food diets and its relation to sleep, and you should remember that the individual experience is different considerably from those who have difficulty sleeping to those who experience their sleep has improved.

The substantial amount of fruits and vegetables will help improve sleep hence promoting the nutrients, but at the same time, there is difficulty in obtaining other crucial nutrients through a raw food diet. Avoiding fatty meats and other heavy meals will help reduce the disruption of sleep.

As the same as the other highly restrictive diets, the raw food diet usually requires significant planning and attention to the detail, as this will add consistency and also avoid the dietary peaks and valleys, which generally interfere with the patterns of sleep.

Foods That Will Help You Sleep

Most of the diets are made up of several individual meals, and the overall diet is what's very crucial for the promoting of the general health. Certain specific foods will be able to aid you to sleep well throughout the night.

- Tart Cherries - the tart cherries usually consist of many specific cultivars of cherries—for example, the Richmond, the Montmorency, and the English Morello, which are generally distinct from the sweeter types of cherries. These cherries usually contain a higher concentration of melatonin and are very useful in the promotion of sleep. The pure tart cherry juice does not mix cherry juice or cocktail juice, as it is an essential way for these fruits to be consumed.

- Kiwi Fruit - Kiwis, which are the small, rounded fruits that are commonly linked with the New Zealand state, have been found to promote sleep when consumed before bedtime. The same machinery is also not known; however, it is linked to the content consisting of the antioxidants, the folate, and the serotonin, which is found in the kiwi fruit.

- Malted Milk - the malted milk is basically linked with James Horlick, who is widely known as its inventor and also a promoter. His recipe consisted of milk, the malted barley, wheat, some sugar, and even an assortment of minerals and vitamins. Studies have found that it helps to improve sleep, and it is also believed that it is related to the vitamins, like vitamin D. The natural, enriched melatonin milk is another milk product which usually gives benefits in the improvement of sleep patterns.

- Oatmeal – A bowl of cereal taken before sleep will be useful in being able to get better sleep. The oats usually contain the tryptophan, an amino acid that is related to sleep, and this is because of how it increases the levels of serotonin and also the levels of melatonin. At the same time, the oatmeal has carbohydrates, which usually help the tryptophan to reach the brain.

- Almonds and Walnuts - The almonds and walnuts are convenient snacks that help in the promotion of sleep highly because of their melatonin content. These nuts usually contain healthy fats hence do not need any advance preparation to have them ready to eat just before bedtime. These nuts may also be taken with other pre-bed foods such as oatmeal.

Foods to Quit Eating Before You Go to Bed

There are specific types of food that, when taken in before you go to bed, would cause insomnia like behavior or just total disruption of your sleep. If you want your sleep to be peaceful and undisrupted, then you are not supposed to consume the following list of foods before bed. It is advisable to do it earlier on during the day.

1. Chocolate - These snacks taste delicious, and to some, it is really addictive; it is made up of caffeine from cacao. Although the intensity of caffeine varies, it is usually highly concentrated in dark chocolates than in milky chocolates. The combination of caffeine and sugar is known to cause sleeplessness at night. It energizes the brain to be more active; hence, sleep is not in question.

2. Hot Sauce - The majority of professionals' advice against the consumption of spicy meals with inclusiveness to hot Sause before going to sleep. Studies have reported that eating hot Sauce may negatively affect your sleep due to the potentiality of indigestion and to avoid the rise in temperatures at night caused by spicy foods. ·

3. Fried Foods - These types of food naturally contain fats and are massive when it comes to digestion. If you are trying to go to bed, metabolism becomes a considerable problem. Fried foods could also stimulate reflux that disrupts sleep. Additionally, many fried foods are in the form of meat, and consumption of proteins may also cause negative impacts on rest.

4. Candy - Nearly all candies contain substantial amounts of sugar, and a lot of sugar does result in pancreases to produce insulin to control your blood sugars. Sadly, these blood sugars spike combined with insulin before sleeping could really disrupt your sleep at night.

5. Alcohol - A bit of alcohol consumption before going to sleep may make you feel sleepy, but generally, it could cause harm to your rest. Studies have reported that the use of alcohol before you sleep disrupts your sleep architecture and could

make you wake up in the middle of the night. Consequently, taking in excessive alcohol results in hangover and drowsiness during the day on the following day.

Nutrition and sleep are highly debated topics, so there are clarifications needed when it comes to the autophagy process and rest. In this book, we will try to clarify some myths that are believed about diets and sleep.

Does Intermittent Fasting Affect Sleep?

Evidence to date is limited but has not shown any clear positive or negative impact of intermittent fasting on sleep.

Intermittent fasting is an approach to dieting that focuses on regular periods with no food intake. Some approaches to intermittent fasting involve only eating for 8 hours each day, creating daily 14-16 hour fasts. Other ways of doing intermittent fasting may include fasting for one full day for every few days without fasting.

It is believed that intermittent fasting may enhance a healthy circadian rhythm. There is no precise data about intermittent fasting in large part because this is a relatively recent dietary approach and because there are various ways of implementing a diet based around intermittent fasting.

Intermittent fasting may affect hunger levels, especially when first becoming accustomed to this pattern of eating. This may influence sleep onset, as some people struggle to fall asleep when hungry. However, studies of people during Ramadan, a religious holiday that involves eating after sundown, have found no substantial disadvantageous results on sleep.

Burning Fats While Sleeping

The bodies usually burn calories during sleep and also while we are awake. Many people typically assume that we burn more calories during the waking hours, but the deprivation of sleep will lead to the metabolism being affected in ways that will decrease the general burning of calories.

The less sleeping usually seems to promote the appetite and also increases the probability that we overeat. Being deprived of sleep can also impact the moods of a person and will result in experiencing emotional eating. Through this, we can burn calories and fat while sleeping and also get a good sleep, which aids in prime the body for the reduction of fat and the general loss of weight.

Sleeping Well Help in Weight Loss

By getting enough sleep, a person can lose weight, as it is an essential part of the weight loss plan. The people who follow the same diets that usually restrict calories had even worse results, whereby they had a 55 percent reduction in their weight loss due to only sleeping for 5 hours a night relative to the others who slept 8 hours. Therefore, sleep is very important to the wellness of various systems in the body and part in promoting healthy metabolism and also helps in weight loss.

The Foods That Help Babies Sleep

No food can assure that a baby will sleep well, let alone be able to sleep through the night. A feeding shortly before an infant goes to bed is usually an essential part of their routine.

When it is possible, transitioning the baby into solid foods will result in positive impacts on their sleeping patterns. A study which was conducted in the UK showed that the babies who were fed with solid food plus breast milk starting at the age of 3 months were able to sleep longer and experienced fewer instances of crying and irritability. But some organizations are against this, claiming that the introduction of the solid food to babies that young is not advantageous as the babies may experience some hardship in being able to digest the food. Therefore, the parents are encouraged to see the doctors for advice.

Food Allergies Causing Sleep Problems

Some food allergies usually cause some issues which are related to sleep, and this is because of the various effects that they typically have on the body. Like food intolerances and allergies generally result in indigestion, nausea, or even diarrhea, which are often discomforting will interrupt sleep patterns. Research has identified an increase in the rates of sleep disturbance in individuals with an allergy to gluten, which is generally known as the celiac disease. Food allergies are also able to cause sleep disruptions since they can be able to overstimulate the nervous system.

The consumption of spicy foods usually results in a lack of sleep. The intake of foods that are very spicy around the period of sleeping usually leads to the disruption of having a quality sleep. Therefore, a person should desist eating spicy foods before going to bed, and this is high because it usually results in indigestion of food and may also increase the temperature of the body hence disrupting the sleeping pattern; this will affect the health of a person negatively due to lack of enough sleep. This will also affect the function of the body during the day as due to the lack of sleep, the person will be worn out.

The Best Time to Eat

The best time to eat dinner is usually some hours before the sleeping period whereby you eat and give the food some time to digest before heading to bed. A person should also be able to limit the intake of snacks in bed, which is not healthy. Through following such a routine, a person will gain a lot, health-wise. A lot of researches has been done on this, and the findings are that the consumption of food just before sleeping usually results in various consequences that are negative to the promotion of the body's health. This can be seen in the individuals that usually consume food just before going to sleep, which affects them negatively in terms of getting a night of quality sleep. Therefore, a person should eat at least 30 to 60 minutes before going to bed hence resulting in some remarkable results.

The Diet for Sleeping Beauty

This is a diet that usually tries to discourse the problem associated with sleeping—for example, lack of sleep and other disorders that are usually associated with sleep. This strategy pays attention to the phrase that the time used for sleeping is the time taken without the consumption of calories. To be able to achieve this, many people who follow this diet plan usually use some sleeping pills so as to be able to have a night of quality sleep. Some people use even painkillers to be able to initiate sleep quickly and for longer periods. The diet of sleeping beauty is not recommended, as it has not been backed by science. This method usually leads to an individual feeling weak and experiencing fatigue in the whole body and may also result in the development of unhealthy eating disorders, which will boost the addition of body weight. You should remember that it is not advised to sleep when feeling hungry highly because it is not healthy for the body. The use of drugs to assist an individual in sleeping for long is not a good idea, as it is dangerous and also may lead a person being addicted to the drugs, whereby they tend to use it every time hence not being able to function without them. This diet program shows us how important having a natural quality sleep is and how it helps the body in its daily functions.

Why Choose Sleep Optimization?

Many people today usually sleep less so as to be able to maximize their work, which will not be able to benefit them health-wise. The best way to be able to achieve waking up with energy and also being ready to tackle the day ahead is usually done through sleeping more, which will result in the individual waking up energetic and also feeling rejuvenated. We need to sleep on a daily basis to be able to give the body some time to rest and boost its function. Therefore, sleeping is usually an important process that aids us in becoming more effective and more efficient. We, at times, have the assumption that when we fall asleep, we just lie, and that is all, as there is nothing happening. However, we are wrong because many processes usually happen when we are fast asleep. Since all the individuals usually get to be exposed to a lot of stimuli and even large quantities of information, therefore, the mind needs time to relax and also process the information and the memories. Even when we are sleeping, the brain still works.

Apart from processing the information by the brain, the body also requires rest to recover from all the activities done during the day. Many types of research have proven that the time you sleep is when the muscles usually grow. When we get quality sleep, the immune system is usually made strong, the cells are rejuvenated, and there is the management of the metabolism and the charging process of the body to be able to wake up without any issues. Therefore, the type of sleep one usually gets will determine how their day will be. Thus, it does not add up when people usually sleep for a small duration of time so as to work more, and this is because when a person does not get enough sleep, they will not be efficient in working, as the simple tasks will take way longer than expected. If a person is interested in boosting their sleep optimization, the person needs to sleep for the whole night, and they should not wake up in the middle of the night. A person should start tracking their sleep at the start so as to be able to know when to sleep and when to wake up. For the tracking process, there are applications and software that can aid in recording such periods. The best way for a person to sleep quickly is basically the change of environment in which they sleep in. For example, people are used to sleeping when there is darkness so as to enable them to sleep well without any distractions. Even the temperature of the room also matters, wherein we get to sleep well when the temperature of our sleeping environment is cooler and not having high temperatures. The final method is to employ a good sleeping routine that you always need to follow. Through this, you will be able to sleep well without waking up in the middle of the night.

Conclusion

Thank you for making it through to the end of the book *Autophagy*! Let's hope it was informative and able to provide you with all of the tools you need to achieve your goals—whatever they may be.

You know the perks of being fit, as well as looking and feeling more youthful. The replenishment of cellular structures means that energy is back to a hundred percent.

It is important to have a better understanding of the benefits of healthy fats and less sugar consumption, which allows you to instill it into your day-to-day activities for generations to benefit.

You have learned about the basics of aerobic training, the process involved, its effects on the brain, its effects on the body, as well as activities that you can perform.

Many important strategies that you require to ensure that your body is less at risk of getting inflammatory diseases, like the ketogenic diet, which lets you gain an array of health benefits.

The next step is for you to get out into the world, equipped with this knowledge, and add the missing ingredient for a healthier body, mind, and soul into your life—both personal and professional—and success will be calling in your favor. The trick is always to work *smarter* and not harder. The best way to get results in the activation of the autophagy process is by being consistent with it. I wish you all the best in your future endeavors!

Finally, if you found this book useful in any way, I wouldn't mind a review on Amazon.

Printed in Poland
by Amazon Fulfillment
Poland Sp. z o.o., Wrocław